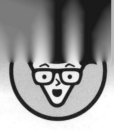

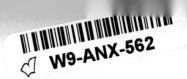

Arthritis

3rd Edition

by Barry Fox, PhD
Nadine Taylor, MS, RD

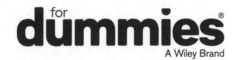

A Wiley Brand

Arthritis For Dummies®, 3rd Edition

Published by: **John Wiley & Sons, Inc.**, 111 River Street, Hoboken, NJ 07030-5774, www.wiley.com

For general information on our other products and services, please contact our Customer Care Department within the U.S. at 877-762-2974, outside the U.S. at 317-572-3993, or fax 317-572-4002. For technical support, please visit https://hub.wiley.com/community/support/dummies.

Wiley publishes in a variety of print and electronic formats and by print-on-demand. Some material included with standard print versions of this book may not be included in e-books or in print-on-demand. If this book refers to media such as a CD or DVD that is not included in the version you purchased, you may download this material at http://booksupport.wiley.com. For more information about Wiley products, visit www.wiley.com.

Library of Congress Control Number: 2022936685

ISBN: 978-1-119-88539-9 (pbk); ISBN: 978-1-119-88540-5 (ebk); ISBN: 978-1-119-88541-2 (ebk)

SKY10034327_050322

Contents at a Glance

Table of Contents

Introduction

Whether it appears as a little bit of creaky stiffness in the hip or knee or as a major case of inflammation that settles in several joints, arthritis is an unwelcome visitor that knocks on just about everybody's door sooner or later. Although we don't have an out-and-out cure for arthritis, there are many techniques for *managing* this disease — that is, controlling its symptoms so that you can get on with your life! Arthritis does *not* mean that you must spend your days relegated to a rocking chair or shuffling from your bed to an easy chair and back again. Most of the time, you can take charge of your disease, instead of letting it take charge of you. By following the simple techniques outlined in this book, you can do much to control your pain, exercise away your stiffness, keep yourself on the move, and slow down or prevent progression of your disease. All you need is a little know-how — and that's what we provide in these chapters.

About This Book

When writing this book, our goal was to provide you with the best and most up-to-date information on arthritis treatments in an easy-to-read format that you could simply thumb through. We have included the best-of-the-best of many different healing systems — ranging from standard Western medicine (including medications and surgery), to Eastern hands-on healing methods (including acupuncture, acupressure, and reiki), to alternative therapies (including homeopathy, herbs, DHEA, hydrotherapy) and such far-out approaches as bee venom therapy.

If you like, you can read this book straight through from cover to cover, but it's not absolutely necessary. We do suggest that you read the first chapter as an introduction, and then zero in on the description of your particular kind of arthritis, found in Chapters 2, 3, 4, or 5. After that, feel free to flip through the book and read whatever catches your fancy.

Because arthritis impacts your life in so many different ways, we have chapters that address the many complex issues that you may face, including the technical aspects of arthritis (tests, medicines, and surgeries), the practical aspects (diet, exercise, and day-to-day living), and the emotional aspects (depression and anger). We also give tips on how to assemble your healthcare treatment team, how to talk to your doctor, and what to do about chronic pain.

Foolish Assumptions

In writing this book, we made certain educated guesses about you, the reader, so that we could figure out what might be most interesting and useful to you and write our book accordingly. We've assumed the following:

- » You either have arthritis yourself or you're close to someone who has it.
- » You're interested in finding out more about arthritis and its treatments.
- » You want to do something to ease arthritis pain and other symptoms.
- » You want to play an active part in managing the disease, rather than just going along with whatever your doctor tells you.
- » You're interested in finding out about some alternative ways to treat arthritis.
- » You'd like to find out how to handle the emotional issues that go hand-in-hand with the disease.

We also don't assume that you're a medical expert! Now and again, the abbreviated forms of several diseases pop up in various parts of this book so let's get a helpful list into the book for you right away. Here's a quick list of the common ones and what they stand for:

- » AS: Ankylosing spondylitis
- » DLE: Discoid lupus erythematosus
- » GCA: Giant cell arteritis
- » JIA: Juvenile idiopathic arthritis
- » OA: Osteoarthritis
- » PMR: Polymyalgia rheumatica
- » PsA: Psoriatic arthritis
- » RA: Rheumatoid arthritis
- » SLE: Systemic lupus erythematosus

And don't worry: We explain in this book what these words mean!

Icons Used in This Book

The icons tell you what you must know, what you should know, and what you may find interesting but can live without.

REMEMBER

When you see this icon, it means the information is essential, and you should be aware of it.

TIP

This icon marks important information that can save you time and energy.

TECHNICAL STUFF

The Technical Stuff icon marks a more in-depth medical passage or gives you further information about confusing medical terms.

WARNING

The Warning icon cautions you against potential problems.

Beyond the Book

In addition to the abundance of information and guidance related to arthritis that we provide in this book, you can find even more help and information online at *Dummies.com*. Check out this book's online Cheat Sheet. Just go to *www.dummies. com* and search for "Arthritis For Dummies Cheat Sheet."

Where to Go from Here

Someone once said, "Knowledge is power." You have the power to take charge of your arthritis; all you have to do is educate yourself and apply what you discover. This book is a good place to start, but you'll have to commit and recommit yourself to maintaining your health on a daily basis. Remember, it's the little things that you do every day that count. As you embark on your journey, we wish you luck, strength, and many active, pain-free years!

1

Making Sense of the Types of Arthritis

Arthritis can really put a damper on your life . . . if you let it. But the good news is that most forms of arthritis and the pain they cause can be managed (if not completely done away with) through medical techniques and lifestyle changes.

Part 1 gives you an overview of arthritis in its many forms: the symptoms, diseases, processes, causes, and most likely victims. You also learn what doctors can do for each type of arthritis and what you can do for yourself. We give special attention to the most common forms of this disease: osteoarthritis and rheumatoid arthritis.

IN THIS CHAPTER

» **Discovering how arthritis affects your body**

» **Becoming aware of the various types of arthritis**

» **Recognizing the signs and symptoms of arthritis**

» **Identifying the major causes of arthritis**

» **Finding out who is most likely to get the various forms of the disease**

» **Considering the treatment options**

Chapter **1**

What Is Arthritis?

O uch! There it goes again! That grinding pain in your hip, those aching knees that make walking from the kitchen to the bedroom a chore, the stiff and swollen fingers that won't allow you to twist the lid off a sticky jar or even sew on a button. Arthritis seems to get to everybody sooner or later — slowing us down, forcing us to give up some of our favorite activities, and just generally being a pain in the neck (sometimes literally!). In more advanced cases, arthritis can seriously compromise quality of life as sufferers surrender their independence, mobility, and sense of usefulness while being relentlessly worn down by pain.

The good news is that you can manage your arthritis with a combination of medical care, simple lifestyle changes, and good old common sense. You don't have to spend your life gritting your teeth from pain, or hobbling around the backyard with a cane. Although you may not be able to run a marathon or do back-flips like you did when you were 13, if you follow the program outlined here, you should be able to do the things you really want to do — such as take a brisk walk in the park, carry a sleeping child upstairs to bed, or swing a golf club with the best of them.

Arthritis may affect a lot of people, but thanks to intensive research over the past several years, we now know a lot more about how to handle it.

Remember that arthritis affects the rich and famous just as much as the rest of us. For a look at how certain celebrities have handled their arthritis, see the sidebar "Stargazing: Famous Arthritis Sufferers" at the end of the chapter.

Understanding How Arthritis Affects Your Joints

So what exactly is arthritis, this disease that brings us so much misery and pain? Unfortunately, we can't provide one easy answer to that question, because arthritis involves a group of diseases — each with its own cause, set of symptoms, and treatments. However, these diseases do have the following in common:

>> They affect some part of the joint.

>> They cause pain and (possibly) loss of movement.

>> They often bring about some kind of inflammation.

As for the causes of these different kinds of arthritis, they run the gamut from inheriting an unlucky gene to physical trauma to getting bitten by the wrong mosquito.

TECHNICAL STUFF

The word *arthritis*, which literally means joint inflammation, comes from the Greek words *arthros* (joint) and *itis* (inflammation), and its major symptom is joint pain. Although the same group of ailments can be called *rheumatism*, it's usually referred to as arthritis, so that's what we call it in this book. The word *arthralgia*, a term used much less frequently, refers to joint pain alone. According to the CDC, arthritis affects some 58.5 million American adults (one out of every four people) and 300,000 children. That's a big chunk of the population. For a look at how many people are affected by some of the most common forms of arthritis, see "Arthritis by the Numbers" later in the chapter.

Saying hello to your joints

Before you can understand what's wrong with your joints, you need to understand what a joint is and how it works. Any place in the body where two bones meet is called a *joint* such as the ball and socket hip joint, or the hinge joint at the elbow or knee. Sometimes the bones actually fuse together; your skull is an example of an area with fused bones. But in the joints that can develop arthritis, the bones don't actually touch. As you can see in Figure 1-1, a small amount of space exists between the two bone ends. The space between the ends of the bones keeps them from grinding against each other and wearing each other down.

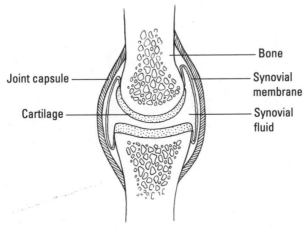

Bone

Synovial membrane

Synovial fluid

Joint capsule

Cartilage

FIGURE 1-1:
Anatomy of
a healthy
synovial joint.

Bones are living tissue — hard, porous structures with a blood supply and nerves — that constantly rebuild themselves. Bones protect our vital organs and provide the supporting framework for the body. Without bones, we would be nothing more than blobs of tissue — like tents without supporting poles!

But bones are more than broomsticks that prop us up; fortunately, they don't leave us rigid and awkward. The 200-plus bones that reside in our bodies are connected together in some 150 joints, giving us remarkable flexibility and range of motion. If you don't believe it, just watch a gymnast, ballet dancer, or figure skater execute a handspring, arabesque, or triple axel. But you don't have to be an athlete or contortionist to enjoy the benefits of joint flexibility. Just think about some of the things you do regularly — such as bending a knee or an elbow. Now imagine how limiting it would be if you had fewer joints, or if they didn't move the way they do! (For a few fascinating facts about your joints, see the sidebar "Strange-but-true joint points" on the next page.)

TECHNICAL STUFF

Other structures surrounding the joint, such as the muscles, tendons, and *bursae* — small sacs of fluid that cushion the tendons like pillows — support the joint and provide the power that makes the bones move. The joint capsule wraps itself around the joint, and its special lining, the *synovial membrane* or *synovium,* makes a slick, slippery liquid called the *synovial fluid.* You can think of the joint capsule as a sealed bag full of WD-40 encasing the joint and filling the little space between the bone ends. Finally, the bone ends are capped by *cartilage* — a slick, tough, rubbery material that is eight times more slippery than ice and a better shock absorber than the tires and springs on your car! Together, these parts make up the joint, one of the most fascinating bits of machinery found in the body.

Cartilage: The human shock absorber

Cartilage is extremely important for the healthy functioning of a joint, especially if that joint bears weight, like your knee. Imagine for a moment that you're looking into the inner workings of your left knee as you walk down the street. When you shift your weight from your left leg to your right, the pressure on your left knee is released. The cartilage in your left knee then "drinks in" synovial fluid, in much the same way that a sponge soaks up liquid when immersed in water. When you take another step and transfer the weight back onto your left leg, much of the fluid squeezes out of the cartilage. This squeezing of joint fluid into and out of the cartilage helps it respond to the off-and-on pressure of walking without shattering under the strain.

Can you imagine the results if we didn't have this watery cushion within our joints? With the rough, porous surfaces of the bone ends pitted against each other, bones would grind each other down in no time. One thing is certain: Nobody would be getting around too easily without joint fluid and cartilage.

Types of joints

To accommodate the bends, twists, and turns that we all perform without even thinking, the skeletal system is made up of different shapes and sizes of bones, which connect to form different kinds of joints. The joints are categorized according to how much motion they allow:

>> **Synarthrodial joints** allow no movement at all. You can find these in the skull, where the bones meet to form tough, fibrous joints called *sutures.* Because they don't move, arthritis doesn't affect them.

>> **Amphiarthrodial joints,** such as those in the spine or the pelvis, allow limited movement. Generally, these joints aren't attacked by arthritic conditions as often as others. (A slipped disc is not arthritis.)

>> **Synovial joints** allow a wide range of movement; most of our joints fall into this class. Synovial joints come in all kinds of interesting variations including those that glide, hinge, pivot, look like saddles, or have a ball-and-socket type structure. (For more on these joints, take a look at the section "Looking at the types of synovial joints" later in this chapter.) Because of the synovial joints, you can bend over and pick a flower, kick up your heels while swing dancing, reach for a glass on a high shelf, and turn around to see what's going on behind you. Unfortunately, these joints are also the ones most likely to be hit with arthritis, precisely because they do move!

STRANGE-BUT-TRUE JOINT POINTS

Here are a couple of things you may not know about your joints:

- By the time a fetus is four months old, its joints and limbs are in working order and ready to move.

- A newborn baby has 350 bones, many of which fuse to form the 206 bones of the adult body.

- Cartilage is 65 percent to 85 percent water. (The amount of water in your cartilage generally decreases as you get older.)

- When you run, the pressure on your knees can increase to ten times that of your body weight.

- Not a single man-made substance is more resilient, a better shock absorber, or lower in friction than cartilage.

Looking at the types of synovial joints

REMEMBER

Because of their tendency to become arthritic, synovial joints are the ones that we discuss the most throughout this book. Synovial joints come in a wide variety of shapes and sizes to accommodate a wide variety of movements.

Gliding joints

A gliding joint contains two bones with somewhat flat surfaces that can slide over each other. The vertebrae in your spine are connected by gliding joints, allowing you to bend forward to touch your toes and backward to do a backbend (well, maybe!). See Figure 1-2 for an example of a gliding joint.

Hinge joints

You can find hinge joints in your elbows, knees, and fingers. These joints open and close like a door. But just like a door, hinge joints only go one way — you can't bend your knee up toward your face, only back toward your rear. See Figure 1-3 for an example of a hinge joint.

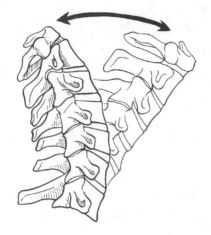

FIGURE 1-2:
A gliding joint.
The gliding joint
helps keep your
vertebrae aligned
when you bend
and stretch.

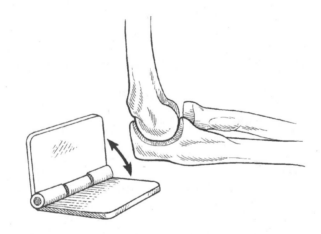

FIGURE 1-3:
A hinge joint.
Hinge joints bend
only one way.

Saddle joints

This joint looks like a horse's back with a saddle resting on it. One bone is rounded (*convex*) and fits neatly into the other bone, which is *concave*. The saddle joint moves up and down and side to side, but it doesn't rotate. Your wrist and your thumb have this kind of joint. See Figure 1-4 for an example of a saddle joint.

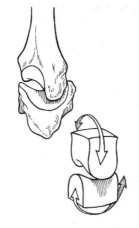

FIGURE 1-4:
A saddle joint.
The saddle joint
moves up and
down and side
to side.

© John Wiley & Sons, Inc.

Ball-and-socket joints

This is truly a freewheeling joint — it's ready for anything! Up, down, back, forth, or around in circles. The bone attached to a ball-and-socket joint can move in just about any direction. The end of one bone is round, like a ball, whereas the other bone has a neat little cave that the ball fits into. Your shoulders and hips have ball-and-socket joints. Swimming the backstroke is a perfect example of the kind of range of motion made possible by these joints. See Figure 1-5 for an example of a ball-and-socket joint.

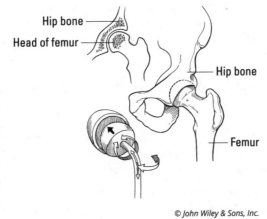

FIGURE 1-5:
A ball-and-socket
joint. These joints
can move just
about any
direction — up,
down, back, forth,
or around
in circles.

© John Wiley & Sons, Inc.

Distinguishing Between Arthritis and Arthritis-Related Conditions

REMEMBER

Some organizations define arthritis as a group of more than 100 related diseases, ranging from bursitis to osteoarthritis. But in this book, we use the following classifications, which conform to those widely accepted by the medical community:

» "True" arthritis

» Arthritis as a "major player"

» Arthritis as a "minor player"

» Arthritis as a "companion condition"

In the following subsections, we go over the various types of arthritis and arthritis-related diseases and their classifications. We also discuss each disease in greater detail in Chapters 2, 3, 4 and 5. (Check out the sidebar titled "Hypersensitive fingers and toes" later in the chapter to find out about Raynaud's phenomenon, a particularly chilling form of arthritis.)

Defining "true" arthritis

True arthritis isn't a medical term; it's just a convenient way of referring to the group of ailments in which arthritis is the primary disease process and is a major part of the syndrome. Osteoarthritis and rheumatoid arthritis are the best-known members of this group, which can cause problems ranging from mild joint pain to a permanently bowed spine.

The following include conditions in which arthritis is the major part of the syndrome and the primary disease process:

» **Ankylosing spondylitis (AS):** A chronic inflammation of the spine, this disease can cause the vertebrae to grow together, making the spine rigid. Although the cause is unknown, heredity seems to be a factor.

» **Gout:** This "regal" form of arthritis is caused by the build-up of a substance called uric acid, which forms sharp crystals that are deposited in the joint. These needlelike crystals cause inflammation leading to severe pain and are most commonly found in the knees, the wrists, and the "bunion" joint of the big toe. Genetic factors, conditions such as high blood pressure, kidney disease, and obesity, a diet high in animal purines, alcohol consumption, and certain drugs may cause gout.

» **Infectious arthritis:** Bacteria, viruses, or fungi that enter the body can affect the joints, causing fever, inflammation, and loss of joint function.

» **Juvenile idiopathic arthritis (JIA):** Formerly known as juvenile rheumatoid arthritis, this is a catchall term for the different kinds of arthritis that strike children under the age of 16. Pain or swelling in the shoulders, elbows, knees, ankles, or toes; chills; a reappearing fever; and sometimes a body rash are typical symptoms of various kinds of JIA. The cause is unknown.

» **Osteoarthritis (OA):** In this, the most common type of arthritis, the cartilage breaks down, exposing bone ends and allowing them to rub together. The result can be pain, stiffness, loss of movement, and sometimes swelling. Osteoarthritis is most often found in the weight-bearing joints, such as the hips, knees, ankles, and spine, but it can also affect the fingers. It may be the result of trauma, metabolic conditions, obesity, heredity, or other factors.

» **Pseudogout:** Like gout, pseudogout is caused by the deposition of crystals into the joint, but instead of uric acid crystals, they're made from calcium pyrophosphate. Pain, swelling, and sometimes the destruction of cartilage can result.

Note: This deposition of calcium pyrophosphate crystals is not related to the dietary intake of calcium.

» **Psoriatic arthritis:** This form of arthritis occurs in people who have the autoimmune skin condition called *psoriasis,* which causes scaly, red, rough patches on the neck, elbows, and knees, as well as nail changes. Psoriatic arthritis can affect joints anywhere in the body, including the spine, the fingers, and the toes, which can swell up like little sausages.

» **Rheumatoid arthritis (RA):** An autoimmune disease, RA causes the body to mistakenly attack its own joints, causing inflammation and swelling of the tissues surrounding the joint, resulting in joint pain and swelling. Over time, there can be a loss of cartilage, causing shrinkage of the space between the bone ends, which increases pain and decreases mobility; irreversible joint deformity can even occur. RA often affects the same joint on both sides of the body (for example, both wrists) and is two to three times more likely to strike women compared to men. (For more on this, see the sidebar "Why are Women More Likely to Get Arthritis," near the end of the chapter.)

ARTHRITIS BY THE NUMBERS

Arthritis affects a surprisingly large number of us, as you can see by the following numbers:

- Over 58 million adult Americans currently suffer from arthritis, or 1 in 4 of us. It is the leading cause of disability among adults in the U.S.

- Women are more likely than men to get arthritis, which currently affects one in four women compared to one in five men. They are also far more likely to develop rheumatoid arthritis than men and to experience worse pain.

- By 2040, it's projected that that the number of U.S. adults with doctor-diagnosed arthritis will have increased by 49 percent to an estimated 78.4 million (nearly 26 percent of the population).

- In 2013, the total national cost of treating arthritis was $140 billion. It is the reason behind more than 100 million outpatient visits and 6.6 million hospitalizations annually.

- Osteoarthritis is by far the most common type of arthritis, affecting more than 30 million Americans, most of whom develop the disease after the age of 45.

- Gout is the second most prevalent form of arthritis in the U.S., affecting 8.3 million sufferers, followed by rheumatoid arthritis at 1.3 million. Sjögren's afflicts 1-4 million and fibromyalgia afflicts 4 million, but not all of them will have arthritis.

- About 1.5 million American adults have rheumatoid arthritis (RA), which mostly strikes women, while gout tends to favor men.

- Some 1 in 1,000 U.S. children under the age of 17 have some form of joint disease, which translates to an astonishing 300,000! Of those, 50,000 have juvenile idiopathic arthritis (JIA).

- Arthritis most often strikes in the knees and the hips, most likely because both are weight-bearing joints and can easily be injured. To fight the pain and disability that can result, there are about 500,000 hip replacements and 750,000 knee replacements performed in the U.S. every year.

Classifying arthritis as a "major player"

In the following conditions, arthritis is present and is usually a major part of the syndrome, but is not the primary disease process:

>> **Lyme disease:** Caused by a certain type of bacteria transmitted to humans via tick bites, Lyme disease brings about fever, a distinctive red skin lesion in

the shape of a bull's-eye, problems with the nerves and/or heart, and arthritis. Antibiotics are the treatment of choice for this disease.

» **Reactive arthritis:** An inflammation of the joints, reactive arthritis strikes along with or shortly after the onset of an infection, often one that is intestinal or sexually-transmitted. The three problems generally associated with reactive arthritis are arthritis, conjunctivitis (inflammation of the eyelid's lining), and urethritis (inflammation of the urethra).

» **Scleroderma:** The word *scleroderma* means hard skin. This is a rare autoimmune condition that involves an attack on tiny blood vessels in many places in the body, and overproduction of collagen in places it doesn't belong. The skin and other organs can stiffen. Joints can become inflamed, and tightness of the skin overlying the joints can make them even harder to move. An autoimmune disease, scleroderma usually attacks adults rather than children.

» **Systemic lupus erythematosus:** This is yet another disease caused by an immune system gone wrong. In lupus, the body attacks its own tissue, causing inflammation, joint pain, stiffness, permanent damage to the joints, and exhaustion. Although lupus most often affects women of child-bearing age, it *does* strike some men and can occur at nearly any age, including childhood and post-menopause.

Describing arthritis as a "minor player"

In these conditions, arthritis may appear, but is a minor part of the syndrome.

» **Bursitis and tendonitis:** Caused by overusing or injuring a joint, *bursitis* is the inflammation of the fibrous sac that cushions the tendons. *Tendonitis* is the irritation of the tendons, which attach the muscles to the bones.

» **Paget's disease:** With Paget's disease, the breakdown and rebuilding of bone speeds up. The resulting bone is larger but also softer and weaker, making it more likely to fracture. These weakened and deformed bones cause arthritis to develop in their respective joints, which typically include those of the hip, skull, spine, knee, and ankle. The cause is unknown.

» **Polymyalgia rheumatica (PMR):** With this condition, severe stiffness can suddenly strike in the lower back, hips, shoulders, and neck, making it difficult even to get out of bed. The pain is similar to that of RA, often without evidence of any active arthritis. PMR can occur by itself or together with a life-threatening inflammation of the blood vessels called giant cell arteritis (GCA). Symptoms of GCA can occur before, after, or at the same time as PMR, and include headaches, scalp tenderness, hearing problems, vision loss or changes, and tongue or jaw pain after prolonged chewing.

HYPERSENSITIVE FINGERS AND TOES

Prompted by arterial blood vessel spasm, Raynaud's phenomenon is a condition that can make the fingers, toes, nose, or nipples extremely sensitive to cold and to emotional upsets, turning them blue/violet or white in color. It sometimes occurs in conjunction with (or as a result of) other arthritis-related conditions including lupus, scleroderma, RA, and myositis, but can also be caused by repetitive trauma or injuries to the nerves of the hands or feet, smoking, certain medications, or chemical exposure. Typical attacks of Raynaud's phenomenon include tingling, numbness and whitening of the fingers (without affecting the thumb), and pain or redness when blood circulation returns.

There's no single blood test for Raynaud's: most doctors diagnose the disease based on signs and symptoms. Treatment generally involves wearing gloves, socks, and hats to maintain total body warmth, and avoiding workplace triggers, such as vibrating tools, freezers, and exposure to air conditioning vents. In severe cases of Raynaud's, doctors prescribe medication to dilate the blood vessels. See Chapter 5 for more on Raynaud's phenomenon.

>> **Sjögren'ssyndrome:** Another autoimmune disease, Sjögren's syndrome (usually referred to simply as Sjögren's) causes inflammation of the tear glands and saliva glands, leading to dryness of the eyes and mouth, hazy vision, cracks at the corners of the mouth, and cavities. Inflammation of the brain, nerves, thyroid, lungs, skin, liver, kidneys, and, of course, the joints may also be present.

Experiencing arthritis as a "companion condition"

These following conditions are linked to arthritis; that is, arthritis may be present, but it constitutes another separate disease process:

>> **Carpal tunnel syndrome:** This syndrome results when pressure on a nerve in the wrist makes the fingers tingle and feel numb. This syndrome is usually caused by overuse of the wrist. Permanent muscle and nerve damage can occur if carpal tunnel isn't treated.

>> **Fibromyalgia:** Also known as fibromyalgia syndrome (FMS), this condition involves pain in the muscles and tendons that occurs without a specific injury or cause. Fibromyalgia can make you "hurt all over," particularly in certain tender points in the neck, upper back, elbows, and knees. Those with

fibromyalgia can suffer from disturbed sleep, fatigue, stiffness, and depression. The cause is unknown. Physical or mental stress, fatigue, or infections may trigger this disease.

>> **Myositis:** This disease causes inflammation of the muscles, which can take one of two forms: *polymyositis* — an inflammation of the muscle that causes muscle weakening and breakdown, as well as pain, and *dermatomyositis* — polymyositis plus rashes that can lead to skin scarring and changes in pigmentation.

Deciding Whether It's Really Arthritis: Signs and Symptoms

With all the different kinds of arthritis, how do you know whether you have one of them? Remember two things: Arthritis can strike anyone at any time, and many times you may find it difficult to tell whether the pain you're experiencing is serious enough to warrant medical attention. Almost everyone has had an ache or pain at some time or has overextended herself physically, but you need to know what is minor and temporary, and what may be serious and long term. Knowing what to watch for can make a difference in your treatment and physical comfort. Typical warning signs of arthritis include:

>> **Joint pain:** This not only includes steady, ever-present pain, but also off-again-on-again pain, pain that occurs only when you're moving or only when you're sitting still. In fact, if your joints hurt in any way for more than two weeks, you should see your doctor.

>> **Stiffness or difficulty in moving a joint:** If you have trouble getting out of bed, unscrewing a jar lid, climbing the stairs, or doing anything else that involves moving your joints, consider it a red flag. Although difficulty moving a joint is most often the result of a muscular condition (like tendonitis due to overuse, or muscle ache), it could be a sign of arthritis.

>> **Swelling:** If the skin around a joint is red, puffed up, hot, throbbing, or painful to the touch, you're experiencing joint inflammation. Don't wait. See your doctor.

REMEMBER

The warning signs may come in triplicate (pain plus stiffness plus swelling), two together, or one all alone. Or, as you find out in Chapters 3 and 4, you may experience other early signs, such as malaise or muscle pain. But if you experience any of these or other symptoms in or around a joint for longer than two weeks, you should see your doctor.

WARNING

You may be tempted to read this book's descriptions of various diseases, pick out the one with symptoms most closely matching yours, and make your own diagnosis. Some people may make the right diagnosis. But a lot of people make the wrong one, because the symptoms of many forms of arthritis overlap with those of other forms of the disease — they can even be confused with entirely different ailments. Making the wrong diagnosis can lead to the wrong treatment, which can be dangerous. Do not self-diagnose. No matter how obvious the situation seems, go to a medical doctor, have a complete examination, and get an "official" diagnosis.

Considering the Causes of Arthritis

Just as many different kinds of arthritis exist, many different causes also exist — and some of them are still unknown. But in general, scientists have found that certain factors can contribute to the development of joint problems:

>> **Heredity:** Your parents gave you your beautiful eyes, strong jawline, exceptional math ability, and, possibly, a tendency to develop rheumatoid arthritis. Scientists have discovered that the genetic marker HLA-DR4 is linked to rheumatoid arthritis, so if you happen to have this gene, you're more likely to develop the disease. Ankylosing spondylitis is linked to the genetic marker HLA-B27, and although having this gene doesn't mean that you absolutely *will* get this form of arthritis, you *can* — if conditions are right.

>> **Age:** It's just a fact of life that the older you get, the more likely you are to develop arthritis, especially osteoarthritis. Like the tires on your car, cartilage can wear down over time, becoming thin, cracked, or even wearing through. Bones may also break down with age, bringing on joint pain and dysfunction.

>> **Overuse of a joint:** What do ballerinas, baseball pitchers, and tennis players all have in common? A great chance that they'll develop arthritis due to the tremendous repetitive strain they put on their joints. The dancers, who go from flat foot to *pointe* hundreds of times during a practice session, often end up with painful arthritic ankles. Baseball pitchers, throwing fastballs at speeds of more than 100 mph, regularly develop arthritis of the shoulder and/or elbow. And you don't need to be a tennis pro to develop *tennis elbow,* a form of tendonitis that has sidelined many a player.

>> **Injury:** Sustaining injury to a joint (from a household mishap, a car accident, playing sports, or doing anything else) increases the odds that you may develop arthritis in that joint in the future. Football players are well-known victims of arthritis of the knee, which is certainly not surprising: They often fall smack on their knees or other joints when they're tackled — then have a ton of "football flesh" crash down on top of them. What's most amazing is that they ever walk away uninjured.

>> **Infection:** Some forms of arthritis are the result of bacteria, viruses, or fungi that can either cause the disease or trigger it in susceptible people. Lyme disease comes from bacteria transmitted by the bite of a tick. The most common cause of bacterial infectious arthritis is a *Staphylococcus aureus* (staph) infection. Staph commonly lives on the skin and can cause infectious arthritis when it enters the body during surgery or trauma, or when a needle is inserted into a joint. It can also result from bone infection or an infection that's traveled from another area of the body. Infection typically strikes in the knee, but can also affect the wrists, ankles and hips. It usually affects only one joint.

Obesity: Carrying too much weight is a big risk factor for OA because it puts undue pressure on the joints, especially the knees, and can cause the cartilage that cushions the joints to wear away faster. Just 10 extra pounds of body weight increases the pressure exerted on your knee joints by 40 pounds every time you take a step on flat ground. Add an incline or a trip up or down some stairs and the pressure easily doubles if not triples. Fat is also a chemically active tissue that constantly releases proteins which cause inflammation. This can increase the likelihood that OA will develop, and can worsen inflammation-related forms of arthritis such as RA, gout, and ankylosing spondylitis.

>> **Tumor necrosis factor-alpha (TNF-alpha):** TNF-alpha (usually just known as TNF, which we'll use in this book) is a substance the body produces that causes inflammation and may play a part in initiating or maintaining rheumatoid arthritis. Although scientists are unsure exactly what triggers RA, they have found that drugs that counteract the effects of TNF-alpha, called *TNF inhibitor,* are often helpful in managing the symptoms of this disease

Understanding Who Gets Arthritis

Statistically speaking, the typical arthritis victim (if there were such a thing) would be a middle-class Caucasian woman between the ages of 65 and 74 who has a high-school education, is overweight, is a city-dweller in the southern United States, and has osteoarthritis.

But arthritis isn't all that picky and doesn't worry too much about statistics. It strikes young and old, male and female, and rich and poor and doesn't seem to care where you live. Arthritis, in one form or another, can affect just about anybody.

However, arthritis does seem to hit women particularly hard. Nearly two-thirds of those who get the disease are women — an estimated 41 million Americans. Some facts about women and arthritis:

>> About 26 percent of the female population have been diagnosed with some kind of arthritis compared to 19.1 percent of males.

Some 16 million women are currently affected by osteoarthritis, a disease that strikes nearly twice as many females as males. Additionally, women are 40 percent more likely to develop knee osteoarthritis and 10 percent more likely to develop hip arthritis compared to men.

Three times as many women as men develop rheumatorid arthritis, a disease in which the immune system attacks joint linings causing pain and disability.

Females make up about 80 percent of those diagnosed with lupus.

>> About 90 percent of those with Sjögren's are female.

>> Of an estimated 5 million U.S. adults with fibromyalgia, only about 10 percent are men.

>> Girls are generally more than twice as likely as boys to develop juvenile idiopathic arthritis.

WHY ARE WOMEN MORE LIKELY TO DEVELOP ARTHRITIS?

It seems unfair, but your chances of developing arthritis are increased — sometimes greatly increased — if you happen to be female. There may be plenty of reasons for this, but the top three appear to be hormones, differences in the female musculoskeletal system, and a greater tendency to gain too much weight:

- **Hormones:** During the menstrual cycle, rising hormone levels promote the loosening of the ligaments (joint laxity), which allows them to bend more than usual. While this might seem great for dancers and gymnasts who need to be super flexible, it increases instability in the joints that can contribute to injuries that could lead to osteoarthritis. This may be the reason that female athletes (but not male) can be two to eight times more likely to suffer from ACL injuries in the knee, which increases their likelihood of developing knee osteoarthritis up to six times.

  Joint pain can also appear or worsen during and after menopause, a time when estrogen levels drop significantly. Estrogen helps protect the cartilage that cushions the joints and also tamps down inflammation of the joints. But these protective effects diminish after menopause, which increases the risk of developing OA.

- **Differences in the Musculoskeletal System:** Because the female body is designed to give birth, there is increased elasticity in the tendons in the body's lower half, causing joint laxity which makes the joints in this area more likely to become unstable. In addition, because women's hip joints are set wider than their knee joints, the femur is aligned at an angle from hip to knee, making the knee less stable and injuries more likely. Both of these causes of joint instability can contribute to OA.

  Giving birth also increases joint laxity to accommodate the birth process, but the joints may not return to normal afterwards. One study found that for each birth a woman's risk of needing a knee replacement increased by 8 percent, while the need for a hip replacement increased by 2 percent.

- **Gaining Too Much Weight:** According to the Center for Disease Control and Prevention (CDC), in 2017–2018, 41.9 percent of U.S. women were obese, as were 43 percent of U.S. men. However, *severe* obesity affected 11.5% of women compared to just 6.9% of men, making women even more likely than men to develop arthritis. While doctors have long known there's a clear connection between obesity and OA, it can also contribute to or worsen RA, psoriatic arthritis, ankylosing spondylitis, gout, and other inflammatory forms of arthritis. Fortunately, just losing a few pounds can not only ease arthritis pain but also improve joint function and increase the quality of life for most arthritis sufferers.

  Women aren't the only ones who are especially prone to developing arthritis and arthritis-related problems. Compared to Causasians, African Americans are twice as likely to have knee OA and 77 percent more likely to develop a condition called multiple large joint OA in their knees and spine. Multiple large joint OA, a disorder that affects more than 27 million American adults, may require joint replacement surgery to ease pain and restore joint function. African American women are also three times more likely than Caucasian women to develop lupus and fibromyalgia, conditions that already target women far more often than men.

Assessing Your Treatment Options

The good news is that, in many cases, arthritis can be managed. It may take some time and effort to find the right treatment(s) for your particular version of the disease, but help is out there. Medications and surgery are only a part of the answer. Following healthful diet, exercising, using joint protection techniques, controlling stress, anger, and depression, and organizing your life can offer relief from pain and a new lease on life. And the worlds of herbs, homeopathy, hands-on healing, and other alternative medicine treatments may offer you additional ammunition in the fight against arthritis pain and other symptoms.

Looking into medications

TIP

When you're in pain, your joints are hot or swollen, and you can hardly walk from one end of the house to the other, you want relief *now*. In many cases, the fastest way to relieve arthritis symptoms is to take medication. Arthritis medications fall into five main classes:

>> **Analgesics:** Analgesics are designed specifically to relieve pain, and include acetaminophen (Tylenol) and opioids (narcotics). Sometimes acetaminophen is combined with an opioid, such as codeine. The analgesics differ from anti-inflammatory drugs (such as NSAIDs) in that they do not interfere with the inflammation process, which makes them easier on the stomach and less likely to cause gastrointestinal bleeding.

>> **Biologics:** The biologics treat specific kinds of autoimmune arthritis (like RA) by turning off certain components of the immune system called cytokines. The cytokines play an especially important part in the inflammation seen in RA, and biologics inhibit their inflammatory action. Enbrel, Humira, Remicade, and Kineret are examples of drugs that fall into the category of biologics.

>> **Disease modifying antirheumatic drugs (DMARDs):** The DMARDs are used to treat autoimmune forms of arthritis (like RA, psoriatic arthritis). DMARDs change the way the immune system works, slowing or stopping its attack on the body. Drugs like sulfasalazine, methotrexate, leflunomide, and hydroxy-chloroquine fall into this category.

>> **Nonsteroidal anti-inflammatory drugs (NSAIDs):** The NSAIDs help relieve pain and reduce inflammation by interfering with an enzyme called COX (cyclooxygenase). The enzyme takes two forms: COX-1 and COX-2. Older, traditional forms of NSAIDs (including aspirin, ibuprofen, and naproxen) block both forms of the COX enzyme, but newer ones (such as Celebrex) block COX-2 only, as COX-1 has been shown to have a protective effect on the stomach lining. Milder versions (aspirin, ibuprofen) are available over the counter, but the more powerful ones (Indocin, Lodine, Celebrex) require a prescription, especially at higher doses.

>> **Steroids:** Also known as corticosteroids, these are man-made versions of naturally-occurring hormones in the body that help quell inflammation. Although they function as powerful anti-inflammatories, they can also have powerful side effects, including elevated blood pressure, thinning of the bones and skin, weight gain, and an increased risk of infection, even when they are injected directly into the joint.

See Chapter 8 for the complete lowdown on arthritis medications.

Considering surgery

If pain is interfering with your ability to lead a happy and productive life, you have to take the maximum amount of pain relievers just to get through the day, and you've tried all other pain-relieving methods with no luck, you may want to consider surgery. Although joint surgery is complex and not to be taken lightly, some people have enjoyed excellent results, to the point of feeling that they've gotten a new lease on life. Surgical techniques can involve flushing a joint with water, resurfacing rough bone ends or cartilage, removing inflamed membranes, growing new bone, or inserting a whole new joint. Turn to Chapter 9 to find out more about surgical treatments.

Making lifestyle changes

Chances are excellent that you can do much to ease your arthritis-related pain, stiffness, swelling, and decreased range of motion just by changing certain things you do every day.

TIP

The following list goes over some options you may want to consider:

>> **Eat a healthful diet.** By this, we mean a diet that includes plenty of fish, fresh fruits and vegetables, and whole grains, with a minimum of processed meats and salad oil (corn, safflower, or sunflower). This healthy, well-balanced diet also has anti-inflammatory effects, which is important as so many forms of arthritis are linked to inflammation. The Mediterranean diet fits the bill perfectly, and has the added bonus of warding off both heart disease and certain types of cancer.

See Chapter 11 to get the skinny on the elements of a healthful diet and how to make it a permanent and delicious part of your life.

>> **Consider taking certain supplements.** Many supplements can help ease the symptoms of different kinds of arthritis, including antioxidants (beta-carotene, vitamins C and E, and selenium), boron, vitamin B6, niacin, vitamin D, zinc, grapeseed extract, flaxseed oil, green tea, glucosamine sulfate, chondroitin sulfate, SAMe, bromelain, and others.

Supplements for arthritis are discussed at length in Chapter 11.

>> **Exercise daily (whenever possible).** Countless studies have shown that exercise can help lubricate and nourish the joints by forcing joint fluid into and out of the cartilage. Underexercised joints don't get much of this in-and-out action, so cartilage can thin out and become dry. Brisk walking and swimming or walking in the shallow end of a pool may be some of the best exercises for those with arthritis, because they don't put undue stress on the joints and are easy and fun to do.

For a look at exercises that help ease arthritis symptoms, see Chapter 12.

» **Watch your joint alignment.** Making sure to stand, sit, walk, run, and lift correctly can help protect your joints from injury or excess wear and tear.

We discuss the best joint-saving techniques in detail in Chapter 13.

» **Control stress, aggression, and depression.** The way you think and feel about your arthritis pain can actually make it worse. So can stress, anger, hostility, aggression, and depression. Luckily, you can reduce your pain just by reducing your stress levels and tapping into your natural potential for relaxation.

In Chapter 14, you'll learn all about positive thinking, biofeedback, controlling your breathing, laughter, prayer, and spirituality — all of which are effective ways of improving your mood, easing your pain, and making you feel better all over.

» **Organize your life for maximum efficiency.** Studies have shown that people who actively manage their arthritis and find new ways to cope with physical problems feel less pain and fatigue.

In Chapter 15, we give you helpful tips for managing arthritis on a day-to-day basis. Included are ideas for conserving your energy, getting a good night's sleep, using assistive devices, making household chores easy, and holding on to your sex life. An occupational therapist and a home health caregiver can you offer valuable assistance with this.

Looking at alternative approaches

Because there isn't any one magic bullet that cures arthritis, a great many people look for help from alternative approaches — either as a substitute for traditional medicine or as that "extra something" that may be exactly what they need.

In Chapters 16 through 19, we discuss the most popular alternative treatments for arthritis — from herbs to homeopathy, from acupuncture to reflexology, from aromatherapy to hydrotherapy. Included are sections describing the therapy, explaining what it can do for you, and tips on how to find a reputable practitioner.

STARGAZING: FAMOUS ARTHRITIS SUFFERERS

Does the idea of having arthritis make you feel like you may as well just give up? Well, many people have felt like this, but gone on to live productive and happy lives. Take a look at what these people have achieved while coping with arthritis:

- **Lucille Ball** was diagnosed with rheumatoid arthritis at the age of 17, but she went on to live a long and healthy life, enjoying a top-notch career in movies and TV and even running her own TV production studio, Desilu.

- **Pierre-Auguste Renoir**, the famous French artist associated with the Impressionist movement developed RA in his late fifties but continued to paint, creating nearly 6,000 pictures during his lifetime, many of them great masterpieces.

- **Paula Abdul**, singer, dancer, choreographer and former *American Idol* judge has both rheumatoid arthritis and osteoarthritis. Yet she recently perfomed for sold-out crowds in Las Vegas and continues to pursue her super fast-paced career. She credits her ability to live a happy, active life to regular workouts based on low-impact strength exercises and Zumba classes.

- **Carrie Ann Inaba**, long-time judge on the popular TV show *Dancing With the Stars* has rheumatoid arthritis, Sjögren's, lupus and fibromyalgia. A strong believer in sharing her journey with others, she has a website dedicated to products and other solutions that have helped her cope with this potpourri of joint diseases.

- **Kathleen Turner**, actress, Academy Award-nominee and winner of two Golden Globe awards was diagnosed with rheumatoid arthritis in 1992. Although the disease temporarily torpedoed her career, she is now back on screen and working harder than ever. She credits twice-weekly Pilates classes to helping her regain her health.

- **Terry Bradshaw**, quarterback for four-times Super Bowl-winning Pittsburgh Steelers teams, was diagnosed with rheumatoid arthritis after pursuing a 14-year pro football career. When his medication caused weight gain, he realized how much he needed and wanted to exercise. He now keeps himself healthy and active, thanks to exercise, a positive attiutde, and an enthusiastc approach to each new day.

- **Tatum O'Neal**, actress, Academy Award winner, and daughter of Ryan O'Neal was diagnosed with rheumatoid arthritis at age 50 and has since undergone back surgery to improve her condition. She continues to take film and TV roles and credits a healthy lifestyle and Pilates with helping her live an active life.

(continued)

(continued)

- **Grandma Moses** had arthritis in her hands at age 76 when she began painting the folksy, whimsical scenes of American life that made her famous. Despite her condition, she created hundreds of paintings, many of which can be found in major museums all over the world.

- **Kim Kardashian**, American media personality, businesswoman, and star of *Keeping Up With the Kardashians* was diagnosed with psoriatic arthritis in 2019 after experiencing pain and stiffness in her hands that made it almost impossible for her to pick up a toothbrush. Taking medication helped her immensely and she has said that she hopes her story will help others with autoimmune diseases realize there is "light at the end of the tunnel."

Armed with a thorough knowledge of arthritis, how to control its symptoms, and all the many techniques you can use to manage this disease (all of which you'll find in this book), you too can be well on your way to taking charge of your condition and getting on with your life!

Chapter **2**

Osteoarthritis: The Most Common Form

Whether you call it osteoarthritis, degenerative arthritis, or degenerative joint disease, osteoarthritis (OA) is the painful result of cartilage breakdown. When the tough, rubbery substance that cushions bone ends no longer does its job, the bone ends can't slide easily across each other within the joint. That's when pain and stiffness can settle into a joint. Suddenly, your knee or lower back aches, your hip burns, a finger joint swells and throbs, or your shoulder stiffens up. You can't bend and flex the painful joint like you used to; its range of movement is limited. Most of all, it just plain hurts!

But what happened to mess up your cartilage in the first place? To understand what went wrong, here's a look at how things work in healthy cartilage.

Considering Cartilage

Healthy cartilage is absolutely essential for joints to function properly and pain-lessly. Slick as polished marble and tough as galvanized rubber, cartilage protects the ends of your bones from wearing each other away where they meet inside a joint. It also provides a smooth, slick surface so bone ends can glide easily across each other. And cartilage is an excellent shock absorber, cushioning the bones and soaking up the impact created by movement and physical stresses. Without intact cartilage, bones grind away at each other and bear the brunt of the impact of movement. Eventually, the joint itself can be damaged or even destroyed.

Four elements help cartilage do its all-important job:

>> **Water:** Sixty-five to 80 percent of cartilage is water — a crucial substance that lubricates the joints, cushions bones, and absorbs shock.

>> **Collagen:** Elasticity and a superb capability to absorb shock make collagen an integral part of healthy cartilage. A connective tissue that helps hold bones, muscles, and other bodily structures together, collagen is the mesh-like framework that provides a home for the proteoglycans.

>> **Proteoglycans:** These large, oblong molecules are covered with centipede-like "arms" that weave themselves securely into the collagen mesh and soak up water like a sponge. Then, when pressured, they release water. Thanks in part to the proteoglycans, cartilage can mold itself to the shape of the joint and respond to the ever-changing amount of pressure within the joint capsule.

>> **Chondrocytes:** These cells follow the principle "out with the old and in with the new" as they break down and get rid of old proteoglycan and collagen molecules, forming new ones to take their place.

Water, collagen, proteoglycans, and chondrocytes all work together to keep your joints moving like well-oiled machinery. When the pressure is released from a joint, say your knee when you lift your leg to take a step, water rushes into the cartilage, nourishing, bathing, and plumping it up. The water-loving proteogly-cans, woven securely into the collagen web, soak up water and hold on to it until pressure is applied to the joint (that is, you take another step). Then the water and wastes rush out of the cartilage. But as soon as the pressure is off, the proteogly-cans thirstily soak up the water again. The resilient collagen stretches and shrinks to accommodate joint pressure and water content, so your cartilage can bounce back after being flattened out.

But if your cartilage loses its ability to attract and hold water, it becomes thin, dry, cracked, and unable to provide a slippery surface (see Figure 2-1). No longer plump and resilient, it makes a poor shock absorber and cushion for the bones, particularly affecting the weight-bearing joints.

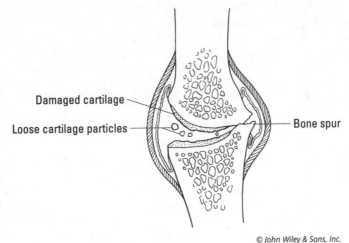

FIGURE 2-1:
Osteoarthritic joints have narrowed joint space, and thin, rough, broken-down, or completely missing cartilage.

Damaged cartilage

Loose cartilage particles

Bone spur

© John Wiley & Sons, Inc.

You can visualize the action of the cartilage by thinking of two cans of soup facing each other end-to-end with an almost-filled water balloon in between them. As you press the soup cans together, the water balloon changes shape to accommodate the pressure, but never lets the cans actually touch. When you release the pressure, the water balloon (like your cartilage) resumes its old shape.

Identifying the Signs and Symptoms of Osteoarthritis

WARNING

Don't assume that you have osteoarthritis just because you have one or more of the following symptoms. Get a thorough examination and diagnosis from a qualified physician. Figure 2-2 shows you the most common sites affected by osteoarthritis.

How do you know if the joint pain you're suffering from is due to osteoarthritis? Most of those with the disease have at least one of the following symptoms:

>> **Joint pain:** Most people experience joint pain as a deep-seated ache radiating from the inner core of the joint. The feeling is distinctly different from a muscular ache and may come and go according to changes in the weather. ("I can feel it in my bones that it's going to rain.") The pain typically increases as the joint is used and eases off with joint rest. As the disease worsens, though, the pain can become fairly steady. If joint pain occurs during the night, poor sleep and next-day fatigue may be two unpleasant side effects.

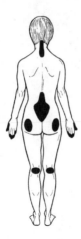

FIGURE 2-2:
The neck, lower back, knees, hips, ends of the fingers, and the base of the thumbs are the sites most commonly affected by osteoarthritis.

Some people really can feel it in their joints when it's going to rain, because as the barometric pressure falls, the lining of an arthritic joint can become inflamed, causing pain and the release of excess fluid (swelling).

» **Stiffness and loss of movement:** Stiff joints, limited range of motion, and, in later stages, joints that freeze into a bent position are all signs of osteoarthritis.

» **Tenderness, warmth, and swelling around the joint:** Although swelling is not usually a big problem with osteoarthritis, some joints do swell in response to cartilage damage and irritation, especially if they've been overused. The finger joints and the knees are most often affected.

» **"Cracking" joints:** If you hear popping or crunching sounds when you move a joint, you may have osteoarthritis. These cracking sounds (doctors call them *crepitus*) can be created by roughened cartilage. (This isn't the same thing as "cracking" your joints by applying pressure to them, which causes a harmless release of nitrogen bubbles and isn't associated with OA.)

» **Bony growths on the fingers:** Bony lumps, either at the ends of the fingers (called *Heberden's nodes*) or on the middle joint of the fingers (called *Bouchard's nodes*) are signs of osteoarthritis. These types of bony growths may be hereditary.

Discovering What Causes Cartilage Breakdown

Sometimes, we really don't know why the cartilage disintegrates. In that case, we designate the problem as *primary osteoarthritis*, or osteoarthritis of unknown cause. Other times we know that the osteoarthritis has been triggered by another problem, in which case we call it *secondary osteoarthritis*.

Considering causes of primary osteoarthritis

The ultimate cause of primary osteoarthritis remains a mystery. Although scientists aren't sure why, the collagen mesh of the cartilage becomes scrambled; it weakens and can't hold its structure. The proteoglycans, once so cozily intertwined in the collagen mesh, suddenly find themselves evicted from their secure homes. As they float off into the joint fluid, they take their water-retaining abilities with them. The cartilage is left high and dry; it thins and may even crack. At the same time, the newly freed proteoglycans draw excess fluid into the joint capsule, causing swelling. (Unfortunately, this fluid can't get back into the cartilage, where it's desperately needed. It's something like dying of thirst in the middle of the ocean.)

Although no one is absolutely certain what causes primary osteoarthritis, here are a few theories:

>> **The chondrocytes become too efficient at breaking down the collagen and proteoglycan molecules.** In healthy cartilage, the amount of breaking down enzymes is equal to the amount of building up enzymes. An overabundance of destructive enzymes leads to weakened collagen and a lack of proteoglycans.

>> **The chondrocytes go wild and start making too many proteoglycan and collagen molecules.** The opposite of the previous condition, these chondrocytes are too good at making new cartilage components. The excess proteoglycan and collagen molecules, in turn, pull extra fluid into the joint, flooding it and washing away most of the chondrocytes. The cartilage, then, is left bereft of cartilage-producing molecules.

Sorting out the sources of secondary osteoarthritis

Although the origins of primary osteoarthritis remain murky, experts are quite sure what causes secondary osteoarthritis: various types of trauma to the joints or an autoimmune arthritis (like RA or gout). That includes sudden, high-velocity trauma (the kind you'd experience in a car accident), as well as little insults to your joints that occur time and again, like repeated poor posture or running on a concrete surface every day for years. The causes of secondary osteoarthritis can be further broken down as follows:

>> **Joint injury:** Weekend warriors beware! Once a joint has been injured, be it through a sports mishap, car accident, household slippage, or anything else, it is much more likely to develop osteoarthritis.

>> **Repetitive motion injury:** Joints that are stressed over and over again in the same way (for example, a ballerina's ankles, a football player's knees, or a data processor's wrists) are more likely to experience a cartilage breakdown than joints subjected to normal use.

>> **Damage to the bone end:** Usually due to trauma or continual stress, a bone may chip or sustain small fractures. In the body's zeal to repair the damage, it may cause an overgrowth of bone in the injured area. The result is a bone end that's bumpy, not smooth, and joint problems can ensue.

>> **Bone disease:** A bone disease, such as Paget's disease, weakens the bone structure, making it more likely to fracture and develop bony overgrowth.

>> **Carrying too much body weight:** The heavier you are, the more stress your knees, hips, and ankles must bear. Osteoarthritis of the knee has been clearly linked to excess body weight. That's not surprising considering that every time you take a step the stress on your knee is roughly equivalent to three times your body weight. Increase that figure to ten times your body weight when you run!

Regarding the repair problem

To make matters worse, once your cartilage is damaged, your body can compound the problem if it repairs itself in certain ways. Like injured bone, injured cartilage can overdo the repair process, piling too much new cartilage into a crack or tear. The result is a lumpy, bumpy surface that doesn't glide smoothly against the cartilage on the opposing bone end. On the other hand, sometimes the cartilage doesn't repair itself at all, and remains in its damaged state — cracked, pitted, frayed, and even worn-through. Pieces of loose cartilage and/or bone may break off and float freely through the joint fluid. The bone ends, no longer well cushioned, start to rub against each other and can develop bony spurs (osteophytes) that further interfere with smooth joint movement. The joint space narrows, and the entire shape of the joint can change. All this from a little damaged cartilage!

TECHNICAL STUFF

You may hear your doctor use some of these technical terms: *eburnation* (increased and abnormal bone density), *subchondral bone* (the bone right below the cartilage), or *subchondral cyst* (an abnormal pocket of fluid in the bone beneath the cartilage or a bone spur).

Recognizing Risk Factors for Osteoarthritis

Although osteoarthritis affects more than 30 million Americans, not everybody suffers from it. Some people actually sail into their golden years with joints unaffected by pain, stiffness, or other symptoms, while others are hobbling around by the time they're 35. So how come one person gets osteoarthritis while another gets away scot-free? And how can you tell if you happen to be particularly susceptible to it?

Your chances of developing osteoarthritis are increased if:

>> **You're past age 45:** Cartilage and other joint structures, like most bodily tissues, tend to degrade and become weaker over time. After decades of use, they start to wear out. Luckily, research has shown that osteoarthritis isn't inevitable as we age. The odds just go up.

>> **You've had a joint injury:** If you've been in a car accident, have played rough-and-tumble sports, or have injured any of your joints in any way, you are more likely to develop osteoarthritis in the joints that were affected by those activities.

>> **Your joints have been repeatedly stressed:** Ballet dancers, assembly line workers, baseball pitchers, grocery checkers, and anyone else who overuses and stresses a joint or joints can suffer from cartilage breakdown in those joints.

>> **You're a woman:** Women are three times more likely than men to develop osteoarthritis. This may be due to smaller joint structures or some link to estrogen; nothing has yet been proven.

>> **Your parents had it:** There appears to be a genetic component to osteoarthritis; in fact, one study concluded that genes were responsible for 50 percent of hip osteoarthritis cases. Osteoarthritis in the hands is also believed to be at least partially due to genetics. An inherited tendency toward defective cartilage or poorly structured joints can certainly put you on the road to osteoarthritis, although you won't necessarily develop it.

>> **You're overweight:** Excess weight puts a great deal of strain on the weight-bearing joints — the hips, knees, and ankles. For every ten pounds of excess weight you carry, you increase the force exerted on these joints anywhere from four to ten times, depending upon the type of activity. Researchers have found a definite link between being overweight and osteoarthritis, especially involving the knee joints.

WARNING

Using chopsticks can actually increase your risk of developing OA of the hand! Researchers studying 2,507 60-year-old residents of Beijing, China found significantly more OA in the first, second, and third fingers of the hand that used chopsticks than the non-chopstick-using hand. Repeated mechanical stress to these joints, via chopstick use, is believed to be the culprit.

Determining Whether It Really Is Osteoarthritis

Nearly 50 percent of those suffering from osteoarthritis don't know what kind of arthritis they have and therefore can't make good decisions about their treatment.

Say your knee hurts. The first time that you visit your doctor complaining of the pain, they put you through the standard round of interviews, examinations, and tests. They review your medical history and makes a detailed list of the injuries you have sustained, especially to your knees. They may palpate your knee to see if it's painful to the touch, carefully bend your knee and straighten it several times (it may hurt a little and seem stiff), and listen for cracking or popping in the joint. If your arthritis appears to be inflammatory, your doctor may send you to the lab to get some blood drawn to rule out other forms of the disease. At this point, all your doctor has to go on is a history of knee injuries, some pain and stiffness upon movement, and a little cracking in the joint. Your symptoms may sound like osteoarthritis, but may not yet be a sure thing.

The next step would be to order an X-ray of your knee to see if one or more of the following signs are present:

>> Cartilage degradation

>> Cartilage overgrowth

>> Narrowing of the joint space

>> Bone spurs

>> Bits of cartilage or bone floating in the joint fluid

>> Joint deformity

Treating Osteoarthritis

After a diagnosis of osteoarthritis is confirmed, you and your doctor can begin to devise a treatment program — confident that you're headed in the right direction. Although the symptoms may not disappear completely, you still have a good chance that, with proper treatment, your pain will diminish significantly and joint degradation can be kept to a minimum. (Check out "Keeping OA at bay: Mark's Story" at the end of the chapter to see how a 35-year-old man successfully took charge of his arthritis.)

A good treatment plan for osteoarthritis should include the following elements to help you manage pain and discomfort on a daily basis.

Muting the pain with medication

Both prescription and over-the-counter remedies are commonly used to relieve osteoarthritis pain. Whether prescription or nonprescription, the drugs usually fall into one or two categories:

>> **Acetaminophen:** These relieve pain and fever, but don't reduce inflammation (for example, Tylenol, Liquiprin, or Datril).

>> **Nonsteroidal anti-inflammatories or NSAIDs:** These relieve pain and fever and *do* reduce inflammation (for example, aspirin, Advil, Aleve, or Motrin). However, NSAIDs may produce side effects that, when combined with other health conditions like heart disease, kidney disease, or stomach ulcersdon't make them the safest choice.

Another medication that has been approved to treat chronic pain, including OA pain, doesn't fall into the above categories. Duloxetine (Cymbalta) is a serotonin-norepinephrine reuptake inhibitor (SNRI) used primarily to treat depression and anxiety. But it is also used to decrease pain due to arthritis, fibromyalgia, or chronic back pain, as well as nerve pain due to diabetes.

If your joints are swollen, your doctor may prescribe an NSAID. If swelling isn't a problem, they may give you acetaminophen. And if you have chronic pain, they may prescribe one of many prescription pain relievers, including Duloxetine.

To avoid drug interactions, overdoses, or side effects, make sure you check with your doctor before taking any over-the-counter medications. (See Chapter 8 for more information on medicines.)

Lubricating your joints with exercise

If you're in pain, you probably want to *stop* moving, and it's certainly advisable for you to rest your joints when you're feeling achy. But too much sitting around can actually be the *worst* thing for you in the long run. Exercise is a great way to "oil and feed" the cartilage. Underexercised joints don't get the lubricating and nourishing benefits of the in-and-out action of the joint fluid, so cartilage can become thin and dry, losing its resilience and capability to cushion the bones.

Include three types of exercises in your overall physical fitness program:

>> **Flexibility exercises:** You should do stretching, bending, and twisting exercises every day to increase your range-of-motion and reduce stiffness. Flexibility exercises help keep your joints loose and flexible.

>> **Strengthening exercises:** Weight lifting or isometric exercises should be done every other day to build your muscles and help keep your joint-supporting structures stable. These types of exercises help increase your muscle strength.

>> **Endurance (aerobic) exercises:** These should be done at least three times a week for at least 20 to 30 minutes each session to increase overall fitness, strengthen your cardiovascular system, and keep your weight under control. Brisk walking (especially up hills), jogging, cycling, dancing, swimming, and so on, all help to increase your fitness and capacity for exercise.

Before starting a new exercise program, get a referral to a physical therapist to find out which kinds of exercise and levels of activity are appropriate for you. Doing the wrong exercises — or doing the right exercises in the wrong way — can cause you further injury. (See Chapter 12 for more information on exercise.)

Protecting your joints through good alignment

Applying the techniques of body alignment, proper standing, sitting, walking and running, and correct lifting can go a long way toward sparing your joints from excessive wear and tear and protecting them from future injury. You may also find it helpful to wrap affected joints with elastic supports or take a load off with assistive devices, such as canes or crutches. Other joint-protective techniques include alternating your activities with rest periods, varying your tasks to avoid too much repetitive stress on any one area, and pacing yourself. Don't try to do too much at once. (See Chapter 13 for more information on joint protection.)

Heating and cooling the pain away

Some people prefer heat, others cold, but use whatever works for you. Hot baths, heating pads, electric blankets, and hot tubs can relax painful muscles, while ice packs can numb the affected area. To avoid damaging tissues, just make sure you don't use either method for longer than 20 minutes at a time. (See Chapter 10 for more information on physical therapy for pain relief.)

TIP

Always give your skin time to return to its usual temperature before reapplying hot or cold packs.

Taking a load off with weight control

If you're overweight, your hips, knees, and ankles are probably suffering. Not only are they subjected to a force equal to three times your body weight each time you take a step, they can be pummeled by ten times your body weight if you jog or run! So that extra 10 pounds around your middle may translate to an extra 100 pounds slamming away on certain joints at certain times. And that's only *one* reason why keeping your weight at an acceptable level is so important. (See Appendix C for more information on diet and weight control.)

WARNING

Fifty percent of patients who develop knee osteoarthritis have been overweight for three to ten years.

Knowing how to help yourself

Strategies for pain management, foods and supplements that may help ease symptoms, positive thinking, prayer, spirituality, massage, relaxation techniques, and alternative healing methods can add to your arsenal in the fight against pain and disability. Don't ignore their enormous potential to improve the quality of your life. (See Chapters 10, 11, and 15 through 19 for more information on these topics.)

Considering surgery

When you have a painful joint that isn't going to get better, and the pain is seriously compromising your level of function and the quality of your life, you may want to consider surgery. These days, routine surgeries like arthroscopic surgery, cartilage transplants, and joint replacement surgery can make a huge difference for those who live in pain. (See Chapter 9 for more information on surgery.)

KEEPING OA AT BAY: MARK'S STORY

Mark, a 35-year-old television executive, had been a hotshot college quarterback in his younger days. But after winding up at the bottom of one too many half-ton pileups, his knees were shot.

"I was a sitting duck for those guys," Mark says ruefully. "They just couldn't wait to pounce on me, no matter what the play. After two years of getting hit over and over again, my body just couldn't take it anymore. I was permanently sidelined."

Sidelined from football, perhaps, but not other sports. Over the next several years he took up jogging, karate, fencing, and weight lifting. "I tried to do something every day," Mark said. "But it wasn't just because I wanted to keep in shape. I would get itchy if I didn't get a certain amount of exercise on a daily basis." In spite of his efforts, though, he managed to pack an extra 20 pounds onto his once rock-hard body. ("Beer and nachos while watching football," Mark explained, smiling.)

Then one day, right in the middle of a fencing match, his right knee began to hurt. "It was a deep pain, way inside my knee, a pretty intense soreness that lasted through the match and really bugged me," Mark said. Afterward, he iced his knee, and the pain went away. But it began to bother him now and again, often during fencing, and also when he was jogging or in the bent-knee stance of karate. When the pain became present more often than not, Mark went to see a sports medicine doctor.

"Sounds to me like osteoarthritis," his doctor said. An X-ray confirmed that the cartilage in his knee was "rough" and quite thin. "Arthritis!" Mark exploded. "But that's for old people. I'm only 35!"

Two years later, Mark's osteoarthritis is pretty well under control. He rarely has pain, unless he stands in line for long periods of time. And although he has given up certain knee-thrashing sports (such as football, karate, and fencing), he has found that he's still physically able to do just about whatever he wants.

"I chalk my recovery up to two main things," Mark says. "Losing weight and switching activities. Once I dropped that extra 20 pounds I'd been lugging around, my knee pain also dropped about 50 percent. Then I started swimming every day — a real boon to my joints since I could keep them loosened up without the slamming impact of jogging or jumping rope. Yoga has also helped me gain some flexibility while getting rid of some tension. And I've been taking a few supplements that seem to help. All in all, I feel like a brand new guy."

Chapter **3**

A War Within: Rheumatoid Arthritis

*R*heumatoid arthritis (RA) is a case of the human body's good intentions gone awry. Your body is equipped with a very effective immune system that fights off bacteria and other foreign bodies. Specialized immune cells attack these invaders, surround them, paralyze them, and destroy them. A strong, intact immune system is absolutely essential to your survival — without it, you would quickly become consumed by infections and disease. But if your immune system should suddenly go haywire and start attacking your body's own tissues, it could become your worst enemy. Such is the case with RA. When you have RA, your immune system attacks the tissues that cushion and line your joints, eventually causing entire joints to deteriorate.

RA doesn't have to be all bad news though; check out the sidebar "Overcoming RA: Lucy's Story" later in the chapter to learn how actress Lucille Ball stayed active and healthy until the end of her life, despite having rheumatoid arthritis.

Turning on Itself: When the Body Becomes Its Own Worst Enemy

For reasons that aren't completely understood, in rheumatoid arthritis the white blood cells of the immune system attack the joint lining (synovial membrane) as if it were a foreign object. And pain, swelling, loss of movement, and joint destruction are the unhappy results. After the immune system goes to work on the joint lining, here's what happens:

1. The assaulted membrane becomes inflamed and painful, the entire joint capsule swells, and the synovial cells start to grow and divide in an abnormal way.

2. Almost as if they're launching a counterattack, these abnormal cells invade the surrounding tissue — mostly the bone and cartilage.

3. The joint space begins to narrow, and the joint's supporting structures become weak. At the same time, the cells that trigger inflammation release enzymes that start eating away at the bone and cartilage, causing joint erosion and scarring.

4. Reeling under this many-sided attack, the joint itself deteriorates, eventually becoming misshapen and misaligned.

See Figures 3-1 and 3-2 for comparison of a healthy joint to one with RA.

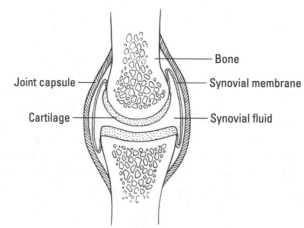

FIGURE 3-1: In the healthy joint, the synovial membrane is thin and free from inflammation; the cartilage is smooth, thick, and even. The joint space is well defined, and the joint capsule assumes a normal shape.

Joint capsule

Cartilage

Bone

Synovial membrane

Synovial fluid

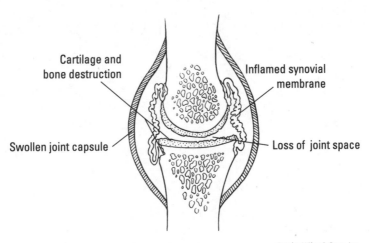

FIGURE 3-2: In the joint affected by RA, the synovial membrane is inflamed and swollen, with infected cells invading both bone and cartilage. The cartilage is thin, the joint space narrowed, and the joint capsule swollen.

Rheumatoid arthritis insidiously makes its way through the body and (in more severe cases) can eventually spread to all of the joints. But the joints are not its only targets. RA is a systemic disease capable of attacking various parts of the body, not just the joints. It can cause inflammation of the eyes, skin, heart, blood vessels, and lungs, generally wreaking havoc on the body as a whole.

WARNING

If the tear and salivary glands partially "dry up," Sjögren's can develop in association with RA. See Chapter 4 for more on this "drying disease."

Some people have RA for just a short time — a few months or a couple of years — and then it disappears forever. Others suffer through painful periods (flares) that come and go, although they can feel quite well in between episodes. Those with severe forms of RA, however, may be in pain a good deal of the time, experience symptoms for many years, and suffer serious joint damage.

Recognizing the signs and symptoms of RA

If you have rheumatoid arthritis, the first thing you may notice is a dull ache, stiffness, and swelling in two matching joints — for example, both elbows, both knees, or both index fingers. The most typical sites for RA are the fingers and wrists, but it can also settle in the hands, elbows, shoulders, neck, hips, knees, ankles, and feet. See Figure 3-3.

WARNING

Although pain and inflammation are early signs of RA, they're not always the first to herald the arrival of the disease. RA typically begins with minor symptoms and slowly makes its presence known. But it can also strike dramatically, causing several joints to become inflamed all at once.

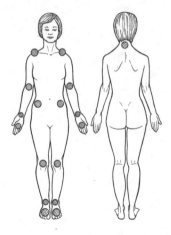

Although the symptoms of rheumatoid arthritis vary, most people with RA experience one or more of the following:

>> Pain, warmth, redness, swelling, or tightness in a joint

>> Swelling of three or more joints for six or more weeks

>> Joints affected in a symmetrical, mirror-image pattern (for example, both knees, both shoulders, and so on)

>> Joint pain or stiffness lasting longer than 30 minutes upon arising or after prolonged inactivity

>> Pea-shaped bumps under the skin (called *rheumatoid nodules*), especially on pressure points like the elbows or the feet, or overlying affected joints. In bedridden patients, they may also occur at the base of the scalp or on the back side of the hip

>> Evidence of joint erosion on an X-ray

>> Loss of mobility

>> General soreness, aching, stiffness

>> A general "sick" feeling *(malaise)*

>> Fatigue

>> Periodic low-grade fever and/or sweats

>> Difficulty sleeping

>> Anemia caused by chronic inflammation in the body

>> Blood tests showing the presence of positive rheumatoid factor (RF) or anti-cyclic citrullinated peptide (anti-CCP) antibody. These are antibodies that are found in up to 80 percent of RA patients.

As RA progresses, the joints enlarge and can become deformed. They may even freeze in a semicontracted position, making complete extension impossible. The fingers can start to curl up, pointing away from the thumb, as their tendons slip out of place. RA may also attack other parts of the body, causing the following conditions:

>> **Pleurisy:** If RA attacks the lungs, it can cause *pleurisy* (inflammation of the membranes around the lungs), prompting difficulty in breathing, chest pain, and scarring and inflammation of the lungs causing chronic dry cough and difficult breathing, especially with exercise.

>> **Episcleritis or scleritis:** If it attacks the tissues covering the white part of the eye, it can cause eye pain, sensitivity to light, and tearing of the eye.

>> **Pericarditis:** If it settles in the membrane surrounding the heart (a condition called *pericarditis*), it can cause chest pain while lying down, or impair the heart's ability to pump blood properly.

>> **Vasculitis:** If it affects the blood vessels *(vasculitis),* the blood supply to other parts of the body can be cut off, causing nerve damage, skin ulcers, gangrene, and other types of tissue death.

REMEMBER

Even though rheumatoid arthritis can have some very serious consequences, this disease can be managed. Many people with RA live long, successful lives, and we now have many FDA-approved medications that can improve quality of life, level of function, and protect the joints from permanent damage and deformity. But remember: Early treatment can make a big difference in RA, so don't wait to see a doctor.The earlier RA is diagnosed and treated, the better the overall prognosis and the higher the likelihood that the disease can be controlled.

Understanding the causes of RA

The truth is that nobody really knows what causes RA, although some believe it is linked to a defect in the immune system. Many people with RA have a particular genetic marker — HLA-DR4 — so it's reasonable to suspect that this gene may be to blame. Yet, not everyone with this gene ends up with RA, and not everyone with RA has this gene. And scientists are certain that more than just one gene is involved: Perhaps HLA-DR4 is only one of several genes that can tip the scales in favor of developing RA. Most likely, genetic markers play a part in the development of the disease but aren't the determining factor. Some researchers believe that RA may be triggered by a virus, or perhaps an unrecognized bacteria, that "wakes up" a dormant genetic defect and sets it in motion. As of yet, no such infectious agent has been discovered, and RA has not been found to be contagious.

Hormones or hormone deficiencies may also play a part, although their possible role is unclear. Women are more likely than men to develop RA, suggesting a possible link to estrogen. But, at present, doctors have more questions than answers about RA.

Pinpointing the most likely victim of RA

Rheumatoid arthritis can strike just about anybody — children, the elderly, the middle-aged, and people of almost all racial or ethnic groups. But RA has a particular affinity for women, especially those between the ages of 20 and 50. Women account for over two-thirds of the 1.5 million Americans who suffer from RA, making them about three times as likely as men to get the disease, although scientists have yet to determine why.

OVERCOMING RA: LUCY'S STORY

Lucille Ball, the famous comedienne and zany star of the *I Love Lucy* television series, was just 17 years old and working as a model in Hattie Carnegie's internationally renowned dress shop when she suddenly developed a fiery pain in both her legs. "It was so bad, I had to sit down," she wrote in her autobiography, *Love, Lucy*. She had recently recovered from a bout with pneumonia and a high fever; now this!

Hurrying to her doctor, she received the terrifying news: She had rheumatoid arthritis, a crippling disease that becomes progressively worse over time. In fact, it was conceivable that she would spend her life in a wheelchair. Lucy's doctor sent her to an orthopedic clinic where she waited for three hours, nearly fainting from the pain, before the doctor informed her that there was no cure. He did ask if she would like to try an experimental treatment, though — injections of a kind of "horse serum." Lucy agreed and received these shots over the next several weeks until she finally ran out of money. Unfortunately, the pain continued.

Discouraged but not about to give up, Lucy went back home to her parents, who massaged her legs, gave her money to continue the horse serum injections, and encouraged her to take better care of her health. Finally, months later, the pain began to ease, and Lucy was able to stand up on weak and shaky legs. Her left leg had shortened a bit during the course of the disease, so she added a 20-pound weight to her corrective shoe to stretch the leg out. (Note: RA is no longer treated with horse serum. We've come a long way since then!)

Lucy's hard work and perseverance paid off. She was able to return to New York; she made several movies and eventually starred in her own television series, one that required vigorous physical comedy, stamina, and energy. She also starred in Broadway plays, performing eight shows a week while managing to sail through energetic song and dance numbers with a seemingly effortless grace and ease. Lucy remained active and healthy until her death in 1989, and in spite of her doctor's ominous prediction, never spent a single day in a wheelchair.

Diagnosing Rheumatoid Arthritis

Unfortunately, no one test can tell your doctor you definitely have RA. Instead, your doctor looks for a tell-tell pattern in the information taken from many sources, such as your medical history, physical examination, laboratory tests, X-rays, a fluid sample taken from affected joints, and, if rheumatoid nodules are present, a biopsy of those nodules.

Searching for clues: The medical history and physical exam

During your initial examination, your doctor will ask about the onset of your symptoms, whether you're experiencing any morning stiffness, the kind and amount of pain you feel, the presence of swelling, whether or not joints are affected on both sides of your body, and so on. Looking into your medical history is a way to see if your symptoms fit the general pattern of RA or suggest another disease instead. During your physical exam, your doctor will also check for tenderness, range of motion, and the presence of rheumatoid nodules.

Taking tests

Three tests typically help diagnose rheumatoid arthritis, all of which involve taking a sample of your blood and sending it to the laboratory for examination:

>> **Rheumatoid factor (RF) test** checks for the presence of a particular antibody that appears in the blood of the majority of people who have RA. But a positive RF test doesn't necessarily mean you have rheumatoid arthritis.

The RF antibody can also appear due to other rheumatic diseases, hepatitis C, and many other medical conditions.

>> **Erythrocyte sedimentation rate (ESR or sed rate)** measures the rate at which red blood cells settle in a test tube, which can indicate inflammation. This is a nonspecific marker of inflammation, which may be due to several factors, including age, obesity, infection, cancer, and autoimmune conditions.

>> **C-reactive protein (CRP)** is another nonspecific marker of inflammation. It checks for a protein that indicates inflammation is present somewhere in the body.

>> **Cyclic citrullinated peptide (CCP) antibody** checks for a type of antibody commonly produced in rheumatoid arthritis as well as certain other autoimmune disorders.

>> **Complete blood count (CBC)** checks for anemia (meaning there are not enough red blood cells) and thrombocytosis (the production of too many platelets), both of which can occur with chronic inflammation and are often seen in RA. These findings are not specific to RA, just a sign of chronic inflammation.

>> **Antinuclear antibody (ANA)** checks for antibodies to components in the nucleus of cells. This is very nonspecific test that is commonly positive in healthy individuals (up to 25 percent at low levels!), but may provide additional clues that you have RA, or another condition such as lupus.

>> **Human leukocyte antigen tissue typing (HLA)** checks for a genetic marker that indicates an increased likelihood for developing an immune-related condition like RA, reactive arthritis, or ankylosing spondylitis. HLAB27 is the test most commonly ordered, but is not routinely needed to evaluate someone for RA.

In addition, your doctor may perform the following tests:

>> **Joint aspiration (arthrocentesis):** The doctor inserts a needle into your affected joint(s) to remove some of the synovial fluid, which is examined under a microscope for evidence of infection or inflammation.

>> **Imaging tests:** A standard X-ray of your joints may be taken to check for bone and cartilage loss and/or serve as a baseline for comparison of future X-rays.

However, X-rays aren't sensitive enough to detect joint damage in the early stages of the disease. Magnetic resonance imaging (MRI) and ultrasound images may be helpful in detecting early signs of RA when the diagnosis is not clear since they can provide more information than X-ray, but aren't always needed to make an RA diagnosis. Computerized technology (CT scans) are rarely used to detect RA because, although they show bone damage, they lack the sensitivity to reveal soft-tissue changes.

>> **Biopsy of rheumatoid nodules:** Rheumatoid nodules are rubbery lumps under the skin that often form near the joints in people who have RA. Occasionally, a biopsy will be done to rule out other conditions, like infections or gout. However, this is not a very common procedure.

Unless the rheumatoid nodules cause pain or impair your range of motion, they usually don't need to be treated. But since other bumps and lumps can look and feel like RA nodules, your doctor may want to take a piece of tissue from one of them and examine it under a microscope to confirm the diagnosis. After carefully cleansing the skin and injecting a local anesthetic, the doctor makes a tiny cut near the nodule and, if possible, shaves off a piece of tissue. Or they may push a thin, hollow needle into the nodule and, using suction, pull out a tissue sample.

Treating Rheumatoid Arthritis

Although RA is often a chronic disease, most people respond well to treatment and lead active, productive lives. A few years back, a victim of RA could look forward to a dreary life spent bedridden or in a wheelchair. But today, they have a better prognosis: Only about one in ten patients progresses to the point of disability, and in a full 70 percent of the cases, symptoms are relieved or controlled for long periods of time.

REMEMBER

Treatment begins with immunosuppressive medications. Not all people respond to the same medicines, so there may be some trial and error while you and your provider find the treatment that works for you and your RA. Sometimes, surgery is needed for permanent deformity, but the goal is to get RA under control before you get to that point. While RA is considered a chronic, lifelong condition, our current treatments can bring about dramatic improvements in the signs and symptoms of the disease.

Relying on rest during a flare

Resting the affected joints during a flare is a must, because using them tends to increase inflammation. Regular rest periods should be worked into the daily schedule, and at times, total bed rest may be necessary during a flare. Immobilizing a severely affected joint with a splint may help, but the joint should be moved from time to time to keep it from locking up. You may want to wear a splint during the most active times of the day, and take it off during the least active times — for example, 12 hours on and 12 hours off.

Mental outlook appears to affect RA symptoms. Stress tends to make flares worse, whereas a positive outlook can help keep complications at bay.

Delving into your diet

What you do and don't eat can make a difference to the arthritis disease process and how much pain you feel. Because many forms of arthritis and arthritis-related conditions involve inflammation, eating foods that help reduce the inflammation response (like fatty fish and fish oil) may make a positive difference. Eating plenty of fruits, vegetables, and whole grains supplies ample amounts of antioxidants like vitamins C and E and selenium, which can fight the cellular damage that contributes to arthritis. (See Chapter 11 to find out more about how what you eat may affect how you feel.)

Easing into exercise and physical therapy

A good overall exercise program helps strengthen joint-supporting structures, increases endurance, and maintains or improves flexibility. Even inflamed joints should be exercised a little to prevent them from freezing up. A physical therapist can provide exercises that gently take the joints through their full range of movement. Exercising in water, especially during flares, may be easier than exercising on land, because it's low impact and the cool water may help ease inflammation. (See Chapter 12.)

Protecting your joints

Not only do you make your mom happy when you stand up straight, but you reduce the pressure on your joints. Maintaining proper posture while walking, standing, and sitting can go a long way toward easing joint stress. And understanding how to lift or move heavy objects correctly is also a must. (See Chapter 13.)

Applying hot or cold compresses

Applying hot or cold packs to inflamed joints may ease the pain and help reduce inflammation. Use heat to ease sore muscles and increase circulation, and try cold to dull the pain and reduce inflammation. (See Chapter 10.)

Taking medication

Many drugs can be used to combat RA symptoms. The following subsections give you the details on the five types of medication commonly prescribed.

Non-steroidal anti-inflammatory drugs (NSAIDs)

NSAIDs (pronounced n-seds) reduce swelling, relieve pain, and are the most commonly used drugs for pain management in RA. While these medicines can help with symptom control, they do not prevent disease progression or stop the immune attack on the joints. Therefore, they should never be the only treatment for your RA.

Ibuprofen (Advil) and naproxen (Aleve) are two well-known over-the-counter NSAIDs, but prescription NSAIDs such as celecoxib (Celebrex) may be preferred because they come in higher doses (which means you take fewer pills) and have longer-lasting results.

WARNING

As with all drugs, certain side effects can occur when taking NSAIDs, including upset stomach, nausea, diarrhea, stomach ulcers, and stomach bleeding. Take this type of medication with food to prevent these reactions. However, if you have kidney disease, high bleeding risk, or heart disease, NSAIDs many not be a good choice. Discuss them with your provider first.

Disease-modifying antirheumatic drugs (DMARDs)

DMARDs are first-line treatments for RA that turn off a part of the immune system that is overactive in RA, addressing the problem at the source. They can alter the course of the disease by reducing inflammation and joint damage, while preserving joint function. DMARDs often used to treat RA include methotrexate, sulfasalazine, hydroxychloroquine, and leflunomide. Some DMARDs are also used to treat autoimmune diseases *such as* lupus.

TECHNICAL STUFF

DMARDs are also known as *remittive drugs* and *slow-acting drugs.* They're called slow acting because you may not see results for 8 to 12 weeks.

These drugs may influence the immune system — whose errant behavior can lead to RA — to slow the formation of joint deformities, affect cell growth, or otherwise lessen the progress of RA. They can even send the disease into remission, at least temporarily.

Typically DMARDs are used for life, although the dose may be reduced once the disease has been in remission for a while. Potential side effects of DMARDs include increased infections, gastrointestinal distress (diarrhea, loss of appetite, vomiting, and so on), liver problems, rashes, and blood cell disorders.

Biologics

Biologics are proteins that are genetically engineered to target specific parts of the immune system that affect inflammation. Each one zeroes in on a particular cause of inflammation and either tamps it down or turns it off completely, or shores up certain immune system components that fight inflammation. Biologics can slow joint damage significantly or actually bring it to a halt.

While they can be used alone, all of them work better in combination with DMARDs such as methotrexate. Two biologics should not be used together. Biologics are quite expensive because they must either be injected or infused. Generally speaking, they take about three months to start working, although some people start to feel better sooner.

Many different types of biologics exist:

>> **Tumor necrosis factor (TNF) inhibitors (Humira, Enbrel, Simponi, Cimzia, Remicade):** All but Remicade are injections given anywhere from once a week to once a month; Remicade is an infusion. Since they have been around the longest, these are typically the first type of biologic used when DMARDs alone fail to provide adequate relief.

When TNF inhibitiors fail, there are several other types of biologics that can be tried next. Which drug is chosen will depend on the patient's health, personal preferences, and insurance coverage.

>> **B-cell inhibitors (Rituxan):** One treatment (two infusions given two weeks apart every four to six months) may provide relief of RA symptoms.

>> **Interleukin-1 (IL-1) inhibitors (Kineret):** A daily injection.

>> **Selective co-stimulation modulators (Orencia):** A once a month injection thought to have the lowest risk of infection.

>> **Interleukin-6 (IL-6) inhibitors (Actemra, Kevzara):** Injection given every one to two weeks. There is also an infusion version of Actemra.

>> **Janus kinase (JAK) inhibitors (Rinvoq, Xeljanz):** Pills taken 1 to 2 times daily.

WARNING

Suppressing the immune system increases your risk of developing infections. Since each biologic partially disables an "arm" of the immune system, you will become more susceptible to certain infections when taking these drugs. For example, the TNF inhibitor biologics can increase your risk of tuberculosis and fungal infections. B-cell inhibitors can cause chest pain, difficulty breathing and flu–like symptoms, and increase your susceptibility to colds and sinus infections. Interleukin inhibitors can cause bowel perforation in rare instances. And selective co-stimulation modulators can contribute to pneumonia, tuberculosis and flu. Ask your doctor about these risks before taking biologics.

Steroids

Steroids, which are technically called *corticosteroids* or *glucocorticoids* and include the drugs prednisone, hydrocortisone and dexamethasone, are powerful weapons against inflammation. They work by suppressing the immune system, which brings about the inflammation seen in RA. Although often prescribed in pill form, steriods can also be injected into the RA-affected joints to relieve pain and swelling. While the relief can be dramatic, unfortunately it doesn't last, and the long term side effects and consequences of chronic steroid use are numerous.

REMEMBER

Steroids are "souped-up" versions of cortisone, the body's natural immune suppressor. Because they act quickly to reduce inflammation and suppress flare-ups, they may be prescribed during early RA in addition to DMARDs and/or other medications which can take weeks or months to produce results. However the routine use of steroids to treat RA, even in early stages, is not recommended because of severe side effects. Steroids are typically reserved for severe cases and used for only short periods of time. Once the DMARDs or other drugs take effect, steroid therapy must be tapered off.

Side effects include high blood pressure, osteoporosis, increased blood glucose, cataracts, accelerated *atherosclerosis* (clogged arteries), weight gain, bruising and thinning of the skin, and a substantially increased risk of infections.

WARNING

If you suddenly stop taking steroids, you may suffer from pain, swelling, critical illness, or even death due to adrenal crisis. Always taper off your use of these drugs.

Saving your joints through surgery

When all else fails and RA becomes severe or disabling, surgery may be an option. Surgeons have different approaches to relieving the symptoms. Some of the approaches are included in the following list:

>> Diseased joint linings can be surgically removed.

>> Joint replacement can correct deformities and ease pain.

>> Fusing or removing joints in the foot may relieve the pain experienced when walking.

>> Fusing vertebrae in the neck may prevent spinal cord compression.

>> Fusing of the thumb joint can aid in grasping.

>> Repairing ruptured tendons can re-enable movement of fingers.

Other sophisticated surgical techniques on the horizon may ensure a healthier and less painful future for RA sufferers who already have permanent deformities.

Reducing the risk factors for heart disease

Many studies have shown that the risk of coronary artery disease is much higher in patients with RA. This is most likely because the chronic inflammation caused by RA speeds up the progression of atherosclerosis, the main cause of heart attack and stroke. Those with RA are also more likely to be smokers and to have high blood pressure, metabolic syndrome, obesity, and abnormal lipid levels than the general population. Most rheumatologists recommend that their RA patients exercise, watch their weight, eat a nutritious diet, keep their cholesterol and blood pressure under control, and stop smoking as part of their routine care. Check out *Preventing & Reversing Heart Disease For Dummies* (Wiley) to find out more.

Predicting the outcome

Predicting how a person with RA will fare is difficult; after all everyone is different. But certain factors can suggest that the course of the disease may be either easier or more difficult. For example, RA may be *less* severe if one or more of the following factors applies to you:

>> **You're female.** Women are more likely to get RA; however the disease often takes a greater toll on men.

>> **You have a college degree or better.** Educated people tend to seek help earlier, are more likely to follow doctor's orders to the letter, often have less physically strenuous jobs, and have better access to care.

>> **You're middle-aged or older when stricken.**

>> **You are diagnosed and treated as soon as possible.** Studies confirm a "window of opportunity" in RA whereby people who are treated sooner and get the disease under control faster do better in the long run.

>> **Your cartilage and bone ends have not been worn away, and you don't yet have joint deformities.**

>> **You don't have rheumatoid nodules.**

>> **Your level of rheumatoid factor is low and/or your anti-CCP test is negative.** Remember, however, that some people who have little or no rheumatoid factor still suffer severely.

>> **You don't smoke.** Smoking has been linked to more aggressive destruction of the joints.

>> **You're pregnant.** Some women enjoy a nine-month period of time with fewer symptoms.

Focusing on the future

Today, rheumatoid arthritis rarely manifests as the crippling, deforming disease of just a few years ago. Researchers in genetics and immunology are constantly uncovering new and fascinating parts of this puzzle, and many new, highly effective drugs have been introduced to treat RA over the past 20 years. Great strides have also been made in surgical techniques, enabling surgeons to offer hope to those with deformed, painful joints. Through our rapidly expanding arsenal of knowledge, our medications, certain lifestyle changes, and new surgical techniques, we should soon be able to tame, if not conquer, the beast known as rheumatoid arthritis.

Understanding the Difference between Osteoarthritis and Rheumatoid Arthritis

RA and OA have two things in common: namely joint pain and damage to certain joint structures, such as the cartilage and the bone. Other than that, they're about as different as night and day. Table 3-1 outlines the differences between RA and osteoarthritis.

TABLE 3-1

Rheumatoid Arthritis Compared to Osteoarthritis

Rheumatoid Arthritis	Osteoarthritis
Joint inflammation and swelling are prominent symptoms.	Joint inflammation and swelling are less common.
Usually begins between the ages of 25 to 50, but can also strike children.	Usually begins after the age of 40. Rarely strikes children.
Settles in a majority of joints, especially fingers, wrists, shoulders, knees, and elbows.	Affects the weight-bearing joints primarily (for example, knees, hips, and spine).
Affects joints symmetrically (for example, both wrists).	Affects isolated joints or one joint at a time.
Morning stiffness lasts more than 30 minutes.	Brief periods of morning stiffness.
Often causes systemic symptoms, such as fatigue, fever, weight loss, and general malaise. In severe cases, they can attack organs outside the joints.	Does not cause systemic symptoms.

Chapter **4**

Investigating Other Forms of Arthritis

The various forms of arthritis all have one thing in common: They produce pain, swelling, and other problems in or near one or more joints. The symptoms may appear suddenly and obviously, or they may sneak up so gradually that you can't remember when they began. They may strike with the force of a jackhammer or feel more like a chilly breeze. Sometimes the diagnosis is obvious; other times it may elude doctors for a year or longer. The varied treatments can be quick and effective, produce delayed reactions or in some cases, not work at all.

Osteoarthritis and rheumatoid arthritis, the subjects of Chapters 2 and 3, are well-known forms of arthritis. This chapter examines some of the lesser-known and less prevalent, but still troublesome, forms of the disease, including pseudogout, juvenile idiopathic arthritis, infectious arthritis, gonococcal arthritis (a form of infectious arthritis), psoriatic arthritis, and ankylosing spondylitis.

Gaining Insight into Gout: It's Not Just for Royalty

Many people think that gout is a disease reserved for corpulent kings and beefy barons, but any one of us can be stricken, even if we're slim and never drink alcohol.

Summarizing the symptoms

More than eight million Americans suffer from gout. In younger populations, gout affects men more often than women, but women catch up to them after menopause. Officially known as *acute gouty arthritis,* the problem usually begins with a sudden, overwhelming "assault" on a joint. You may go to bed feeling fine with no inkling of trouble ahead only to wake up in the middle of the night with excruciating pain in the "bunion joint" of your big toe. The joint is stiff and warm to the touch, and swelling lends a shiny, tight, reddish or purplish look to the skin, which is tightly stretched over the area. Sometimes the joint is so inflamed and tender that even the touch of a bed sheet causes agonizing pain. You may also have a fever, chills, a rapid heart rate, and a general blah feeling.

Gout is linked to excess levels of uric acid in the blood (known as *hyperuricemia*). When the blood has more uric acid than it can handle, the body may convert the excess into sharp, pointed urate crystals and store them in one or more joints. Since these urate crystals don't belong in the joints, the immune system tries to clean them up, resulting in pain and inflammation. See Figure 4-1 for an example of what these crystal deposits look like in a joint.

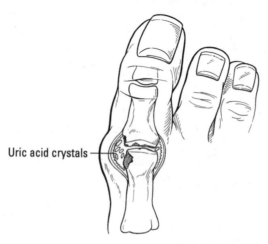

Uric acid crystals

FIGURE 4-1: Crystal deposits in a gouty joint.

© John Wiley & Sons, Inc.

The joint at the base of the big toe is quite often the first site that gout strikes. The elbows, wrists, fingers, knees, ankles, heels, and instep may also be attacked during the first or subsequent bouts, while the shoulders, spine, and hips are rarely touched. No matter where gout strikes first, there's about a 75 percent chance that it will affect the big toe at some point.

Your first attack of gout may also be your last. Or, it may herald the beginning of a series of attacks on that joint and/or others, leading to progressive and irreversible joint injury. Fortunately, medical treatment can help ward off recurring attacks while preventing or minimizing permanent joint damage. In this sense, gout is really the only curable form of arthritis — so long as you take your medicines as directed every day! If you want to guard against gout, your best strategy is probably to be born female. Women's uric acid levels are naturally lower than men's until they reach menopause. Then their uric acid levels start to rise, although it can take up to 20 years before they equal the levels seen in men.

Several situations are linked to an excessive amount of uric acid in the blood, including the following:

>> Genetics — Approximately 20 percent of those with gout have a history of the disease in the family.

>> Taking drugs that can lead to increased uric acid (such as diuretics, aspirin, nicotinic acid, levodopa, and cyclosporine).

>> Blood cancer or other diseases that cause the rapid multiplication and destruction of body cells, leading to higher levels of purines and uric acid.

>> Chronic kidney disease which hamper the kidneys' ability to filter out uric acid.

>> Drinking too much alcohol (beer or grain liquors, including whiskey and vodka) and/or eating or drinking foods that contain high-fructose corn syrup may also play a role in initiating gout.

To a lesser extent, eating lots of foods containg a high amount of purines such as red meat, lamb or pork, organ meats, shellfish, and certain fish (including anchovies, sardines, mussels, codfish, and herring), may stimulate the body's production of uric acid. Gout is also associated with high blood pressure, heart disease, diabetes, high levels of cholesterol, and obesity.

Though the disease becomes apparent when excess uric acid in the blood is converted into a crystalline form and deposited in the joints, elevated uric acid alone doesn't cause gout. Many people with excess levels of uric acid never get the disease, while others who suffer from terrible gout-related pain may have fairly standard amounts of uric acid. It's also possible to have fully formed uric acid crystals deposited in a joint or two yet feel no pain at all.

Diagnosing and treating gout

Sometimes the symptoms of gout "speak" loudly, making diagnosis fairly easy. Other times, they can be vague, making diagnosis a real head-scratcher.

REMEMBER

The best, most reliable test for gout is joint aspiration (arthrocentesis) — that is, using a needle to drain fluid from the affected joint, and when examining it under the microscope, finding it contains uric acid crystals. Your doctor will also look for *tophi* (lumps of uric acid underneath the skin that appear chalk-like), and tender and swollen inflamed joints. If tophi are present, your gout is considered severe and chronic. Your doctor may also X-ray the afflicted joint.

Gout is curable with medications, so long as you take them daily and your doctor adjusts the dosage of your medication to ensure that your uric acid levels stay below a certain threshold.

For treatment of a gout flare, high doses of NSAIDs (see Chapter 8) are used to ease pain and inflammation. Steroids may also be injected directly into the joint to reduce inflammation, and your doctor may insert a needle into the joint and draw out the excess joint fluid to relieve the pain and pressure.

If you have more than two gout flares per year, you have tophi, and/or an X-ray shows that your have permanent joint damage due to gout, your doctor will likely recommend chronic urate lowering therapy (for life), using a medicine such as allopurinol or febuxostat that lowers uric acid to levels where crystals cannot form.

Helping yourself heal

You can help heal gout and prevent its recurrence by:

>> Losing weight if you are overweight

>> Eliminating alcohol intake, especially beer or grain liquors, which contain purines

>> Eliminating foods containing purines (detailed earlier in this chapter)

>> Working with your doctor to keep your blood pressure under control, if it's a problem, as well as heart disease and/or diabetes

>> Consulting with your doctor to make sure you're not taking any medicines or supplements that encourage gout or interfere with your treatment

>> Exercising regularly

Studying Pseudogout: The Royal Pretender

Although gout is an ancient disease that has ruined many a day in a medieval VIP's life, pseudogout is a relatively "new" affliction. Although it's probably been around as long as "regular" gout, doctors didn't realize it was a separate problem until it was first described in 1962.

The official name for pseudogout is *calcium pyrophosphate deposition disease (CPPD)*, although "pseudogout" is still used by both doctors and patients.

Summarizing the symptoms

The symptoms of pseudogout are similar to those of gout but without the needlelike uric acid crystals in the joint. Instead, pseudogout is characterized by rhomboid-shaped crystals made up of calcium pyrophosphate dihydrate. And although gout typically affects the big toe joint, pseudogout more often targets the knee.

The disease itself may be acute or chronic. Acute attacks are likely to strike suddenly, settle in, and last for several days or even weeks. (Fortunately, they are usually not as painful as acute attacks of "true" gout.) The chronic form of pseudogout produces attacks that last longer, typically targets more than one joint at a time and, with time, severely damages those joints.

The causes of pseudogout are unknown. Surgery, a hormonal imbalance, or a metabolic upset may touch it off. Sometimes it strikes in conjunction with other diseases or conditions, such as low blood levels of magnesium or excessive blood levels of iron or calcium. Pseudogout strikes men and women at about the same rate and prefers older folks, especially those over the age of 60. Trauma to a joint will also increase the risk of developing pseudogout in that joint.

Diagnosing and treating pseudogout

Because pseudogout can masquerade as gout, rheumatoid arthritis, or another ailment, diagnosis is usually made by inspecting fluid taken from the affected joint. If you have pseudogout, your fluid will contain calcium pyrophosphate dihydrate crystals. (These crystals can also be picked up on X-rays.)

Unfortunately, there's no way to cure the disease completely and no method for removing the offending crystals from the joints. Instead, doctors will try to relieve the symptoms, typically by prescribing NSAIDs or the gout drug, colchicine, to reduce the pain and inflammation. In difficult cases, steroids such as prednisone may be needed to get the inflammation under control. Your doctor may also "tap" the joint and draw out the excess fluid to relieve the pain. Any of these treatments can bring relief during attacks but they can't prevent joint damage. Unlike gout, there is no curative long-term treatment for pseudogout. But, fortunately, most sufferers will do well if their pain and inflammation are kept under control by medication.

Understanding Juvenile Idiopathic Arthritis

Arthritis is bad for everyone, but it seems worse when it strikes children. *Juvenile idiopathic arthritis* or JIA (formerly called juvenile rheumatoid arthritis or JRA) is a broad term for childhood arthritis diseases that appear before the age of 17 and are characterized by joint inflammation that lasts more than six weeks. Nearly 300,000 children in the U.S. are affected by arthritis or other rheumatic conditions; more children than are currently affected by cystic fibrosis, sickle cell anemia, and muscular dystrophy combined.

TECHNICAL STUFF

The word "idiopathic" means the disease has no known cause. JIA is an autoimmune disease that causes the body to turn on itself and destroy its own joint tissue. It can cause pain and stiffness that comes and goes and changes from morning to afternoon or day to day. When the symptoms worsen, it's called a *flare* or *flare-up*. Sometimes JIA goes away on its own for a short or long period of time, or even forever; these periods of time are called *remission*. Fortunately, many teens eventually experience full remission and end up with little to no joint damage.

Summarizing the symptoms

There are seven kinds of JIA that can be differentiated by their symptoms:

>> **Enthesitis-related arthritis (ERA):** ERA causes pain and swelling in the joints and the points where tendons and ligaments attach to the bone. The hips, knees and feet are the most likely sites of this form of JIA, although the back and the sacroiliac joint (the triangular bone between the lumbar spine and the tailbone) can also be affected, usually later in the disease process. ERA occurs most often in boys older than age 10.

WARNING

The presence of the HLA-B27 gene and eye inflammations called *uveitis* or *iridocyclitis* are commonly seen with ERA. These forms of eye inflammation can cause irreversible eye damage, so it's important for children with JIA to be routinely screened by an ophthalmologist.

- » **Oligoarthritis:** Around half of all children with JIA have oligoarthritis, which usually involves less than five joints, strikes in the knees and other large joints, and may only strike one of a pair of joints (one knee rather than both, and so on). In 20 to 30 percent of cases, oligoarthritis can trigger the eye inflammations uveitis or iridocyclitis. Fortunately, many children outgrow oligoarthritis, although eye problems can continue into adulthood.

- » **Polyarthritis, rheumatoid factor-negative or -positive:** Polyarthritis strikes some 40 percent of those with JIA and attacks five or more joints during the first six months of the disease. It usually appears in children younger than 5 and settles in the fingers and other small joints, although the large joints are not immune. The disease is usually symmetrical, which means it attacks the fingers on both hands, rather than just one. There may also be a fever and rheumatoid nodules. Polyarthritis is further divided into those that test positive for rheumatoid factor (RF) and those who do not. Of all the types of JIA, polyarthritis with a positive RF is the one that is the most like adult RA.

- » **Psoriatic arthritis:** This form of arthritis is much like the adult form of the same disease, both of which are combinations of psoriasis and arthritis. Usually involving the knees and/or the small joints of the hands and feet, psoriatic arthritis starts with a few joints then spreads to others. In 50 percent of sufferers, severe inflammation of the finger joints and toe joints can make the digits look like sausages.

- » **Systemic JIA:** The systemic form of JIA affects the entire body, causing trouble wherever it settles. The least common form of the disease, systemic JIA may produce fever, pale red spots on various parts of the body, anemia, swollen lymph nodes, inflammation of the linings of the lungs and heart, joint swelling, pain and stiffness, and other problems.

- » **Undifferentiated arthritis:** This is the catchall category for various kinds of arthritis that don't fit into any of the other categories, or belong to more than one category.

REMEMBER

Regardless of the form JIA takes, it always causes joint stiffness, pain, and swelling that is usually worse upon awakening from a night's sleep or even just a nap. Symptoms usually come and go. Sometimes a child may be lucky — the symptoms arise only a few times and then disappear forever — but a large percentage of children continue to have arthritis into adulthood. Luckily, most experience only mild forms.

Diagnosing and treating JIA

To be considered JIA, the disease must produce joint inflammation and stiffness in at least one joint for at least six weeks in a person under the age of 17.

JIA is similar to adult rheumatoid arthritis, with a few key differences:

>> Many children with JIA outgrow the problem, while most adults with RA don't.

>> JIA may affect bone development and growth in children, causing slow, rapid, or uneven growth in the afflicted joints.

>> Less than 50 percent of children with JIA test positive for rheumatoid arthritis factor, compared to 70 or 80 percent of adults.

Doctors diagnose and treat JIA in much the same way they do the adult version. But in addition to the medical treatment, children with JIA need special emotional and social support.

Investigating Infectious Arthritis

Infectious arthritis is caused by viruses, bacteria, or fungi that enter the body and settle into one or more joints. Depending upon which germs have invaded, they joint(s) they inhabit, the strength of the immune system, and the speed and accuracy of the treatment, a bout with infectious arthritis may be brief and relatively easy to take, or serious and painful.

TECHNICAL STUFF

Technically speaking, infectious arthritis is an infection of the joint tissues and/or fluid, or an autoimmune response to an infection in the joints. Several different germs, ranging from staphylococci to HIV to tuberculosis, can infect a joint or trigger an autoimmune inflammatory response in a joint.

Summarizing the symptoms

With infectious arthrtitis, symptoms include joint pain to the touch or with movement, as well as swelling and stiffness. The skin around the joint may be red and puffy. If the infection spreads beyond the joint, a fever or other symptoms may accompany it (although fever can occur for other reasons). Some forms of infectious arthritis hit hard and fast, so it's important that you see your doctor immediately if you have any symptoms. If left untreated, infectious arthritis may seriously damage joints within just a few days or weeks.

Diagnosing and treating infectious arthritis

If your doctor suspects infectious arthritis, they will call for various tests to firm up the diagnosis. Blood, urine, and joint fluid samples will be analyzed for infectious organisms. But even before the lab results come back, your doctor may begin giving you antibiotics, starting with those that kill the "usual suspects." Other medicines may follow once the doctor is sure what's ailing you, including additional or other antibiotics, antifungal medicines, or antiviral medications.

In addition, your doctor may drain pus from the joint, splint the joint, if necessary, and arrange for you to get physical therapy. Certain infections may also require surgery to clean out the joint.

Getting a Grip On Gonococcal Arthritis

Caused by the *gonococci* bacterium — the same culprit responsible for gonorrhea — gonococcal arthritis is the most widespread form of infectious arthritis.

Summarizing the symptoms

Gonococcal arthritis typically strikes hard and fast, and the pain seems to move from one joint to another. Small blisters can appear on the skin in some or many parts of the body, and the tendons may swell and ache.

Diagnosing and treating gonococcal arthritis

Both men and women can develop gonococcal arthritis. Men are much more likely to know that something is wrong because of the penile discharge and painful urination experienced with gonorrhea. Thus, they're more likely to receive treatment for the disease before it progresses to gonococcal arthritis. Women, who don't have such obvious symptoms, are less likely to receive early treatment for gonorrhea and more likely to develop gonococcal arthritis, and to suffer from pain in the abdomen and fever related to the disease.

The typical patient with is a young, sexually active person with the signs and symptoms of venereal disease, so the doctor can often zero in on a possible diagnosis of gonococcal arthritis during the medical history and physical examination. The doctor will then check for skin blisters and wait for lab reports on samples of various body fluids before making a definitive diagnosis.

Treatment with standard antibiotics used to be successful, although in recent years certain strains of gonorrhea have become resistant to many drugs. Today, gonococcal arthritis is treated with an injection or infusion of ceftriaxone, a broad spectrum antibiotic that will stop the infection, possibly together with another antimicrobial agent. These medications should knock out the infection but they won't be able to repair any permanent damage caused by the disease.

Surveying Psoriatic Arthritis

Psoriatic arthritis (PsA) adds insult to the injury of psoriasis because it strikes those who are already suffering from this inflammatory disease of the skin. According to the National Psoriasis Foundation, about 30 percent of psoriasis sufferers go on to develop psoriatic arthritis.

Summarizing the symptoms

In PsA, the joints of the fingers and toes become inflamed, swollen, stiff and, in more severe cases, deformed. There can be pitting of the nails or separation from the nail bed, as well as eye pain and redness. Psoriatic arthritis can also affect the spine, shoulders, or hips.

Diagnosing and treating psoriatic arthritis

A specific test for PsA doesn't exist, so the diagnosis is based on patient history and a physical exam. Typical signs of PsA (besides joint pain) include skin psoriasis, a family history of psoriasis, nail psoriasis, swelling of the fingers or toes (dactylitis), and inflammation of the areas where tendons insert on bone (enthesitis). Psoriatic arthritis is also particularly likely to occur in the joints at the end of the fingers near the fingernails.

Treatment is important, because psoriatic arthritis can cause severe damage to the joints. Unfortunately, it has no cure, but just like RA there are many medicines that have revolutionized its treatment. Standard treatment for PsA includes DMARDs such as methotrexate or biologics such as Humira to slow the progression of the disease and protect the joints from permanent damage.

Though many of the treatments for PsA and RA overlap, they are very different diseases. During the past few years, the FDA has approved several new drugs to treat psoriatic arthritis that don't work for RA, like secukinumab (Cosentyx) and guselkumab (Tremfya). Chapter 8 tells you more about these medications.

Anlalyzing Ankylosing Spondylitis

Ankylosing spondylitis (AS) attacks and inflames the cartilage, ligaments, and tendons of the spine. The back becomes stiff and sore and as the disease progresses, its ligaments and tendons can become more like bone tissue, forming bony bridges between the vertebrae and locking them into place. In more severe cases, AS can turn the spine into an unbending rod, although the disease usually doesn't advance to that point. Figure 4-2 shows the difference between a normal spine and one with AS.

A. Normal vertebra

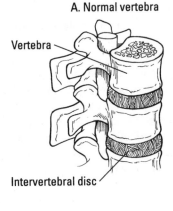

Vertebra

B. Vertebrae with ankylosing spondylitis

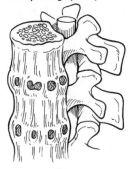

Intervertebral disc

FIGURE 4-2:
Normal vertebrae
compared to
those with
ankylosing
spondylitis.

© John Wiley & Sons, Inc.

AS currently affects some 300,000 Americans, with its favorite targets being Caucasian men between the ages of 16 and 35. The disease often runs in families and has been linked to a certain genetic marker (HLA-B27), although 80 percent of those with this gene never develop the disease. Something else (perhaps an infection) is undoubtedly triggering it.

Summarizing the symptoms

AS generally comes on gradually, as pain or stiffness settles into the lower back or hips, and the places where tendons and ligaments attach to the spine. Problems can also develop with the neck, shoulders, hips, knees, and back of the heel. The pain may be worse at night or upon arising, then recede once the person begins to move around. AS symptoms can be fairly constant or come and go.

A systemic disease, AS can cause compression fractures to the vertebrae, eye problems, loss of appetite, fatigue, and fever. There may also be difficulty in taking a deep breath, damage to the aorta (the body's largest artery), and problems caused by pressure on the nerves.

Diagnosing and treating ankylosing spondylitis

No one, single test can detect AS, so diagnosis is usually made from a combination of symptoms and family history, a physical examination, blood tests showing inflammatory markers and/or the HLA-B27 gene, and MRIs or X-rays, which can reveal characteristic joint damage or extra bone in the spine or sacroiliac joints of the pelvis.

Treatment is aimed at relieving pain and inflammation and preventing or correcting deformities of the spine to preserve spinal flexibility. NSAIDs are prescribed to ease inflammation, pain and stiffness. But one of the most exciting developments in rheumatology over the last few years is the effectiveness of biologics in treating ankylosing spondylitis, including tumor necrosis factor (TNF) inhibitors such as adalimumab (Humira) and etanercept (Enbrel), and interleukin-17 (IL-17) inhibitors such as secukinumab (Cosentyx) and ixekizumab (Taltz). These and other biologics have been found to improve mobility and possibly fight the progression of AS (you can read more about them in Chapter 8).

REMEMBER

Though AS has no cure, most who have the disease suffer from mild to moderate symptoms and do fairly well. Physical therapy can be very helpful in preserving spinal strength and flexibility. More extreme cases of AS may require surgical replacement of one or more joints, but spinal surgery is rarely indicated as the spines of AS patients are so fragile.

Chapter **5**

Exploring Other Conditions Linked to Arthritis

Millions of people have been struck by symptoms ranging from joint stiffness to skin rashes to difficulty swallowing. Sometimes their conditions are diagnosed quickly. Other times, they're forced to endure countless tests and bounce from doctor to doctor until they find out what's wrong. Along the way, they may be mistakenly told that their problems are caused by stress, lack of sleep, or depression, when in reality they're suffering from a condition related to arthritis. That is, arthritis is a major or minor part of the syndrome, but not the primary disease. Or arthritis may accompany another illness, while being a completely separate disease process.

These conditions that are somehow linked to arthritis can be categorized in one of three ways:

>> Arthritis is a major player in the disease.

>> Arthritis is a minor player in the disease.

>> Arthritis is a companion condition to the disease.

Experiencing Arthritis as a Major Player

In ailments such as systemic lupus erythematosus and scleroderma, the joint problems that characterize arthritis are a major part of the syndrome. But even though arthritis is present — often in a big way — it isn't the primary disease process.

Systemic lupus erythematosus: The wolf disease

Systemic lupus erythematosus (commonly known as *lupus* or *SLE*) is an autoimmune disease that can affect any part of the body. Even though we only have one name for this disease, it has hundreds of versions, and every person who has lupus also has their own set of symptoms.

Lupus can attack the joints, heart, nervous and vascular systems, skin, kidneys, lungs, and other parts of the body. The symptoms strike because the body produces large numbers of antibodies — called *autoantibodies* — that attack bodily tissue for no apparent reason. Those with lupus are at a higher risk of heart attacks, strokes, and kidney failure than those without the disease. Ninety percent of lupus patients are women, and most of them are in their childbearing years (ages 15 to 45). Perhaps as many as 1.5 million Americans suffer from the disease, which strikes women of color (African Americans, Hispanics/Latinos, Asian Americans, Native Americans, Native Hawaiians, and Pacific Islanders) two to three times more often than Caucasians. One study found that women of color develop lupus at an earlier age, experience more serious complications, and die from the disease more often than white women.

Summarizing the symptoms

Because everyone who has lupus has their own individual version, it may just affect the outside parts of the body, causing symptoms like joint pain, rashes, fatigue, and mouth ulcers. Or it can affect the inside of the body, attacking organs like the heart, lung, brain, and/or kidneys. Lupus settles in for the long haul but it tends to hit and run, causing symptoms to flare up and then retreat. For many people, the "good" periods can last for weeks, months, or even years.

Diagnosing and treating lupus

Lupus can cause a bewildering variety of symptoms that may mirror those of other diseases, making the diagnosis difficult. Blood tests are used to look for antibody abnormalities, abnormal blood chemistries, problems with blood clotting, immune system abnormalities, kidney damage, and so on. Biopsies of the skin and kidneys may be required, as well as X-rays, CT scans, MRIs, electrocardiograms, and more.

REMEMBER

The gold standard for lupus care is the anti-malarial DMARD hydroxychloroquine, routinely recommended for lupus patients unless there is a contraindication because it helps prevent lupus from becoming more severe. It also helps ease certain mild symptoms like joint pain, fatigue, mouth ulcers, and mild rashes.

For symptoms that persist in spite of hydroxychloroquine, treatments are tailored to the patient's needs. DMARDs may be prescribe for arthritis symptoms, aspirin or stronger blood thinners may be given to prevent blood clots, and other drugs may be used for skin problems. In some cases, steroids may be need to tamp down inflammation, stronger immunosuppressants may be usedto keep the haywire immune system in check, and blood thinners administered to lower the risk of clots.

TIP

Fortunately, you can do several things to cope with lupus. You can't make the symptoms disappear, but you can certainly improve the quality of your life by doing the following:

>> If you tire easily, cut back on your work or home duties.

>> Look for ways to reduce stress. (See Chapter 15 for tips on coping with stress.)

>> Protect yourself from the sun. This is crucial, because excessive sun exposure leads to the worsening of skin disease and disease flares. Complete sun avoidance is advisable; for short exposure, the use of sunblock *and* protective clothing is recommended.

>> Follow your doctor's dietary instructions carefully.

Cutaneous lupus erythematosus: A less dangerous form

A form of the disease that is more common than SLE, *cutaneous lupus erythematosus* (DLE) generally confines itself to the skin and doesn't venture into the body to attack the organs. There are several different kinds of cutaneous lupus rashes, including *discoid lupus erythematosus* (DLE). Five to 25 percent of those with DLE will go on to develop the systemic form of lupus, and, conversely, about one quarter of those with SLE demonstrate discoid disease at some time during their disease course.

Summarizing the symptoms

Like SLE, discoid lupus tends to attack women and produces a characteristic skin rash. The rash begins with little, reddish, disc-like patches, about as big around as the circumference of a drinking straw. Typically appearing above the neck (on the face, scalp, and ears), the patches may also appear on the upper chest and back, the backs of the arms, and even the shins. Untreated, these rashes may begin to grow outward, and a scar may develop in the central area of each rash. In skin that is not treated early and promptly, there can be scarring, hair loss, and depending on the skin tone, there can be hyperpigmentation or hypopigmentation changes.

The patches can come and go or remain in place, and may be accompanied by joint aches. A drop in the white blood cell count, indicating immune system depression, is also common.

Diagnosing and treating discoid lupus

DLE is difficult to diagnose because the primary symptom — the rash — can lead doctors to suspect other causes such as psoriasis, actinic keratosis, seborrheic dermatitis, SLE (in fact, tests may confirm that the condition *is* SLE), or other diseases. Because there is no single, conclusive test for discoid lupus, much of the diagnostic workup is aimed at eliminating other diseases as the cause, then diagnosing discoid lupus by default. (A biopsy is often helpful in determining the diagnosis.)

Treatment usually consists of sun avoidance and the use of anti-malarial drugs to control the disease. If an active rash is present, topical or oral steroids and/or eczema treatments called topical calcineurin inhibitors (TCIs) may be prescribed to quiet things down. If the disease is detected and treated early, scarring can be kept to a minimum.

Systemic scleroderma: When the skin hardens

Although it attacks various parts of the body, *systemic scleroderma,* an autoimmune disorder that affects the skin and internal organs, is best known for its effects on the skin. In fact, the disease's name comes from the Greek words for *hard* and *skin*. There are two kinds of scleroderma: *localized*, which only affects certain parts of the body; and *systemic*, which affects the skin, blood vessels, and internal organs.

It's the systemic version that causes the joint or muscle pain and stiffness that is sometimes mistaken for rheumatoid arthritis, as well as digestive problems, skin changes, and an increased sensitivity to the cold known as Raynaud's.

TECHNICAL
STUFF

Technically speaking, systemic scleroderma is a collagen vascular disease: *collagen* because excessive deposits of collagen (the main structural protein found in the skin, bones and cartilage) damages body tissue, and *vascular* because the blood vessels wind up suffering.

No one knows why but in the 300,000 Americans who have scleroderma (all types), the body produces too much collagen. Unable to dispose of it properly, the body starts storing the excess collagen in body tissues in harmful ways. In the localized form of scleroderma, too much collagen deposited in the skin makes the skin tight and hard. In the systemic form, too much collagen stored in the organs makes it difficult — if not impossible — for them to work properly. To make matters worse, systemic scleroderma prompts the cells in the lining of the blood vessels begin to grow abnormally. With these vital delivery and waste routes hampered, the body has even more difficulty operating effectively.

We don't know exactly why scleroderma develops in any form. Most likely it's due to a combination of immune system errors, genetics, and environmental triggers. Hormonal upsets are also possible culprits, which would explain why as many as 80 percent of those diagnosed with scleroderma are women.

Summarizing the symptoms

The symptoms of systemic scleroderma vary from person to person. The disease often begins with joint pain, but sometimes the first symptom is difficulty swallowing. It may progress rapidly and fatally, or it may confine itself to the skin for years or decades before moving on to attack other parts of the body.

Symptoms of systemic scleroderma include:

>> **Skin problems:** Thickening, hardening, roughness, and/or dryness of the skin on the fingers, arms, face, and elsewhere. There may also be "spider veins" on the face, tongue, chest, and fingers, as well as lumpy calcium deposits under the skin.

>> **Joint pain, swelling, and locking:** Pain in the joints can make scleroderma appear to be rheumatoid arthritis. As the disease advances, the elbows, wrists, and fingers may become locked in a closed position.

>> **Difficulty swallowing:** If collagen is deposited in the esophagus, you may experience trouble swallowing.

>> **Shortness of breath:** Systemic scleroderma can cause scar tissue to accumulate in the lungs, making it difficult to breathe It may also cause changes in the blood vessels that service these vital organs.

>> **Digestive difficulties:** If the intestines are strewn with collagen, you may have trouble digesting food and absorbing nutrients.

>> **Raynaud's phenomenon:** Many systemic scleroderma patients develop this extreme sensitivity to cold in the fingers and/or toes.

WARNING

Systemic scleroderma patients can also suffer from a host of other problems, depending upon which organs are overrun with collagen, including abnormal function of the heart, lungs and kidneys. These diseases, if left untreated, can be life threatening.

Diagnosing and treating scleroderma

Diagnosing systemic scleroderma can be difficult in the early stages, especially if joint pain and tenderness are the only symptoms. However, with the appearance of skin changes or difficulty swallowing, the identification process becomes much easier.

After a medical history and physical examination, the doctor may order blood tests to determine if autoantibodies are in the blood, pulmonary tests to assess lung function, echocardiogram (heart ultrasound) to assess heart function, X-rays to check for changes in the bones or soft tissues, tests to assess GI function, and other tests to determine the extent of the problem. Sometimes a kidney biopsy is needed if there is concern for kidney involvement. A CT scan might be ordered if there is concern for lung involvement. Interestingly, skin biopsies are rarely needed to make this diagnosis. Medications are usually prescribed to treat or slow skin changes, dilate the blood vessels, fight inflammation and suppress the immune system. Other medications that may be used are NSAIDs for pain and inflammation, anti-hypertensives to lower elevated blood pressure, antacids or histamine-blockers for heartburn, and so on. Exercise and physical therapy can help strengthen muscles and "oil" the affected joints. For severe problems with swallowing, placement of an artificial feeding tube may be necessary. The good news is that sometimes systemic scleroderma needs no meds at all, just montoring for progression or worsening.

The good news is that there are several lifestyle changes you can adopt to help relieve the problems systemic scleroderma produces and improve the quality of your life:

>> Help protect your skin by limiting yourself to short showers or baths, keeping it moist with creams and lotions, and avoiding strong soaps and household chemicals.

>> Use a humidifier if indoor heaters are drying out your skin.

>> If you smoke, stop! This is important for blood vessel health and the prevention of Raynaud's attacks.

>> Diligently perform the flexibility and strengthening exercises that your doctor or physical therapist prescribes. The exercises may be difficult to do, but they will help you maintain joint function.

>> If swallowing is difficult, chew your food well, avoid foods that are hard to swallow, and drink plenty of liquids with your meals.

>> If nighttime heartburn is a problem, elevate your head by buying an adjustable bed or place blocks under the legs of the bed frame at the head of the bed. You might also try eating dinner earlier than usual or having a lighter meal so you'll have less in your stomach at bedtime.

The symptoms of systemic cleroderma are daunting, and doctors have yet to find a way to stop the overactive "collagen factories." Still, many people with the disease do well for years or even decades, and some even have spontaneous remissions, especially when the disease first appears in the joints and skin rather than in the organs. Also, the FDA recently approved a medication called Ofev (nintedanib) which slows the rate of systemic scleroderma-related lung disease (SSc-ILD) and the resulting decline in lung function. Ofev is the first medication for this rare lung condition approved by the FDA.

Reactive arthritis: From a stomach ache to arthritis

Like gonococcal arthritis, reactive arthritis usually develops after you've contracted a sexually transmitted infection such as chlamydia, although it isn't always the unhappy result of unprotected sex. Reactive arthritis can also develop after a gastrointestinal infection caused by salmonella or another kind of bacteria, or the disease may strike without any preceding infection at all.

Summarizing the symptoms

Reactive arthritis has three classic groups of symptoms:

>> **Arthritis** that takes the form of mild to severe pain and inflammation, often in the feet, hips, ankles, and knees, although it can also appear in the wrists,

fingers, and other joints. The arthritis may completely vanish or return episodically for years.

>> **Eye inflammation**, also known as *conjunctivitis*, that manifests as eyes that are red and swollen, burning, itching, and watering excessively.

>> **Urethritis**, an inflammation of the urethra, which is the "pipe" that conducts urine from the bladder to the outside of the body. This causes increased frequency of urination and discomfort when urinating.

In addition, patients may have thick, crusty rashes on the soles of their feet or the palms of their hands, sores affecting the mouth, vagina, tongue or penis, yellowish deposits under the fingernails and toenails, and problems with the heart. Young adults age 20 to 40 are the most likely group to be struck by reactive arthritis, which affects women and men equally when it's caused by a gastrointestinal infection. But men are 9 to 10 times more likely than women to develop the disease following a sexually acquired infection.

TECHNICAL
STUFF

Chlamydia trachomatis is the bacteria responsible for the largest number of reactive arthritis cases associated with sexual contact. As for reactive arthritis linked to gastrointestinal infections, the major culprits are campylobacter, salmonella, shigella, and yersinia.

Diagnosing and treating reactive arthritis

The diagnosis of reactive arthritis can be difficult and delayed, because doctors have no single symptom or definitive test to rely on. The presence of the three classic symptoms is an important clue, but they don't necessarily appear at the same time. Doctors generally send samples of a patient's joint fluid, plus samples swabbed from the urethra, to the laboratory for analysis.

Part of the diagnostic workup is designed to rule out diseases such as lupus (a negative ANA would do this), whereas other parts are designed to "rule in" reactive arthritis. For example, finding the presence of the HLA-B27 gene and an infectious agent such as chlamydia will increase the likelihood that reactive arthritis is the culprit. X-rays showing damage to the cartilage or bone, bony deposits where the bones and tendons meet, soft tissue swelling, and other signs can also point to reactive arthritis.

Your doctor can prescribe antibiotics to treat the infection and NSAIDs to ease the arthritis symptoms. They may also prescribe stronger drugs, such as steroids or immunosuppressives. The conjunctivitis usually isn't treated directly, although eye drops or an ointment may be prescribed for symptomatic relief. Bed rest and exercise are also helpful.

The outlook is generally positive for reactive arthritis patients. Many recover substantially within five or six months, although mild to moderate arthritis symptoms may linger. Some 15 to 50 percent will develop symptoms again after the initial flare, and about a fifth of the patients wind up with chronic, generally mild arthritis. Only a small percentage suffer from severe, ongoing symptoms and joint deformity.

Lyme disease: When you're the bull's-eye

This new version of arthritis popped up during the 1970s in the town of Lyme, Connecticut. Local doctors were puzzled when individuals, groups of friends, and even entire families began developing a disease that looked a lot like arthritis, but didn't fall into any of the known categories.

Fortunately, doctors realized that more people developed the disease during the summer than in any other time of the year, that many patients had developed a large, round bull's-eye rash, and that the town of Lyme was surrounded by wooded areas harboring deer and other wild animals. By putting these and other facts together, they discovered that they were looking at a new disease caused by bacteria called *borrelia burgdorferi,* which were carried by certain ticks hitching rides on deer in the nearby woods. When these ticks bit people, the bacteria passed into their bodies. And you needn't go into the woods to contract Lyme disease — your dog or cat can bring the offending ticks into your home. (See the sidebar, "Staying in the clear(ing): Avoiding Lyme disease" to learn how to steer clear of Lyme disease.)

Summarizing the symptoms

The first symptom of Lyme disease is likely a large red spot on your rear end, thigh, trunk, or armpit. The rash may have a "blank" spot area in the center, making it look like a bull's-eye. It may itch and be painful or hot. However, some people with Lyme disease never develop a rash.

Sometimes the rash may be so insconsequential that it isn't even noticed (by the patient or the doctor), and other times patients never see a doctor about the rash because it went away. Whatever the reason, Lyme disease is often untreated, and about 60 percent of those with untreated Lyme disease develop recurrent attacks of arthritis. These manifest as swelling and pain in one or both knees and/or other joints, including the shoulders, elbows, wrists, and ankles. These arthritis attacks may last for several months. Unfortunately, 5 to 20 percent of those infected may go on to suffer from chronic arthritis. Early treatment and identification of Lyme disease can prevent this as the arthritis typically occurs during the second phase of illness many months after initial tick bite.

Other common symptoms of Lyme disease include fever, fatigue, chills, joint pain, muscle aches, headache, and stiff neck. Less common symptoms include sore throat, swollen lymph nodes, nausea, vomiting, backaches, and other problems that may come and go.

Diagnosing and treating Lyme disease

The presence of the classic rash is the first clue that a patient has Lyme disease. The personal history will then become a very important part of the diagnostic procedure. Knowing that the patient went hiking in the woods and the problems began in the summer, for example, are significant clues.

Diagnosis can be confirmed by the results of two blood tests that look for the presence of antibodies to *Borrelia burgdorferi*. In patients exhibiting nervous system disorders, doctors may perform a spinal tap to look for the antibodies in the spinal fluid.

Arresting the spread of Lyme disease is often fairly easy if treatment is started early. Antibiotics, taken orally or given intravenously, can often halt the progress of the disease and prevent the appearance of arthritis and other later-stage symptoms. More severe cases can require treatment with IV antibiotics for several weeks. The doctor may also prescribe NSAIDs for pain and swelling, as well as crutches or other assistive devices, depending on the parts of the body affected. In some people, years may pass before all the symptoms of Lyme disease vanish.

STAYING IN THE CLEAR(ING): AVOIDING LYME DISEASE

The best way to keep clear of Lyme disease is to make your body a "tick-free zone." If you go into the woods or other areas where deer or other wild animals roam, you should remember the following precautions:

- Use insect repellent.

- Use your clothing as a shield over exposed areas of skin.

- Wear light-colored clothes so the dark-colored ticks stand out if they get on you.

- Walk on trails if possible, and stay in the center of the trails, giving a wide berth to ticks in the grass and brush.

- Admire any animals you come across from a distance.

- Afterward, carefully check yourself and your children for ticks. Pay special attention to the hairy areas of the body.

- If you live in a tick-infested area or near the woods, make sure your pets have flea and tick collars.

- Watch for the telltale bull's-eye spot on your trunk, rear end, thighs, or in your armpit. If you find one, see your doctor immediately.

- If a tick is found and a rash develops, bring the tick to your doctor, because only a certain species of tick carries the bacteria that cause Lyme.

Experiencing Arthritis as a Minor Player

In bursitis, polymyalgia rheumatica, and the other diseases in this category, arthritis is not the major disease process, although symptoms of arthritis (joint pain, inflammation, limitation of movement) are often present in varying degrees. Thus, the arthritis shows up as a *symptom* rather than a cause of the disease.

Bursitis: When the bursae become swollen

Bursae are little fluid-filled sacs strategically placed throughout the body. They're designed to help reduce the friction caused by movement in the joints. Unfortunately, a bursa can become inflamed if injured or overused. Infections or certain forms of arthritis, such as gout, can also prompt this inflammation.

Summarizing the symptoms

When one or more of the bursae become inflamed, you have *bursitis*. The normally flat sacs swell with excess fluid, producing pain and often limiting movement. The shoulders are common targets of bursitis; the elbows, the *trochanteric bursa* (the bony knob near the top of the outside of the thigh bone), and other joints can also be struck. See Figure 5-1 for an example of where the bursae are located in the shoulder.

The pain and resulting movement limitation can range from mild to severe. You may have a nagging little pain in one hip or such severe shoulder pain that dressing is difficult.

Diagnosing and treating bursitis

Ultrasounds and MRIs are very good at identifying bursitis. Your doctor may also rely on your history and symptoms, as well as a physical examination of the affected areas. In many cases, treatment is limited to NSAIDs, rest, and perhaps joint immobilization. If a bursa is infected, your doctor may drain it and give you antibiotics. Very rarely, in the case of chronic and severe bursitis, prednisone or another steroid may be required. Exercise can help restore the joint's range of motion and rebuild weakened muscles, with physical therapy and foam rolling particularly helpful in cases of trochanteric bursitis.

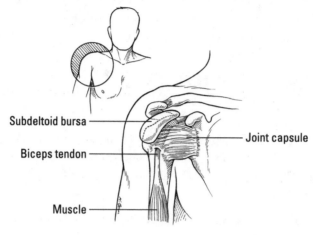

Subdeltoid bursa

Joint capsule

Biceps tendon

Muscle

FIGURE 5-1:
Placement of the bursae and tendon in the shoulder.

Tendonitis and tenosynovitis: Inflammation of the bone-and-muscle link

When certain muscles contract or relax, our bones move accordingly. But the bone-and-muscle, contract-and-relax-system depends on the connecting link: the tendons, which join muscle to bone.

Summarizing the symptoms

Tendons are the tough, fibrous extensions at the ends of the muscles that attach themselves to the bones. *Tendonitis* occurs when one or more of these tendons become inflamed. Most often associated with repetitive motions, impingements, strenuous activity, and advancing years, this ailment can leave tendons red, raw, and painful to the touch or upon movement.

TECHNICAL STUFF

The sheaths surrounding the tendons may also become inflamed, producing a condition known as *tenosynovitis.* If the sheaths dry out and rub against the tendon, they produce a grating sound or sensation. Various diseases, including scleroderma, gout, and gonorrhea can cause tenosynovitis.

Diagnosing and treating tendonitis and tenosynovitis

A diagnosis is based on symptoms, medical history, and the physical examination. The doctor may prescribe medications such as NSAIDs to counteract pain and inflammation. If the tendonitis or tenosynovitis is caused by rheumatoid arthritis, psoriatic arthritis, gout, or a similar condition, treatment should be directed toward the original condition (such as DMARDs or gout medication).

Steroids or local anesthetics are sometimes injected right into the sheath surrounding the tendon. Chronic problems may require surgery to remove calcium deposits or release contracted tendons.

The outlook for those with tendonitis and tenosynovitis is good, and the problem often clears up on its own.

TIP

A few easy, inexpensive things can help alleviate the pain. You may want to try the following:

>> Stop the activity that caused the inflammation.

>> Rest.

>> Apply hot or cold packs to the area.

>> Immobilize the involved joints.

Raynaud's: A chilling problem

Raynaud's phenomenon involves changes to the small blood vessels in the hands and feet (or less commonly, the nose, lips, or ear lobes) when the patient gets cold.

Summarizing the symptoms

The hallmark of Raynaud's is discoloration in one or more fingers or toes, the nose, the lips, or the ear lobes. The color changes (with affected areas turning white or blue, followed by red) can occur on their own or be accompanied by tingling, burning pain and/or numbness. Although many people have cold hands and feet, the characteristic color changes indicate Raynaud's.

Spasms of the small arteries that supply blood to these areas cause these symptoms by diminishing the blood supply. Brought on by cold temperatures and/or emotional stress, the spasms can last a few minutes or go on for hours. Recurrent and severe episodes of Raynaud's can compromise blood flow to the ends of the fingers or toes, causing sores in those areas or even gangrene and/or loss of the affected digits.

Raynaud's comes in two forms:

>> **Primary Raynaud's:** The more common form of the disease, it's also typically milder. It acts alone when it attacks and its cause is unknown.

>> **Secondary Raynaud's:** This is a more serious form of the ailment that involves short-term interruption of blood flow to the fingers and toes and other extremities. It may be a sign of an underlying autoimmune disorder, such as scleroderma or lupus.

TIP

Certain types of work increase a person's vulnerability to Raynaud's. Those who operate vibrating tools, are exposed to vinyl chloride, and type, play the piano, or otherwise subject their fingers to repetitive stress are more likely to develop this problem.

Diagnosing and treating Raynaud's

Diagnosing Raynaud's can be easy, but distinguishing the primary from the secondary type can be more problematic. Diagnosis and differentiation are made on the basis of the person's symptoms and laboratory tests, such as the antinuclear antibody test and erythrocyte sedimentation rate. Much of the laboratory testing is done to rule out other diseases. Treatment for Raynaud's may be as simple as teaching you what you can do for yourself and monitoring the situation, or it may include administering powerful drugs. In very severe cases, nerves to the afflicted areas may be cut to provide temporary relief.

TIP

Your Raynaud's may be here to stay, but you needn't be a helpless victim. You can fight back in several ways:

>> Stay warm all over. Dress warmly, layer your clothing, and wear absorbent socks and underwear to draw perspiration away from your skin.

>> Immerse your fingers and toes in warm water to help keep them warm during a flare.

>> If you smoke, stop. Nicotine constricts blood vessels, a major problem with Raynaud's.

>> Speak to your doctor about the possibility of switching medicines if you are taking beta-blockers or other drugs that constrict blood vessels. Decongestants like Sudafed are common offenders.

>> Work on controlling your reaction to stress.

>> Exercise regularly.

Sjögren's syndrome: Dry mouth, eyes, and maybe more

Sjögren's syndrome (typicalled referred to just as Sjögren's) is a disorder of the immune system that typically causes dry eyes and a dry mouth and affects up to 3.1 million Americans, 90 percent of whom are women. No one knows what brings on Sjögren's, but the immune system's affect on the salivary and tear glands is clearly involved. It can occur alone (known as *primary Sjögren's*) or as a part of another autoimmune disease (known as *secondary Sjögren's*). The latter form occurs most commonly in conjunction with RA, and about 10 to 15 percent of RA patients develop the annoying dry eye/dry mouth symptoms of Sjögren's. Other diseases associated with Sjögren's include lupus, dermatomyositis, and scleroderma.

Summarizing the symptoms

The characteristic dryness in the mouth and eyes occurs when those mainstays of the immune system, the white blood cells, invade and damage the salivary and tear glands. The same problem can also cause dryness of the trachea, vagina, the lining of the gastrointestinal tract, and other parts of the body.

About one-third of Sjögren's sufferers develop arthritis that is similar to, but usually less severe than, rheumatoid arthritis. Those with Sjögren's are also 5-44 times more likely than the normal population to develop non-Hodgkin's lymphoma, a 5–10 percent lifetime risk.

Diagnosing and treating Sjögren's

The combination of dry mouth, swollen salivary glands, dry eyes, and joint distress can make diagnosis a simple matter. Tests can confirm that the level of tears and saliva production is sub par. Further clues can be found in the abnormal blood tests. Antibody abnormalities and possibly anemia, fewer white blood cells, and an elevated erythrocyte sedimentation rate (ESR) may be found.

Sjögren's can't be cured, but many of the symptoms can be alleviated. By chewing sugar-free gum (it must be sugar free, because one of the most serious side effects in this disease is severe dental cavities), sipping fluid, and using a mouth rinse and artificial teardrops, you can help keep your eyes and mouth moist. Frequent dental visits are also necessary. The drugs pilocarpine (Salagen) and cevimeline (Evoxac) may be given to increase the production of saliva. Pain and swelling of the salivary glands and joints can be treated with painkillers, but stronger drugs may be needed to deal with any trouble arising from damage to the internal organs. For patients with severe joint or salivary symptoms, NSAIDs, anti-malarials, immunosuppressive agents, or steroids are sometimes used.

The outlook depends upon which parts of the body are affected. Most people find they are able to live normal lives with a few adjustments. But a small number succumb to kidney failure or other problems that arise when a key part of the body becomes too dry.

Polymyalgia rheumatica: The pain of many muscles

No one knows what causes *polymyalgia rheumatica*, which means *pain in many muscles.* It typically attacks people over the age of 50 and strikes more women than men. The older you are, the more likely you are to wake up one morning with the muscle pain and stiffness that are the hallmarks of this disease.

Summarizing the symptoms

In the typical scenario, a woman goes to bed at night feeling fine and wakes up the next morning with tremendous pain and stiffness in her neck, shoulders, upper arms, lower back, hips, and/or buttocks. She may say, "It feels like I worked out too much yesterday, like I really overdid it — but I didn't do anything!"

However, not everyone develops polymyalgia rheumatica overnight. Sometimes it comes on gradually. Pain and stiffness, fever, weight loss, and a general feeling of the blahs are common.

Although the pain can be severe and may resemble that of rheumatoid arthritis, the muscles involved don't show signs of inflammation, and the joints rarely show signs of arthritis. However, inflammation of the joint linings may be present.

Diagnosing and treating polymyalgia rheumatica

With no characteristic joint damage, antibodies, skin rashes, or other obvious signs to look for, doctors must make the diagnosis of polymyalgia rheumatica by eliminating other causes of the pain and stiffness. The patient's age is one clue, with those over 50 most likely to be affected. Another clue is a sudden onset of symptoms. People with the disease also have a high erythrocyte sedimentation rate, which is virtually required for this diagnosis.

Sometimes the diagnosis is clinched by the patient's response to the standard treatment: low doses of prednisone or other steroids. Almost all polymyalgia rheumatica patients respond well to low doses of these drugs.

This "pain of many muscles" often disappears on its own or improves dramatically with treatment. And a significant number of patients do so well after a couple years that they can cut back on their medication.

WARNING

Fifteen percent of those with polymyalgia rheumatica may develop a life-threatening inflammation of the blood vessels called giant cell arteritis (GCA). Symptoms of GCA can include headaches, scalp tenderness, vision changes/loss, jaw or tongue pain after prolonged chewing. Fevers, unintentional weight loss, chest pain, and a severe case of the "blahs" are also possible signs of GCA. If you experience these symptoms, see a medical professional immediately.

Paget's disease: Becoming too bony

Bones grow throughout life. They may not grow longer after a certain point, but they are constantly being broken down and restored, right up until the end of life.

With Paget's disease, the normal breakdown/rebuild system shifts into overdrive, causing excessive destruction of the bone and poor-quality bone repair. As a result, bones may become bulkier, softer, and weaker, with a greater tendency to fracture.

Summarizing the symptoms

Many people with Paget's have no idea anything is wrong, whereas others suffer from gradual joint stiffness and fatigue. Sometimes the bones may become enlarged, deformed, and painful. And there can be secondary damage, such as pain, osteoarthritis, loss of height, and bowleggedness.

Diagnosing and treating Paget's disease

Making the diagnosis of Paget's is fairly simple: X-rays of the bones show the abnormal areas of growth, and a laboratory test detects elevated blood levels of alkaline phosphatase, an enzyme necessary for bone formation.

Treatment will depend upon the symptoms — if you don't have symptoms, perhaps nothing may be done. Surgery may be needed if nerves are being pinched or if a joint is no longer functioning properly. In more severe cases, your doctor may prescribe drugs that slow the disease, such as calcitonin, or drugs used to strengthen bones, such as alendronate.

Experiencing Arthritis as a Companion Condition

In these conditions, the disease is centered in the structures that surround the joint (muscles, tendons, ligaments, and nerves) instead of in the joints themselves. Although the joints are painful, these maladies don't begin in the joints and aren't classified as "true" arthritis.

Carpal tunnel syndrome: Nerve compression

You may have seen office workers or supermarket checkers wearing splints on their hands, wrists and lower arms to immobilize their wrists. Or perhaps you've noticed people rubbing and shaking their hands, complaining of pain and tingling in their thumbs and fingers.

They may be suffering from carpal tunnel syndrome, a problem caused by compression of the nerve and tendons that pass through the *carpal tunnel* (a corridor between the ligaments and bones in the wrist). This syndrome causes pain, numbness, decreased sensation, and tingling in the thumb, index, and middle fingers. If left untreated, carpal tunnel syndrome can cause the muscles on the thumb side of the hand to waste away, making it difficult to make a fist or grasp objects.

Your doctor bases the diagnosis on your symptoms, medical history, and physical examination and looks for weakness and decreased sensation in your hand.

Treatment often begins with a splint, followed by medication to reduce pain and inflammation. Steroid injections into the afflicted nerve can be temporarily helpful. If the problem is related to water gain, you may be given diuretics to help rid your body of excess fluid. More advanced cases may by helped by surgery.

TIP

In addition to these medical measures, look for ways to cut back on — or completely eliminate — any repetitive motion that may bring on the pain. Also, do whatever you can to ease joint stress. For example, if you type a lot, consider getting an ergonomically designed keyboard.

The outlook for those with carpal tunnel syndrome is generally positive. Most will recover, and only a very small percentage of those who are treated will develop permanent nerve injury.

Fibromyalgia: The pain no one can find

It's an odd situation: You hurt, perhaps all over, but the doctor can't find any inflammation or damage to explain the pain. He or she may even suggest that "it's all in your head" and say that you're stressed, depressed, or need more sleep.

Pain and stiffness in the muscles, ligaments, and tendons are the primary signs of fibromyalgia. Both generally occur throughout the body, although the pain and stiffness can begin in one area and spread (see Figure 5-2). Fatigue is also a major problem, with as many as 90 percent of fibromyalgia sufferers experiencing moderate to severe fatigue.

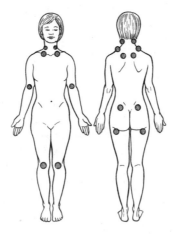

FIGURE 5-2: Common areas that are painful with fibromyalgia.

© John Wiley & Sons, Inc.

Symptoms may come and go, and are often associated with sleep disturbances. Sufferers may also experience mood changes, numbness and tingling in the extremities, and headaches. No one knows what causes fibromyalgia, but it is often triggered by stress, injury, lack of sleep, infections, and other diseases. A history of prior trauma or abuse is also common, as are co-morbidities with irritable bowel syndrome, insterstitial cystitis, migraines, depression, and/or anxiety. Although it can be painful, fibromyalgia is not life threatening or otherwise dangerous. For some people, however, the symptoms can become so severe that work beomes impossible.

The Centers for Disease Control estimates that 4 million Americans suffer from fibromyalgia, with women twice as likely as men to be struck, especially during their childbearing years. Risk factors for fibromyalgia include advancing age and suffering from lupus or RA. Other suspected risk factors include repetitive injuries, obesity, family history, illnesses, and stressful or traumatic events.

The diagnosis can be difficult to make because the symptoms of fibromyalgia are similar to those of other diseases. Finding the location and pattern of your pain can help your doctor make the diagnosis. Fibromyalgia is a diagnosis of exclusion based on symptoms and the presence of tender points. As appropriate, the doctor might order other tests to rule out other conditions. Increasing physical activity improves the symptoms of fibromyalgia and is possibly the most important component of therapy. Treatment may include medicines to ease pain, local anesthetics injected directly into painful areas, and antidepressants to aid in sleep. Your doctor may also prescribe massage therapy, along with the application of heat to the affected areas. Stress management, relaxation techniques and good sleep habits can also help you manage your pain.

REMEMBER

Fibromyalgia is *not* all in your head; it's not a hysterical response to stress or a cry for help. It's a real disease that also has an important psychological component. That's good news, in a sense, because it means you can begin doing something, right now, to help relieve your symptoms by controlling stress. (See Chapter 14 for methods of dealing with stress.)

TIP

For immediate relief, try taking a warm bath or applying compresses to your sore muscles. And you may have a little more luck sleeping with a different mattress, a white noise machine to block disturbing sounds, blackout curtains, and a more comfortable pillow. (See Chapter 15 for the basics of good sleep.) Overall, the outlook for fibromyalgia patients is positive. It causes no long-term damage to the joints or the rest of the body and can be eased with medications and stress reduction. Check out *Fibromyalgia For Dummies*, 2nd Ed. (Wiley) to find out more.

Polymyositis: A rare sapping of strength

An uncommon disease affecting less than 0.1 percent of the population, polymyositis is an inflammation of the muscles closest to the trunk (meaning shoulders, upper arms, neck, hips, and thighs) that saps the victim's strength.

Summarizing the symptoms

In severe cases, those with polymyositis may have trouble just getting out of a chair or brushing their teeth. The large muscles closest to the torso — those found in the shoulders, upper arms, thighs, and hips — are usually the ones that suffer. But the neck muscles may also be stricken, as well as those that are used to breathe and swallow. In addition, patients may experience fever, weight loss, pain in the joints, Raynaud's phenomenon, and the blahs.

Polymyositis can strike at any age but usually targets adults between 30 and 50 years of age. The disease prefers women, striking them about twice as often as men and is seen more often in African Americans than Caucasians. It rarely affects children. No one knows what causes polymyositis, although it is an autoimmune attack on the muscles and infections and immune system disorders are suspected.

Diagnosing and treating polymyositis

Lacking a quick-and-easy test for polymyositis that can provide a definitive diagnosis, doctors look for identifying signs and symptoms. These include unexplained muscle weakness, certain microscopic changes in the structure of the muscle tissue, the presence of autoimmune antibodies and inflammation, and unusually high levels of muscle enzymes in the blood. Electromyography (EMG tests) and nerve conduction tests can show abnormalities commonly seen with polymyositis and help rule out other diseases. Muscle biopsies may also be conducted.

A steroid called prednisone, which is given to quell inflammation, is the first-line treatment of choice for polymyositis. Ironically, when used over time, prednisone can cause muscle weakness and a host of other side effects ranging from the unpleasant to the serious. Thus your doctor may prescribe a steroid-sparing agent to be taken along with prednisone to decrease its dosage and side effects. Azathioprine (Imuran), mycophenolate mofetil (Cellcept), and methotrexate (Rheumatrex) are the three most commonly used medications for this purpose. Physical therapy is also an important treatment.

While as many as one in five people suffer from symptoms that grow progressively worse and die within five years of developing polymyositis, most are able to keep the disease under control and live fairly normal lives.

Dermatomyositis: Polymyositis plus

Dermatomyositis is a disease that causes all the symptoms of polymyositis, plus rashes and other skin problems.

Summarizing the symptoms

There may be a reddish rash on the face and elsewhere on the body, and reddish-purple swelling about the eyes. Typically appearing on the knuckles, the rash can be raised, smooth, or scaly. With time, the rash fades but may leave behind areas with brownish pigmentation or no pigmentation at all, as well as scarred or shriveled skin.

Diagnosing and treating dermatomyositis

Dermatomyositis is diagnosed and treated in much the same way as polymyositis. Doctors look for unexplained muscle weakness, certain microscopic changes in muscle tissue structure, and changes in the levels of certain blood enzymes.

Dermatomyositis is treated in the the same ways as polymyositis. Prednisone or other steroids are used to decrease the inflammation and suppress autoimmune responses, with a steroid-sparing agent like azathioprine or methotrexate taken in conjunction with the prednisone to decrease its dosage and side effects. Topical medicines (creams, ointments, gels, solutions, sprays, or foams) can also be applied to the skin to bring some relief, and sunscreens and/or antimalarial medications are used to manage persistent rashes.

2

Tests and Treatments: What to Expect

It would be great if a single test could tell you whether or not you have arthritis, which type, and which treatment is appropriate for your condition. Unfortunately, such a test doesn't exist. Diagnosis can be quick and easy, a long and drawn-out process, or anything in between. And making the treatment decisions can sometimes be quite difficult.

In this part, we explain how doctors go about diagnosing the many forms of arthritis and the high-tech and low-tech tests they may use. We also discuss the medicines they may prescribe and surgeries they may recommend. And, equally important, we show you how to work with your doctor to make treatment decisions and manage any pain you may experience.

Chapter **6**

Your Doctor and You: Allies Against Arthritis

I n the old days — let's say 40 or 50 years ago — when the doctor said, "Jump," the patient said, "How high?" In other words, the doctor was completely in charge, ordering tests, deciding how aggressively or conservatively to attack the disease, pushing the patient toward surgery or drugs, taking a dim view of alternative approaches, and so on.

Fortunately, a new approach to health care exists today: Doctors and patients work together as a team with you, the patient, being in charge. Research has shown that patients who take an active role in their treatment tend to fare better than those who stay in passive roles. So selecting your doctor carefully, helping to draw up the treatment program, and following that program to the letter are very important. Your odds of recovery improve if you believe in your treatment and play an active part in your recovery efforts, doing everything you can to get well.

Positioning Yourself for Treatment Success

Doctors are experts who are well-trained in diagnosis and treatment. They'd better be, because we put our health (and our lives) in their hands. Still, doctors are only human, which makes them subject to limitations and foibles just like the rest of us.

TIP

To make sure you get the best treatment, follow these three cardinal rules:

» **Select your doctor carefully.** Find someone who is not only thoroughly familiar with and experienced in treating your kind of arthritis, but is also up on the latest research and treatments. You don't want to miss out on an effective therapy because your doctor is uninformed. The following section, "Choosing a Good Doctor," tells you how to find the right person for the job.

» **Thoroughly research your condition.** How can you gauge whether or not your doctor is following correct procedures and doing everything possible to treat your condition unless you know something about the topic? Information about every type of arthritis, its symptoms, treatments, alternative healing methods, and so on is available from the Arthritis Foundation (see their online help page: https://www.arthritis.org/i-need-help or their web site https://www.arthritis.org) and similar organizations. Appendix B has more information on resources.

» **Be a team player with your doctor.** After you've decided on a doctor, regard them as the expert — your trusted advisor. Ask any questions you can think of, but try to work with them not against them. Unless something feels wrong about the advice you're getting, follow it to the letter. Get behind your treatment and do all you can to make it successful. Only then will you reap the best possible results.

Choosing a Good Doctor

How do you find a good doctor? Ideally, you begin by getting recommendations from doctors or other people in the medical field, including your own general practitioner or internist (if you're searching for a specialist), or perhaps a highly regarded nearby hospital or medical center. You can also ask friends for their recommendations. You then need to check the candidates' credentials on the Internet or by contacting your local chapter of the American Medical Association (www.ama-assn.org) to narrow the field. Finally, you should personally interview those left on your list and select the doctor who seems to suit you best. Of course, you may not have the opportunity to select your doctors quite so freely — you may be restricted to the ones on the list provided by your insurance company, HMO, or PPO.

Luckily, you have a good chance of finding an excellent doctor on these lists. Still, some will undoubtedly be a better match for you than others. Assuming that you do have some choice, searching for the physician best suited to your needs will be well worth your while.

Determining whether the doctor is knowledgeable

Almost every doctor has an office wall covered with diplomas and certificates, and although you may find them interesting to look at, most of these fancy, framed pieces of paper can't offer you much useful information. Not even a diploma from Harvard Medical School, you ask? Isn't a diploma from a super-prestigious school better than one from Tiny Town Med? Not necessarily. Plenty of brilliant doctors have graduated from little-known medical colleges.

What about the official-looking paper that the state issues proclaiming that the doctor is licensed to practice medicine? Remember that every practicing physician *has* to have one of those to treat patients. (Think of it as a driver's license for doctors.)

As for membership in the American Medical Association, the AMA is primarily a trade association. If Dr. Smith can pay the dues, they can join the AMA, but that doesn't necessarily mean they're better than a non-AMA doctor.

And what about the certificates indicating that the doctor is a member of various medical societies? Again, these documents guarantee nothing. A doctor can belong to an organization that offers wonderful seminars and educational materials without ever taking advantage of them. On the other hand, a doctor who doesn't belong to a medical organization may spend hours studying medical journals and swapping tips with colleagues. What if the doctor is a diplomate in a medical society? Sometimes this title can mean something. Certain medical societies require that their members pass rigorous written tests before allowing the doctors to call themselves diplomates. On the other hand, some societies offer diplomate tests that aren't so difficult.

The one thing that *does* mean something is board certification. *Board certified* means that the doctor has passed difficult written and/or oral tests in their field. Certification is generally considered an impressive credential, because it isn't required to practice. Being board certified is an extra stamp of validation that not every doctor receives.

For a quick look at the difference between a general practitioner and a rheumatologist, see the sidebar "General practitioner versus rheumatologist" later in the chapter.

Sharing the same treatment philosophy

Many people think of medicine as a science, but it's often just as much an art. For example, doctors frequently follow hunches during their diagnostic workups. And although standard approaches to treating most diseases exist, doctors know that everybody responds a little differently. Therefore, most treatment programs must be individualized and then changed as time goes on — anywhere from slightly tweaked to radically altered.

Because everyone responds to treatment differently, physicians have some leeway when diagnosing and treating patients — some wiggle room that also allows for the expression of personality. Some doctors are more aggressive than others; some like the idea of alternative approaches, and others are determined to stick strictly to Western medical techniques. Some doctors want to tell you exactly what to do, but others are more willing to involve you in the decision-making process.

Although no diploma hanging on the wall is going to let you in on a doctor's treatment philosophy, these framed documents *can* offer you some clues. Framed certificates of membership in medical or nonmedical organizations dedicated to nutrition or exercise, for example, suggest that the doctor is open to alternative therapies. But the best way, by far, to figure out a doctor's philosophy about diagnosis and treatment is simply to ask.

Interviewing a prospective doctor

When you're ready to interview those on your "short list" of prospective doctors, call and make an appointment with each one, explaining that you simply want to talk about the possibility of becoming a patient. Yes, it will cost whatever the doctor wants to charge — which can be hefty. And no, your insurance company probably won't pay for it. But it can mean the difference between finding a doctor who's just right for you or getting stuck with one who isn't right. Your future health is worth the investment.

REMEMBER

Your primary goal for the interview is to get a feel for what the doctor is like, how they respond to you and your questions, and what makes up their general treatment philosophy.

You may want to bring a list of questions, such as the following:

>> What is your background and training in arthritis treatment?

>> Which kinds of cases (osteoarthritis, rheumatoid arthritis, and so on) do you typically treat?

>> Do you like to work as part of a team (rheumatologist, physical therapist, massage therapist, and so on) or do you prefer to handle the treatment alone?

>> If you do like to work as a team, who is in charge of the treatment?

>> Do you think medication is always, or almost always, the best treatment for arthritis?

>> How valuable are diet, exercise, and stress reduction in treating arthritis?

>> Do you favor the use of vitamins, herbs, and other supplements as adjuncts to treatment? If so, which ones?

>> How do you feel about using other alternative therapies (massage, homeopathy, magnets, acupuncture, and so on) in conjunction with standard treatment? Which do you feel are best?

No right answers to these questions exist. Look for a doctor whose attitude dovetails with yours.

Considering compatibility

After you're sure that your prospective physician is qualified, you must try to predict whether the two of you can work together. Don't automatically assume that the answer is *yes*. You, the patient, should be considered a member of the treatment team — the most important member — rather than a passive pincushion who acquiesces to whatever medicines and surgeries your doctor deems necessary. How can you find out if your prospective doctor seems like a team player?

After you visit with a doctor for either an interview or an appointment, think carefully about what went on during your time together. Did the doctor:

>> Try to rush you through the interview?

>> Keep looking at their watch?

>> Solicit your opinions?

>> Give you ample time to express your thoughts, wishes, concerns, and fears?

- >> Listen carefully?

- >> Give you thoughtful, complete responses in plain English (instead of confusing medical speak)?

- >> Invite you to ask questions?

- >> Ask about your preferred approach to treatment? (For example, whether you wish to begin treatment with strong painkillers or prefer to give exercise and a back brace a chance before moving on to medication?)

- >> Push you to pursue much more aggressive or conservative treatment than you prefer?

- >> Brush aside your concerns by saying, "Trust me," or, "I know what's best"?

- >> Focus on drugs and surgery for treatment and downplay your desire to work with a physical therapist or other alternative healer?

REMEMBER

You can gather a lot of information by asking questions, listening carefully, and observing the doctor's behavior. If you aren't comfortable, find another doctor.

Working with Your Doctor

Nothing can be quite as educating, enlightening and reassuring as a long talk with your doctor about your condition. But for many people, the time actually spent with the doctor seems all too short. Certain things you wanted to report can slip your mind, and you might miss the opportunity to ask important questions or clarify confusing explanations. But you can make the most of your appointments by doing a little advance planning.

TIP

Before your first appointment, gather the information your doctor will need and come prepared. Bring the following information along with you to your appointment:

- >> Medical records from other doctors or health professionals: Have them forwarded to your doctor's office.

- >> A log of your arthritis symptoms: Describe how each symptom felt, the intensity of the pain, when it occurred, and what you were doing when you noticed it.

- >> A list of all prescription and non-prescription medications you're currently taking, plus all herbs, vitamins, minerals and other supplements.

- >> A list of all the treatments you've used (including home remedies) to ease your arthritis symptoms.

>> A list of the questions you'd like your doctor to answer. For example:

- How did you determine that I have this particular kind of arthritis?
- What's causing my arthritis?
- Do I have any joint deformity?
- What kinds of treatment do you recommend?
- What outcome can I expect?
- Which non-medication kinds of treatment do you recommend?
- Will physical therapy help? Which kinds?
- Will I need surgery? If so, how long can I wait before I have it?
- What will happen if I do nothing?
- What will my treatment cost?

>> A notepad: Take notes so that you can review your doctor's answers at home when you have no distractions.

TIP

If, when you get home and review your notes, you find that you don't understand an answer or you've forgotten to ask a question, don't be afraid to call the doctor's office and ask for a phone consultation. The more you know, the better prepared you'll be to tackle your condition head-on.

GENERAL PRACTITIONER VERSUS RHEUMATOLOGIST

Whether you need a specialist depends upon the kind of arthritis you have. If you have osteoarthritis (see Chapter 2), you may do well under the care of a general practitioner or internist. But if you have a more complicated kind of arthritis, one that involves entire body systems (such as rheumatoid arthritis — check out Chapter 3), you probably need to see a rheumatologist.

Rheumatologists specialize in diseases of the joints, muscles, and bones. They treat arthritis, musculoskeletal pain disorders, osteoporosis, and various autoimmune diseases. An important part of the rheumatologist's job is proper diagnosis of the disease, because symptoms can point to many different conditions. After the rheumatologist pinpoints the disease, proper treatment can begin, so early and accurate diagnosis is crucial. If you don't have a clear-cut case of osteoarthritis, or if your family physician or internist seems baffled by your symptoms, consult a rheumatologist.

Speaking Your Doctor's Language

Although you're not expected to know everything (any more than an orchestra conductor has to play every instrument proficiently), you do need to know enough to communicate with your doctor(s) and the other members of your medical team. Doing so requires a certain amount of education. You don't have to become an expert, or stay up all night mastering arcane medical terms and memorizing medical books. However, you should read all you can about the type of arthritis you have and the medications you're taking to become well-informed about your disease.

TIP

Some good information sources include the following:

>> **The Merck Manual Home Health Handbook, 3rd Ed. (Merck Publishing).** This is the layman's version of the technical manual that doctors use.

>> **The PDR Pocket Guide to Prescription Drugs, 10th Ed. (PDR Consumer).** This is a slimmed-down and simplified version of the *PDR (Physician's Desk Reference),* the doctor's reference guide to medications. In regular, nonmedical English, *The PDR Pocket Guide* spells out important issues concerning each medication, such as:

- Why it's prescribed

- The most important facts about the drug

- Tips on how you should take the medication

- Side effects

- Tips for when you shouldn't use the drug

- Clues concerning how the drug may interact with foods and other drugs

>> **Arthritis support groups.** Consider joining an arthritis support group. The other members understand what you're going through, so they listen sympathetically, and they've been in your situation, so they can give you helpful advice. Likewise, if you join the group, at some point you become a regular, which gives you the great satisfaction of helping others. You can find support groups by asking your doctors, nurses, or the community support staff at your hospital.

You can also find arthritis support groups through the National Mental Health Consumer Self-Help Clearinghouse at 800-553-4539 or 215-751-1810, or check out its web site at https://www.amhselfhelp.org or email them at info@mhselfhelp.org.

>> **The Internet.** Three great places to begin your search are the Arthritis Foundation (www.arthritis.org), the National Institute of Arthritis and Musculoskeletal and Skin Diseases (NIAMS) (ww.niams.nih.gov), and the American College of Rheumatology (https://ww.rheumatology.org). You can find more web sites in Appendix B of this book.

WARNING

The Internet is a great place to find information. Unfortunately, you can't treat everything you find there as gospel. Before accepting what you read, ask yourself who is offering the material, who wrote the material, and why and when it was written. If the information is offered by well-known, reputable organizations, such as the Arthritis Foundation, the National Institute of Arthritis and Musculoskeletal Diseases, or the American College of Rheumatology, it's undoubtedly good information. However, if an organization devoted to selling products that are mentioned in the literature prepares and posts the information you find, take what you read with a grain of salt.

No matter where you find information, ask yourself who wrote it: A physician or other health professional? A respected nonmedical educator? Some guy off the street? Is the author qualified to present information or give advice? Ask yourself whether the article is offered to provide information or to sell a product. There's nothing wrong with selling products, and some pieces that are written with the idea of selling are packed with unbiased, useful information. However, others aren't. Also, be sure to check the date the information was posted. Even a well-researched article may contain erroneous information if it hasn't been updated in several years.

Figuring Out When You Should Find a New Doctor

Not every marriage is made in heaven, and not every patient/doctor partnership works out for the best. If you're wondering whether you ought to switch to a different doctor, take a look at the following list (adapted from the article "Red Flags" by Doyt Conn, MD) and see if the situations ring any bells for you:

>> **Feeling the progress of your treatment is too slow.** It may take a while before your doctor finds the right treatment for you, and medications can take three to six months before they really kick in, especially for autoimmune forms of arthritis. In addition, complete relief of your symptoms may not be possible. If your doctor is still trying to adjust your treatment, you may want to stick it out a little longer. If not, find someone else.

>> **Noticing that your treatment consists of medication only.** Treatment of arthritis is multifaceted and should include nondrug therapies, such as exercise, diet, joint protection techniques, rest, and so on.

>> **Realizing that your doctor relies solely on NSAIDs.** At one time, NSAIDs (see Chapter 8) were the treatment-of-choice for arthritis and were better at relieving the pain of hip and knee OA than acetaminophen (Tylenol). But it may be a better choice to start with acetaminophen and then escalate to NSAIDs, if necessary, because NSAIDs are notorious for causing stomach problems. Topical NSAIDs, however, don't cause stomach problems and can work well. As for RA, treatment may require the use of more aggressive drugs, such as methotrexate or sulfasalazine, in addition to NSAIDs. In some cases, waiting too long to use these drugs can result in irreparable damage to the affected joints.

>> **Finding that your doctor gives you too many "cortisone" injections.** Injecting steroids into an inflamed joint is a fast way of stopping an RA flare or decreasing the pain associated with OA. But overuse of injectable steroids (most experts recommend no more than four injections per joint per year) can have serious side effects, including tendon rupture, destruction of the joint, and, occasionally, high blood pressure, diabetes, cataracts, and osteoporosis. As long as the injections aren't performed too frequently and are used in combination with other therapies, they can be safe and effective.

REMEMBER

Generally, the best advice is to go with your gut feeling. If something feels wrong or you and your doctor don't seem to click, find someone with whom you do feel comfortable. Having confidence in the type and quality of medical care that you receive can make a positive difference in your recovery.

Chapter **7**

Judging Joint Health with Low- and High-Tech Tests

Diagnosing arthritis can be as easy as 1-2-3. Or it may take months or even years of following up on clues and running endless tests. With osteoarthritis, the diagnosis is usually pretty clear: The patient is typically over 40, has pain in a single joint but no swelling, and an X-ray shows the narrowing of the joint space. But with other forms of arthritis, such as infectious arthritis, the symptoms can be much vaguer: fatigue, chills, fever, rash, inflammation of the heart, meningitis, and joint aches that may come and go for years. However, doctors have many tests available to narrow the long list of possibilities and pinpoint a diagnosis.

Checking In for a Check-Up

No one test can determine for sure whether you have arthritis. Instead, your doctor must go through several procedures, such as taking a thorough medical history, examining you carefully, and performing a series of tests. Together, these clues should provide a pretty accurate picture of what's going on in your body.

Presenting the past: Your medical history

Your doctor will need to assemble a great deal of information about your overall health, as well as your specific complaints. The medical history includes that questionnaire you answer in your doctor's waiting room and questions your doctor asks you in person. Medical histories commonly include general information, such as your age, sex, and occupation, as well as specific information about

>> Any accidents or injuries that you've sustained

>> Diseases that run in your family

>> Illnesses you've had (especially recently)

>> Allergies you have (especially those that bother you)

>> Medications you take (bring a list, plus your pill bottles, if possible)

>> Other problems, including recent weight loss, depression, sleep disturbances, aches and pain, skin changes, and fatigue

Your doctor will also review your activities at work and at home. Knowing that you type eight hours a day, for example, may help the doctor connect your hand pain and tingling to carpal tunnel syndrome. Likewise, knowing that you drink a lot of alcohol may point them to the possibility of gout. You may help guide your doctor to the diagnosis of Lyme disease by revealing that you went camping in the woods and discovered a rash on your back shortly before your joints began hurting. And of course, you should always tell your doctor about any and all of your symptoms.

TIP

Don't hold back information because you think it's not important. You may not mention that you've had some difficulty in swallowing because you don't think it's related to your joint and muscle pain. But if you have scleroderma or polymyositis (see Chapter 5 for information on both of these conditions), it may very well be relevant.

From head to toe: The physical exam

Even if you have pain in just a single joint, you should be examined from head to toe. Your primary physician (internist or family practitioner) is the doctor most likely to do perform this examination. If you see a rheumatologist or other specialist, they probably won't look you over from stem to stern, but *should* carefully examine all affected and related areas.

How important is the head-to-toe examination? Well, urinary difficulties in men can be due to reactive arthritis, gonococcal arthritis, or something totally different, such as an enlarged prostate gland. Without a thorough examination, the proper diagnosis may be missed.

At some point, the examination will focus on your painful joint(s). Your doctor should be particularly interested in the following key symptoms:

» How many joints are affected?

» Does the pain affect the same joints on both sides of the body?

» Do any of your joints feel stiff?

» Do redness, swelling, and warmth surround the joint, and is it tender to the touch?

The doctor will check for redness, warmth, swelling, and excessive fluid in the affected joints. You may be asked to bend and straighten these joints several times to determine the range of motion. The doctor will then manipulate your joints, checking for crackling and pain upon bending and flexing, examine any related areas, and may check your reflexes and muscle strength.

The doctor may ask you to walk, sit, rise from a chair, bend, and do other movements to assess the way you use your joints. You may be asked to reach for something or make a fist around a pencil to gauge the impact of your condition on your ability to perform daily activities.

You and your doctor will need to discuss in detail the kind and amount of pain you're experiencing, and you will need to answer questions that are specifically geared to the pain itself. You may want to pay special attention to these issues before you see your doctor so that you can have your answers ready.

TIP

The following is a pain checklist you can use to check off symptoms, add your own comments, and take with you to your doctor's appointment:

❑ Is it an ache, a burn, a throb, or a stabbing pain?

❑ Does it come and go, or is it constant?

❑ What activities or movements make the pain worse?

❑ What makes the pain recede?

❑ Are you stiff in the morning?

❑ Do your joints lock up?

❑ Is the pain more intense at a certain time of day?

❑ How does your condition affect your work and home life?

You may also be asked to rate your pain on a scale of one to ten, with ten indicating intolerable pain. If you keep a pain diary or a symptom diary for several days or weeks before visiting your doctor, you will be able to paint a more accurate picture of your pain and other problems.

Explaining Imaging Tests

In order to understand what's making your knee hurt, your hip ache, or your finger swell, your doctor needs to take a peek inside the affected joint. Luckily, looking inside your joint is painless; your doctor has sophisticated equipment designed to do just that via X-rays and various types of scans, while you relax on a table.

Examining the benefits of an X-ray

An X-ray is often one of the first tools that a doctor uses when gathering information to make a diagnosis. X-rays are useful in distinguishing between two of the most common forms of arthritis, osteoarthritis (Chapter 2) and rheumatoid arthritis (Chapter 3), and may be useful in diagnosing gout (Chapter 4), ankylosing spondylitis (Chapter 4), and reactive arthritis (Chapter 5).

REMEMBER

X-rays are particularly helpful in confirming that cartilage and/or joint damage does exist, and in distinguishing between osteoarthritis and rheumatoid arthritis. In OA,an X-ray can reveal roughened bone ends, uneven narrowing of the joint space indicating cartilage deterioration, bone spurs, and thickened bone-ends, while in RA it can show, decreased bone density, narrowing of the joint space in an even manner and, possibly, bone erosion. In ankylosing spondylitis, an X-ray can show the inflammation, small bone growths, and changes in the sacroiliac joints commonly seen with this condition. In reactive arthritis, it can reveal characteristic joint damage.

TIP

X-rays can be helpful in detecting rheumatoid arthritis, osteoarthritis, ankylosing spondylitis and reactive arthritis, but aren't so useful in diagnosing Raynaud's phenomenon or bursitis.

Seeing more with a scan

Sometimes a standard X-ray can't tell the doctor what they need to know, because X-rays can't produce images of soft tissue or give the doctor a three-dimensional view. That's where CT, MRI, and ultrasound scans come in handy. All three of these show different things in different ways, with each one providing needed information:

- » **MRI scans:** MRI stands for magnetic resonance imaging (MRI). Magnetism, radio waves, and a computer are used to create detailed images of body structures. MRIs are especially helpful in diagnosing ailments that affect soft tissues and may detect OA even before symptoms are present. Some experts use MRI scans when they suspect a case of early RA, to detect erosions in the joints that are too subtle to be seen on X-rays. For a traditional MRI scan, you lie on a narrow table that is wheeled inside a tunnel-like scanner. Unfortunately, you must lie perfectly still, you can feel claustrophobic while squeezed inside the tunnel, and the machine makes a great deal of noise. Plus the scan can go on for as long as an hour and a half! The new open-MRI scanner is more comfortable, less noisy, and less likely to cause claustrophobia because it's similar to a tanning bed that's open on all sides.

- » **CT scans:** The CT scan (which stands for computerized axial tomography) is a marriage of X-rays and computer technology in which a series of X-rays of one area are taken from different angles. The computer builds these images into three-dimensional pictures, which can be helpful for examining organs, such as the lung or GI tract that can be affected by diseases like lupus. Unlike MRIs, CT scans are completed in 15 to 30 minutes, make minimal noise, and, because the machine isn't tunnel-shaped (CT machines are shaped more like doughnuts), they don't cause claustrophobia.

- » **Ultrasound:** An ultrasound scan (also known as a sonogram) uses high-frequency sound waves to create images of certain parts of the interior of the body. Ultrasounds are useful for imaging soft tissue structures and can help provide early diagnosis of several forms of arthritis including OA, RA, inflammatory arthritis, gout, psoriatic arthritis, ankylosing spondylitis, and infectious arthritis, among others. Ultrasounds are also quick and affordable, especially compared to MRIs, and unlike X-rays and CT scans, they don't use radiation.

Backing Up a Diagnosis with Blood Tests

Sometimes the best way to figure out what's going on inside the body is to take samples of the blood for an up–close look. Blood tests can help confirm a tentative diagnosis or rule out other causes of joint pain. Certain substances found in the blood can indicate inflammation, infections, muscle damage, or other signs of a particular type of arthritis. For example, the presence of rheumatoid factor suggests rheumatoid arthritis; certain antibody abnormalities can suggest lupus; and the presence of antibodies to *Borrelia burgdorferi* indicate Lyme disease. However, blood abnormalities can point to many different diseases, so these tests are usually used to supply diagnostic clues only.

Common blood tests for the various kinds of arthritis include:

>> **Anti-DNA and anti-Sm:** If the ANA test is positive, your doctor may want to obtain further antbody testing to better understand what kind of antibody you are making. For example, tests can be sent for antibodies to double-stranded DNA (anti-dsDNA) and Smith (anti-Sm), which are proteins found in the nucleus of the cell. Anti-dsDNA antibodies are found in half of those with lupus, while anti-Sm antibodies are found in 30 to 40 percent of them. Because these antibodies are rarely present in the blood of people without lupus, this test can be a reliable diagnostic tool. If the ANA test is negative, however, these extra tests are unnecessary.

>> **Antinuclear antibody (ANA):** Antibodies can trigger the immune system to attack the body's own tissues, which is the problem behind autoimmune diseases. All lupus patients and 40 to 50 percent of those with established RA have *antinuclear antibodies* (ANA) in their bloodstreams. (In fact, a negative ANA test rules out lupus.) Those with scleroderma, Sjogren's, and Raynaud's disease may also test positive for ANA.

>> **Blood chemistries:** Some basic blood tests provide further clues. A high level of uric acid, for example, can be a sign of gout. High levels of creatinine can indicate disturbed kidney function (which may point to lupus) or another disease of the connective tissue. High levels of C-reactive protein can indicate inflammatory forms of arthritis such as RA, infectious arthritis, or gout.

>> **C-reactive protein (CRP):** C-reactive protein is produced by the liver in response to inflammation in the body to help regulate immune reactions. High levels of CRP can indicate inflammation is present somewhere in the body and can be a sign of inflammatory diseases such as RA, infectious arthritis, obesity, cancer, or heart disease.

>> **Complement:** A group of blood proteins activated as part of the immune process, the *complement system* releases substances that kill bacteria and send white blood cells rushing to fight invaders. A low complement level suggests that the immune system is working in overdrive, perhaps the result of lupus or another autoimmune disease.

>> **Complete Blood Count (CBC):** Although the presence of arthritis can't be confirmed by a complete blood count test, it may be indicated. For example, a low red blood cell count (anemia) or abnormally high levels of blood platelets can be signs of chronic inflammation, which is found in RA, Sjögren's syndrome (usually referred to simply as Sjögren's), and polymyalgia rheumatica, among others. A high white cell count may signal some kind of infectious

arthritis, such as Lyme disease or gonococcal arthritis, while low levels of blood platelets can be an indication of lupus.

» **Cyclic citrullinated peptide (CCP) antibody:** The CCP antibody, which is found in more than 75 percent of those who have RA, targets healthy tissues in the joints. Testing for CCP antibodies is usually combined with the rheumatoid factor test. That's because RF can be found in people with other autoimmune diseases or even healthy people. Combining the RF test with the CCP antibody test is a more accurate method of diagnosing rheumatoid arthritis.

» **Erythrocyte sedimentation rate (ESR):** During inflammation, the red blood cells (*erythrocytes*) clump together, becoming heavier than normal. When left to stand in a test tube, these heavy red blood cells fall faster than normal. The rate at which your red blood cells settle during a one-hour period is called the *erythrocyte sedimentation rate*, or ESR, or the sed rate. A high sed rate indicates inflammation, although it can be due to aging, obesity, infections, cancer, and many other conditions.

» **Human leukocyte antigen B27 (HLA-B27):** This test looks for a protein found on the surface of white blood cell called HLA-B27. A positive test suggests a greater-than-average risk of developing reactive arthritis, psoriatic arthritis, or ankylosing spondylitis.

» **Rheumatoid factor (RF):** Some 50 to 80 percent of patients with RA have an antibody called *rheumatoid factor (RF)* in their blood. No one is quite sure whether RF causes the disease or results from the immune system's reaction to the disease. Although rheumatoid factor is a pretty good indicator of rheumatoid arthritis, some people with RA don't have it, and some who do have the factor don't have RA. Like most blood tests, this one must be considered in conjunction with other symptoms before an accurate diagnosis can be made.

These are not the only blood tests your doctor may order, and the examples given are not the only reasons for using them. They are, however, commonly used to help diagnose various forms of arthritis.

Taking Other Tests on the Road to Diagnosis

Doctors often have a good idea of what may be wrong after listening to you describe your symptoms, examining you, and considering your medical history. With many forms of arthritis, they may need nothing more than an X-ray or scan, a blood test or a biopsy to confirm the diagnosis. However, sometimes more testing is necessary. If, for example, your doctor suspects you have gout, a sample of your joint fluid may be taken to be examined in the laboratory. If ankylosing spondylitis is likely, genetic testing may be required.

Joint aspiration

Your doctor may want to insert a needle into one or more of your affected joints to withdraw a small amount of fluid for examination under a microscope. They may draw out additional fluid to help relieve pain and pressure inside of your joint, if the swelling is intense.

Called *joint aspiration* or *tapping a joint,* the process consists of the doctor sterilizing the area, applying or injecting a local anesthetic, then inserting a needle to pull out a small amount of fluid (as little as a couple of drops or as much as a tablespoon or two). The joint fluid is then sent to a laboratory for analysis. Healthy joints contain light yellow to clear fluid; anything else usually indicates a problem. Blood in the fluid may be the result of a substantial injury to the joint. Cloudy fluid or the presence of large numbers of white blood cells can indicate either infectious or inflammatory arthritis. Crystals in the fluid are probably due to gout or pseudogout. Bits of cartilage or bone usually indicate osteoarthritis.

Arthroscopy

An *arthroscope* (a fiberoptic camera about as big around as a straw) is inserted into your joint through a small incision, allowing the doctor to check out your joint's insides in all their glory. The doctor may use the arthroscope as a diagnostic tool or even as a way to help perform surgery inside your joint by repairing torn cartilage, cutting away inflamed or diseased tissues, removing bits of bone or cartilage, or reconstructing ligaments. Only orthopedic surgeons perform arthroscopy.

WARNING

Recent studies have stirred up controversy by showing that arthroscopy as a surgery for degenerative knee disease compared with sham surgery (the patient had arthroscopic tools inserted into the joint but no corrections were made) had similar effects in pain relief and joint function. That is, neither seemed to do much for the patients. So although it's still used for diagnostic and surgical purposes, the role of arthroscopy has yet to be defined.

Genetic testing

Scientists have discovered that certain genes may be associated with certain types of arthritis. The genetic marker HLA-B27, for example, is often found in those with ankylosing spondylitis. The marker HLA-DR4 has been found in 60 to

70 percent of people of European ancestry who have RA. Still, doctors can't rely solely on genetic testing because many people who have these genes do *not* get arthritis, and many who do have arthritis don't have these genes. However, these tests can show an inclination toward developing a particular kind of arthritis.

Urine testing

In this test, your urine is examined for protein, red blood cells, or other abnormal substances. Protein or red blood cells in the urine may be an indication of kidney disease, which is often seen in lupus.

Chapter **8**

From Aspirin to Steroids: Medicines for Arthritis

M any of the medicines that doctors prescribe for arthritis are briefly described in this chapter. Naturally, which, if any, of these medications may be right for you is a decision that you and your doctor should make together.

TECHNICAL STUFF

In this chapter and throughout the book, you'll see the abbreviated forms of various classes of drugs. Here's a quick list of what they mean:

- » COX-2 inhibitors: Cyclooxygenase-2 inhibitors

- » DMARDs: Disease-modifying antirheumatic drugs

- » IL-1, IL-6, or IL-17 inhibitors: Interleukin-1, interleukin-6, or interleukin-17 inhibitors

- » JAK inhibitors: Janus kinase inhibitors

- » NSAIDs: Non-steroidal anti-inflammatory drugs

- » SNRI: Serotonin-norepinephrine reuptake inhibitor

- » TNF-alpha inhibitors: Tumor necrosis factor-alpha inhibitors

Talking to Your Doctor

Your doctor's job is to diagnose and treat you, but this important task can't be done without your help. In order to diagnose and treat your condition properly, they must be thoroughly familiar with all of your symptoms — and you're the only one who can supply that information.

TIP

Your doctor will need to ask a lot of questions to build a "knowledge database" but probably won't think of everything. So, if you haven't already been asked, be sure to compile this information for your doctor:

» List everything that's bothering you. You should relate every little symptom and problem, whether physical, mental, or emotional.

» Give a complete list of all of your allergies and any allergic reactions you've ever had to any medications over the years.

» List every prescription and nonprescription medicine you're currently taking, including vitamins, minerals, amino acids, herbs, weight loss products, muscle builders, and so on. It's important to write down the dose you take and how often you take it. For some it might be easier to bring in the pill/supplement bottles. (See the sidebar, "Generic name, brand name, generic equivalent: I'm so confused!" later in the chapter.)

» List every medicinal cream or ointment you're currently using.

» If you're pregnant, planning to become pregnant, or nursing, be sure to mention this to your doctor.

» Inform the doctor if you're on hormone replacement therapy.

» List the foods that you like to eat. (Grapefruit, for example, can interfere with the workings of some medicines.)

» Tell your doctor which chemicals, liquids, or fumes you're exposed to at work and at home.

» Explain the tasks you handle at work and home, and tell your doctor about your hobbies and recreational activities.

» Make a list of any recent trips you've taken overseas, any hiking you've done recently, and any exposures you may have had to ticks and animals of any kind. This could be important when diagnosing certain diseases such as Lyme disease.

In short, tell your doctor all about yourself, your job, your habits, and everything you're ingesting. Relate your previous experiences with medicines, even if they were good. (Knowing that you tolerated a certain drug well may help your doctor choose a similar medicine for you or they even decide to stick with the same one.) The more your doctor knows about you, the better off you will be. If you're not asked for the information, volunteer it.

The following questions are good ones to ask your doctor concerning any medications prescribed for you:

>> How do I take this drug, exactly? (With or without food, in the morning, at bedtime, with fluid, after thoroughly shaking the bottle, and so on.)

>> Which activities are unsafe while I'm taking this medication? (For example, can I drive? Take other medicines? Take my vitamins?)

>> Are there any drugs, supplements, foods, or anything else I should avoid while I'm taking this medicine?

>> What is my pill or capsule going to look like? Look for a picture of it in the *PDR* (*Physician's Drug Reference*), the *Pocket Guide to Prescription Drugs* or a similar book. Compare what the doctor or pharmacist gives you to the description or picture of the drug to be sure you have the right thing.

GENERIC NAME, BRAND NAME, GENERIC EQUIVALENT: I'M SO CONFUSED!

A *generic name* is a medication's official moniker, bestowed upon it by the United States Adopted Names Council. A *brand name,* on the other hand, is a proprietary name given to the medication by the pharmaceutical company that owns it. Generic names often tell you something about the drug's structure or chemical formula. As far as lay people are concerned, generic names tend to be dull and unpronounceable. But brand names are often chosen with an eye toward "sales sizzle." For example, the drug with the generic name of methotrexate is sold under the brand name Rheumatrex.

You can quickly distinguish generic from brand names by looking at how they're written: Generic names begin with lowercase letters; brand names start with capitals. (This rule doesn't apply when the drug name appears at the beginning of a sentence, of course, where it is always capitalized.)

A *generic equivalent* is a drug whose active ingredients are chemically identical to the drug your doctor prescribes under its brand name, although the inactive ingredients (binders, fillers, etc.) may not be the same.

TIP

Doctors love to use big words, especially when talking about drugs. When you talk to your doctor, you're likely to hear words like *analgesics, biologics, anti-malarials, NSAIDs,* and *immunosuppressants* tossed around. If your doctor uses any word that you don't understand, ask for a definition. You may also want to ask your doctor to spell it for you.

Exploring the Five Classes of Drugs for Arthritis

Before deciding which drug to prescribe, doctors must first consider which class of medication is best. Doctors can prescribe from five primary classes: analgesics, nonsteroidal anti-inflammatory drugs (NSAIDs), disease modifying antirheumatic drugs (DMARDs), biologics, and steroids (corticosteroids).

For a quick look at how to take medications to get the best possible results, see the sidebar, "It's not just gulp and swallow," later in the chapter.

Analgesics

If you have arthritis pain without inflammation (as is often the case with osteoarthritis or fibromyalgia), your doctor may recommend an analgesic. Analgesics change the way the body and brain sense and respond to pain. But they do nothing to interfere with the inflammation process, which makes them easier on the stomach than the NSAIDs (see the next section). The best-known and most commonly used analgesic for osteoarthritis pain is acetaminophen, brand names for acetaminophen-containing analgesics include:

>> Tylenol

>> Percogesic

>> Aspirin-free Excedrin

Prescription varieties of analgesics include the following, all of which contain opiates:

>> Vicodin

>> Percocet

>> Codeine

A combination of acetaminophen plus a prescription analgesic, such as codeine, may be used for more intense pain. If you still hurt after taking an analgesic or NSAID alone, your doctor may prescribe a combination of the two, which may be more effective.

WARNING

Opiate-containing analgesics are potentially addicting, even when properly prescribed and properly taken by those with no tendency toward substance abuse. Ask your doctor about the addiction potential of any opiate-containing medications that are prescribed for you.

Nonsteroidal anti-inflammatory drugs (NSAIDs)

NSAIDs (pronounced EN-seds) help relieve pain and reduce inflammation by interfering with an enzyme called COX (cyclooxygenase). (Though technically considered analgesic drugs, for the purposes of this explanation we have separated them according to their effects on inflammation: NSAIDs do relieve inflammation, while analgesics do not.)

Widely used for many forms of arthritis, NSAIDs come in prescription and non-prescription (over-the-counter) forms, running the gamut from ibuprofen to Naproxen. The over-the-counter vareties come in lower dosages and are generally well-tolerated, while the more powerful prescription forms come in higher dosages and can trigger numerous side effects, often centered in the stomach. That said, over the counter NSAIDs can also cause these side effects if taken for long periods of time or in larger doses.

Perhaps the best known of the NSAIDs, asprin, which is also available under several brand names, works by interfering with the body's manufacture of the inflammatory substances that cause swelling, pain, and other problems. Aspirin's side effects are similar to those seen with the other NSAIDs, plus a few more that are all its own.

If traditional NSAIDs cause stomach upset, doctors often prescribe cyclooxygenase-2 (COX-2) inhibitors. COX-2 inhibitors (generic name celecoxib) tamp down the inflammatory COX-2 enzymes in the stomach, while sparing the stomach's protective COX-1 enzymes. The COX-2 inhibitors seem to be just as effective at relieving pain and inflammation as traditional NSAIDs, but are less damaging to the stomach and possibly the kidneys.

Disease modifying antirheumatic drugs (DMARDs)

DMARDs are generally reserved for autoimmune/inflammatory forms of arthritis — such as rheumatoid arthritis, psoriatic arthritis, and ankylosing spondylitis and are now the standard care early in treatment. DMARDs work by altering the way the immune system works, slowing or halting its disastrous attack on the body. Because they take time to work — in some cases, months — DMARDs may be prescribed along with an NSAID or a steroid, which can ease inflammation until the DMARDs kick in. Methotrexate, sulfasalazine, hydroxychloroquine are a few examples of DMARDs.

Biologics

For those with autoimmune/inflammatory arthritis (moderate to severe RA, ankylosing spondylitis, psoriatic arthritis, lupus, scleroderma, or myositis) who haven't improved when using traditional DMARDs, *biologics* are often prescribed.

TECHNICAL STUFF

First introduced in 1998, the biologics are genetically-engineered proteins that interrupt the immune system signals that bring on inflammation. They do this by lessening the action of pro-inflammatory substances called *cytokines* which play major roles in autoimmune/inflammatory conditions. Two of the major cytokines are *tumor necrosis factor* (TNF) and *interleukin* (IL-1), although there are many others. Many of the biologics used to treat these diseases are tumor necrosis factor (TNF) inhibitors such as Cimzia, Enbrel, Humira, Remicade, and Simponi, or interleukin-1 (IL-1 inhibitors) such as Kineret. Other drugs that target different kinds of pro-inflammatory interleukins, T-cells, or B-cells may also be used.

The biologics, which are usually injected or infused, can be taken alone or with other non-biologic medications. While they can be quite pricey, researchers are currently working on less expensive versions of these drugs that can be taken by mouth rather than by injection or infusion.

WARNING

Because the biologic drugs used for RA and other autoimmune/inflammatory disorders suppress the immune system, they increase your risk of developing serious infections such as tuberculosis or pneumonia. Tell your doctor if you have tuberculosis, pneumonia, hepatitis B or C, a current infection, a history of serious infections, or asthma before taking a biologic. Other possible side effects of biologics include redness, pain, or bruising at the injection site, and infections.

Steroids

Steroids (short for corticosteroids or glucocorticoids) are man-made versions of certain hormones that your body naturally produces. And just like the "real thing," they can be quite powerful in both good and bad ways. Steroids, including prednisone, hydrocortisone, and methylprednisolone, are powerful anti-inflammatories that can quickly reduce damaging inflammation of the joints or organs. Unfortunately, they can also increase your risk of infections, diabetes, high blood pressure, skin thinning, easy bruising, weight gain, osteoporosis, fluid retention, cataracts, coronary artery disease, and glaucoma.

WARNING

Because of these dangerous side effects, doctors typically prescribe the lowest effective dose of these medicines for the shortest amount of time. The goal should never be to treat your arthritis with steroids indefinitely. If this is your doctor's plan, see a different doctor. Steroids may be used to treat rheumatoid arthritis, lupus, psoriatic arthritis, polymyositis, and certain other forms of arthritis.

Uncovering Specific Medicines for Specific Types of Arthritis

In addition to analgesics, NSAIDs, DMARDs, biologics, and steroids, doctors may prescribe muscle relaxants, sleeping pills, or anti-anxiety drugs, among other drugs, to treat arthritis and its symptoms. Certain medications may be prescribed for problems that extend beyond the joints. For example, Raynaud's phenomenon is often treated with drugs normally thought of as blood pressure medicines, such as *vasodilators,* which open up the blood vessels and increase circulation to the extremities. Other drugs may be necessary to counteract or ameliorate the side effects of arthritis medicines.

WARNING

No matter which medications you take, remember to get complete instructions for their use from your doctor, and follow those instructions carefully. If anything seems amiss or if you have any questions, call your doctor immediately.

Following is a list of some of the drugs doctors may prescribe for arthritis and arthritis-related conditions. In most cases, they are listed under their brand names, with their generic names included in parentheses and in the discussions that follow.

Actemra

Actemra (generic name, tocilizumab) is a biologic that blocks the receptor for an inflammatory protein called interleukin-6 (IL-6). Actemra is used to treat adults with moderate to severe RA when at least one DMARD has produced unsatisfactory results. It is also used to treat adults with giant cell arteritis (GCA) and to slow the rate of decline in lung function in adults with scleroderma-associated interstitial lung disease (SSc-ILD). In children, Actemra may be used to treat certain forms of juvenile idiopathic arthritis. Actemra is given as an injection under the skin or an infusion into a vein.

Possible side effects include headache, weight gain, high blood pressure, swelling of the sinuses and throat, upper respiratory infections (such as the common cold), and high levels of liver enzymes (which can indicate liver problems).

Actonel

Actonel (generic name, risedronate) is used to prevent and treat osteoporosis and belongs to a class of drugs called bisphosphonates. Those who have Paget's disease or those who take medications that can cause osteoporosis (such as prednisone) may take Actonel to inhibit bone breakdown.

Possible side effects include upset stomach, flatulence, constipation, diarrhea, heartburn, and bone or joint pain, among others. Actonel must be taken with a full glass of plain water while sitting upright at least 30 minutes before eating or drinking anything else.

IT'S NOT JUST GULP AND SWALLOW

Medicines are tricky. Some are best absorbed on an empty stomach, so you must be sure to take them between meals. Others can irritate the stomach, so you should take them with food. You take some long-lasting medicines once a day; others only work for a brief period of time and must be taken several times a day. Sometimes it's necessary to have a constant level of the drug in your body, so you need to take it according to a rigid schedule. Other drugs may be taken whenever you feel they're necessary. Some medicines mix well with others, and some don't.

The point is that there's more to taking medicines than gulp and swallow. Ask your doctor for precise instructions regarding the taking of all your medicines: when, how (for example, with or without food), how often, and so on. Ask what to do if you forget to take a dose. Ask what side effects you can expect, which of them are dangerous, and which are not.

If your doctor doesn't tell you all about the medicine(s) you're taking, don't be afraid to ask!

Amoxil

Amoxil (generic name, amoxicillin) is an antibiotic used to treat a wide variety of bacterial infections including Lyme disease. It's available under the brand names Amoxil and Larotid.

Some possible side effects include agitation, anxiety, confusion, diarrhea, hives, hyperactivity, insomnia, rash, nausea, and vomiting.

You should not take this medication if you're allergic to penicillin or cephalosporin antibiotics (for instance, Cefaclor). If you've had asthma, hives, hay fever, or other allergies, make sure your doctor knows this before you take this drug.

Anaprox-DS

Anaprox-DS (generic name, naproxen sodium), also available as Naprelan and Aleve, is an NSAID used for osteoarthritis, rheumatoid arthritis, tendonitis, bursitis, gout, juvenile idiopathic arthritis, ankylosing spondylitis, and other forms of the disease. It reduces joint pain, swelling, inflammation, and stiffness.

Some possible side effects include difficulty breathing, drowsiness, skin eruptions, bleeding in general, stomach ulcers, itching, abdominal pain, bruising, and constipation. See your doctor regularly to monitor for possible internal bleeding, ulcers, and stomach ulcers.

Ansaid

Ansaid (generic name, flurbiprofen) is an NSAID used for osteoarthritis and rheumatoid arthritis that reduces joint pain, swelling, inflammation, and stiffness.

Some possible side effects include infection of the urinary tract, gastrointestinal upset, the "blahs," anxiety, an altered sense of smell, skin eruptions, bleeding in general, stomach ulcers, itching, abdominal pain, bruising, and constipation. See your doctor regularly to monitor for possible internal bleeding and stomach ulcers.

Arava

Arava (generic name, leflunomide) is a DMARD that blocks the formation of DNA, which is necessary for replicating cells, including those in the immune system. In this way it suppresses the immune system, which translates to a reduction in the inflammation, pain, and swelling seen in rheumatoid arthritis.

Arava produces the same kind of relief seen with methotrexate in those who haven't been helped by methotrexate, can't tolerate methotrexate's side effects, or have pre-existing kidney failure. While Arava doesn't cure rheumatoid arthritis, it can help relieve its symptoms and slow the rate at which the disease progresses.

Some possible side effects include liver problems, thinning or loss of hair, and stomach and digestive problems. Careful monitoring is required in those who have elevated blood pressure, problems with the immune system, or kidney disease. Arava may also cause birth defects and should be used with caution by women in their childbearing years.

WARNING

Women taking Arava leflunomide must not get pregnant while taking the drug, which takes about 18 months to wash out of the system. Fortunately, there is a medication (cholestyramine) that can wash Arava out of the system much sooner (although it does so via severe diarrhea).

Arthrotec

Arthrotec (diclofenac sodium/misoprostol), is a combination of the NSAID diclofenac plus the anti-ulcer medication misoprostol that is used to treat osteoarthritis and rheumatoid arthritis in people at high risk of developing stomach ulcers. The diclofenac helps relieve the pain and inflammation seen in these kinds of arthritis, while the misoprostol reduces stomach acid and replaces the protective substances in the stomach that are normally decreased by NSAIDs.

Some possible side effects include difficulty breathing, drowsiness, skin eruptions, bleeding in general, stomach ulcers, itching, abdominal pain, bruising, and constipation. Arthrotec may also cause heart attacks, stroke, and birth defects, miscarriage, and premature labor in pregnant women. See your doctor regularly to monitor for possible internal bleeding, ulcers, and stomach ulcers.

Aspirin

Aspirin (generic name) is an NSAID used to reduce pain, inflammation, and swelling in certan forms of arthritis, including osteoarthritis and rheumatoid arthritis. It's available over-the-counter under various brand names, such as Bayer, Empirin, and Entercote.

Some possible side effects include difficulty breathing, drowsiness, skin eruptions, bleeding in general, stomach ulcers, itching, abdominal pain, heartburn, bruising, and constipation. Aspirin may also cause complications during pregnancy. See your doctor regularly to monitor for possible internal bleeding, ulcers, and stomach ulcers.

Azulfidine

Azulfidine (generic name, sulfasalazine), a DMARD, is an anti-inflammatory sulfa drug that can be used to treat autoimmune diseases such as RA, ankylosing spondylitis, lupus, and others to decrease pain and swelling, prevent joint damage, and lower the risk of long-term disability. RA patients often take this medication in delayed-release form, Azulfidine EN-Tabs, to lessen the stomach upset seen with sulfasalazine.

Azulfidine should not be taken if you are allergic to sulfa drugs, PABA-containing sunscreens, or local anesthetics. It may cause increased sensitivity to the sun or bright light. Use sunscreen and wear sunglasses and protective clothing while taking this drug. Some possible side effects include headache, nausea, abdominal discomfort, loss of appetite, sun sensitivity, and rashes.

Celebrex

Celebrex (generic name, celecoxib) is an NSAID and a COX-2 inhibitor. It's used to relieve the pain, inflammation, and stiffness of osteoarthritis and rheumatoid arthritis with fewer of the gastrointestinal side effects seen with standard NSAIDs. Still, like other NSAIDs, it can cause diarrhea, abdominal pain, indigestion, ulceration, bleeding, and other problems. It may also increase the risk of serious cardiovascular events like heart attack and stroke. It can be dangerous to use Celebrex while you're on other medications or if you have liver or kidney disease, asthma, allergies to sulfa drugs, or you're pregnant. Celebrex is also much more expensive than standard NSAIDs.

Cimzia

Cimzia (generic name, certolizumab pegol) is a TNF inhibitor biologic used to reduce inflammation in rheumatoid arthritis, ankylosing spondylitis, and psoriatic arthritis in adults. Cimzia is given as an injection under the skin, usually every other week for three sessions before switching to one injection every other week or a larger dose every month. If it is well-tolerated, it may be used long term.

Side effects include an impaired ability of the immune system to fight infections, which may result in the development of tuberculosis and/or viral, bacterial or fungal infections. TNF inhibitors such as Cimzia may also increase your risk of developing a serious infection, including tuberculosis. Tell your doctor if you have ever had tuberculosis, recurrent infections, a nervous system disorder, a neurologic disorder such as multiple sclerosis, impaired heart function, or recent bouts of cancer, as TNF inhibitors can make these conditions worse.

Clinoril

Clinoril (generic name, sulindac) is an NSAID used to reduce joint pain, swelling, inflammation, and stiffness in osteoarthritis, rheumatoid arthritis, bursitis, tendonitis, gout, and ankylosing spondylitis.

Some possible side effects include headache, nervousness, ringing in the ears, swelling, difficulty breathing, drowsiness, skin eruptions, bleeding in general, stomach ulcers, itching, abdominal pain, and constipation. See your doctor regularly to monitor for possible internal bleeding, ulcers, and stomach ulcers.

Cochicine

Colchicine (generic name) is an anti-inflammatory this is used to prevent and treat gout flare-ups in adults and a genetic disease called Familial Mediterranean Fever in both children an adults. Sold under the brand names of Colcrys, Gloperba, and Mitigare, colchicine is taken orally in pill or capsule form or as an oral solution. It works by killing a type of white blood cell that comes into the gout-stricken joint to "clean up" the uric acid crystals by releasing inflammatory substances. But inflammation causes pain, so colchicine is used to kill the neutrophils and turn off inflammation. Cochicine works best if taken at the first sign of gout (redness, swelling and pain).

Possible side effects include fever, sore throat, muscle weakness and cramps, loss of appetite and hair loss or thinning. Taking too much colchicine can cause stomach pain, diarrhea, nausea, vomiting and/or a burning feeling in the throat, stomach, or skin.

ColBenemid

ColBenemid (generic name, probenecid/colchicine) is an antigout medicine. It contains both colchicine, an antigout medicine that slows the movement of white blood cells to the joints, and probenecid, which removes extra uric acid from the body. It doesn't cure gout but can prevent gout attacks. However, relief lasts only as long as you take it.

Some possible side effects include muscle weakness, nausea, vomiting, diarrhea, and blood and kidney problems. Probenecid can trigger dizziness, headaches, fever, and blood problems.

Cosentyx

Cosentyx (generic name, secukinumab) is a biologic categorized as an interleukin-17 (IL-17) inhibitor. Given in the form of an injection, it's used to treat psoriatic arthritis, ankylosing spondylitis, and certain other forms of spondyloarthritis.

Cosentyx works, in part, by lowering the body's ability to fight infections, which means side effects such as cold symptoms, diarrhea, upper respiratory infections, and serious infections such as tuberculosis can occur. Your doctor may want to give you a medicine for TB before treating you with this drug. In rare cases, Cosentyx may cause inflammatory bowel disease or flare-ups of this disease.

Cymbalta

Cymbalta (generic name, duloxetine) is a serotonin-norepinephrine reuptake inhibitor (SNRI) that is used to treat a potpourri of conditions including depression and anxiety, pain due to the nerve damage related to diabetic neuropathy, chronic musculoskeltal pain, and fibromyalgia. It is taken in capsule form.

Side effects of Cymbalta can range from grogginess, decreased appetite, fatigue, headache, insomnia, digestive problems to more serious effects, including liver damage, changes in blood pressure, agitation, changes in vision, and suicidal thoughts or behaviors, although the serious side effects are rare.

Cytoxan

Cytoxan (generic name, cyclophosphamide), is a DMARD and an anticancer drug used to treat serious cases of scleroderma, lupus, polymyositis and dermatomyositis, and sometimes rheumatoid arthritis. A potent immunosuppressant, Cytoxan works by slowing or stopping cell growth and decreasing the immune system's response to certain diseases.

Some possible side effects of Cytoxan include severe nausea and vomiting, bladder damage, loss of appetite, hair loss, mouth ulcers, darkening of skin and fingernails, low white blood cell counts, and an increased risk of developing shingles, lymphoma, skin cancer, and bladder cancer. But for those in their childbearing years, the biggest issue may be adverse effects on fertility, including a permanent decrease in egg supply in women and a temporary decrease sperm quality in men. And even small amounts of the taken during pregnancy can cause miscarriages and severe birth defects.

Daypro

Daypro (generic name, oxaprozin) is an NSAID used for osteoarthritis and rheumatoid arthritis to reduce joint pain, swelling, inflammation, and stiffness.

Some possible side effects include difficulty breathing, drowsiness, skin eruptions, bleeding in general, stomach ulcers, itching, abdominal pain, bruising, and constipation. See your doctor regularly to monitor for possible internal bleeding, ulcers, and stomach ulcers.

Decadron

Decadron (generic name, dexamethasone) is a steroid used to treat rheumatoid arthritis, ankylosing spondylitis, juvenile rheumatoid arthritis, gout and lupus by blocking the immune system's response to inflammation.

Decadron can increase your susceptibility to infections and make them harder to treat. It can also "hide" the presence of infections, making it difficult for your doctor to diagnose and treat the problem. Other possible side effects include high blood pressure, thinning of the skin, easy bruising, weight gain, loss of muscle, osteoporosis,nausea, vomiting, mood changes, high blood glucose, and glaucoma.

Deltasone

Deltasone (generic name, prednisone) is a steroid used to decrease inflammation in rheumatoid arthritis, lupus, ankylosing spondylitis, juvenilerheumatoid arthritis, gout, and many other conditions.

Deltasone can increase your susceptibility to infections and make them harder to treat. It can also "hide" the presence of infections, making it difficult for your doctor to diagnose and treat the problem. Other possible side effects include high blood pressure, thinning of the skin, easy bruising, weight gain, loss of muscle, osteoporosis,nausea, vomiting, mood changes, high blood glucose, and glaucoma.

Disalcid

Disalcid (generic name, salsalate) is an NSAID used for osteoarthritis, rheumatoid arthritis, and other forms of arthritis to relieve pain, inflammation, and joint stiffness.

Some possible side effects include difficulty breathing, drowsiness, skin eruptions, bleeding in general, stomach ulcers, itching, abdominal pain, bruising, constipation, ringing in the ears, and hearing problems. Disalcid contains salicylate, which has been linked to Reye's syndrome in children. See your doctor regularly to monitor for possible internal bleeding, ulcers, and stomach ulcers.

Doryx

Doryx (generic name, doxycycline) is a tetracycline antibiotic used to treat bacterial infections including gonococcal infections and Lyme disease. Also available as Vibramycin and Vibra-Tabs, it works by killing certain bacteria or inhibiting their growth and multiplication.

Some possible side effects include serious allergic reactions causing swelling of the face, difficulty swallowing, inflamed tongue, and chest pain. Other side effects include serious sun sensitivity and abdominal discomfort.

Enbrel

Enbrel (generic name, etanercept) is a TNF inhibitor biologic used to reduce the pain, swelling and stiffness seen in rheumatoid arthritis, juvenile rheumatoid arthritis, psoriatic arthritis, and ankylosing spondylitis. Enbrel works by blocking the activity of TNF, a substance that causes arthritis-related swelling and joint damage. Enbrel is typically given twice a week as injections in the thigh, stomach, or upper arm.

Some possible side effects include redness, pain, swelling, itching, or bruising at the injection site, and infections of the upper respiratory tract. Though rare, symptoms of lupus have also occurred with Enbrel treatment. TNF inhibitors like Enbrel may also increase your risk of developing a serious infection, including tuberculosis. Tell your doctor if you have ever had tuberculosis, recurrent infections, a nervous system disorder, a neurologic disorder such as multiple sclerosis, impaired heart function, or recent bouts of cancer, as TNF inhibitors can make these conditions worse.

Etodolac

Etodolac (generic name) is an NSAID used to reduce the joint pain, swelling, inflammation, and stiffness seen in osteoarthritis and rheumatoid arthritis.

Some possible side effects include blurred vision, chills, pain or difficulty upon urinating, more frequent urination, asthma, fever, black stools (a sign of stomach bleeding), rapid heartbeat, and congestive heart failure. See your doctor regularly to monitor for possible internal bleeding or stomach ulcers.

Feldene

Feldene (generic name, piroxicam) is an NSAID used to reduce the joint pain, swelling, inflammation, and stiffness seen in osteoarthritis and rheumatoid arthritis.

Some possible side effects include abdominal pain, anemia, dizziness, nosebleed, elevated blood pressure, sweating, stomach ulceration, the "blahs," headache, itching, and nausea. See your doctor regularly to monitor for possible internal bleeding or stomach ulcers.

Fosamax

Fosamax (generic name, alendronate sodium) is used to treat Paget's disease and postmenopausal osteoporosis (thinning of the bones). It prevents or slows the weakening of the bones and helps maintain bone integrity. Fosamax (which comes in tablet form) must be taken once a week, first thing in the morning, with a full glass of water 30 minutes before anything is eaten. During that time, you should stand or sit upright to reduce the risk of developing heartburn or injuring your esophagus due to medication that isn't sufficiently "washed down" to the stomach.

Some possible side effects of Fosamax include bloating, diarrhea, constipation, stomach irritation, muscle or bone pain, difficulty swallowing, and ulcers in the esophagus. Be sure to get plenty of calcium and vitamin D as a part of your osteoporosis treatment to help Fosamax work as effectively as possible.

Humira

Humira (generic name, adalimumab) is a TNF inhibitor biologic used either by itself or with other medications to reduce the pain, swelling, and difficulty in moving caused by rheumatoid arthritis and certain forms of JIA. Humira works by blocking the activity of tumor necrosis factor (TNF), which causes arthritis-related swelling and joint damage. Humira is given in the form of injections, usually every other week, to those who have not been helped by other rheumatoid arthritis medications. It's more common than not that Humira is given in combination with methotrexate or another DMARD as this makes both more effective.

TNF inhibitors such as Humira may increase your risk of developing a serious infection, including tuberculosis. Tell your doctor if you have ever had tuberculosis, recurrent infections, a nervous system disorder, a neurologic disorder such as multiple sclerosis, impaired heart function, or recent bouts of cancer, as TNF inhibitors can make these conditions worse. Rarely, symptoms of lupus have occurred with treatment with Humira.

Hymovis

Hymovis (generic name, hyaluronan) is a thick, gel-like substance that acts as a shock absorber and lubricant inside the knee joint. Intended for those who suffer from osteoarthritis-related knee pain that has not been helped by pain relievers, exercise or physical therapy, Hymovis is injected directly into the knee joint and may provide relief from knee pain for up to six months. It is typically given as two injections, one week apart.

Common side effects of Hymovis treatment including joint pain, stiffness, swelling, itching, or numbness; headache; dizziness; back pain; and pain, redness or swelling at the injection site. Those with bleeding disorders, certain allergies, or infections in the knee area should not be treated with Hymovis.

Ibuprofen

Ibuprofen (generic name) is an NSAID used to relieve the pain and swelling seen in osteoarthritis, rheumatoid arthritis, juvenile rheumatoid arthritis, and carpal tunnel syndrome. It's available under several brand names, including Advil and Motrin.

Some possible side effects include headache, itching, nervousness, ringing in the ears, and abdominal problems including pain, bloating, constipation, diarrhea, and flatulence.

Motrin and Advil are available over-the-counter without a prescription, but there are also prescription forms of ibuprofen, including Brufen, Calprofen, and Nurofen. Some possible side effects include difficulty breathing, drowsiness, skin eruptions, bleeding in general, stomach ulcers, itching, abdominal pain, bruising, and constipation. See your doctor regularly to monitor for possible internal bleeding, ulcers, and stomach ulcers.

Ilaris

Ilaris (generic name, canakinumab) is a biologic that falls into the category of interleukin-1β (IL-1β) blockers. Ilaris is used to treat systemic juvenile idiopathic arthritis (SJIA), and adults with conditions including Still's disease and Familial Mediterranean Fever. FDA approved as a once-a-month injectable medicine to treat children with SJIA aged 2 or older, Ilaris works by targeting IL-1β, a potent mediator of the inflammatory response. By suppressing the activity of IL-1β, the activity of the immune system is also suppressed, which reduces inflammation.

One study showed that when 190 children with SJIA symptoms were given Ilaris, eight out of ten of them experienced improvement in symptoms such as fever and painful or swollen joint in just 15 days.

Because Ilaris works by impairing ability of the immune system to fight infections, there is a heightened risk of developing tuberculosis and/or viral, bacterial or fungal infections when taking it. Tell your doctor if you have current or recurrent infections, a weakened immune system, diabetes, HIV-1, or hepatitis B before taking Ilaris.

Imuran

Imuran (generic name, azathioprine) is a DMARD used to treat rheumatoid arthritis and lupus. It decreases the body's response to infections, and interferes with the action of the white blood cells that worsen the symptoms of rheumatoid arthritis and lupus.

Some possible side effects seen with Imuran include infection, suppression of the bone marrow, loss of appetite, liver damage, hair loss, skin rashes, diarrhea, nausea, vomiting, and pancreatitis. Long-term use increases the risk of developing cancer.

Indocin

Indocin (generic name, indomethacin) is an NSAID used to reduce the joint pain, swelling, inflammation, and stiffness seen in osteoarthritis, rheumatoid arthritis, bursitis, ankylosing spondylitis, gout, and tendonitis.

Some possible side effects include difficulty breathing, drowsiness, skin eruptions, hair loss, hepatitis, vaginal bleeding, vertigo, stomach ulcers, itching, abdominal pain, bruising, and constipation. See your doctor regularly to monitor for possible internal bleeding, ulcers, and stomach ulcers.

Keflex

Keflex (generic name, cephalexin) is an antibiotic used to treat bacterial infections, including those found in infectious arthritis. If you have an infected joint, your doctor may give you an intravenous form of Keflex as a first-line treatment. After two weeks of this treatment, your doctor may then switch to the oral form of Keflex. (Other brand names include Bio-Cef and Panixine DisperDose.)

Some possible side effects of Keflex include upset stomach, diarrhea, vomiting, mild skin rash, colitis, yeast infections, fatigue, fever, hallucinations, joint pain, and joint inflammation.

Ketoprofen

Ketoprofen (generic name) is an NSAID used to treat the joint pain, swelling, inflammation, and stiffness seen in osteoarthritis, rheumatoid arthritis, ankylosing spondylitis, Reiter's syndrome, bursitis of the shoulder, and gout. Over-the-counter versions of this medication have been discontinued in the United States. Although usually taken in capsule form, ketoprofen can also be used topically in the form of a cream or a patch, both of which can provide effective pain relief for certain people with osteroarthritis.

Some possible side effects include difficulty breathing, drowsiness, skin eruptions, bleeding in general, stomach ulcers, itching, abdominal pain, bruising, and constipation. In rare cases, there may be liver disease, kidney problems, meningitis symptoms, or signs of infection. See your doctor regularly to monitor for these and the internal bleeding and stomach ulcers that may develop with any NSAID use.

Kevzara

Kevzara (generic name, sarilumab) is a biologic in the category of interleukin-6 (IL-6) receptor blockers that is used to treat adults with moderate to severe rheumatoid arthritis who have not experienced relief from other medications. Kevzara targets the receptor of the IL-6 protein, which is produced by the white blood cells and plays a major role in causing the pain, swollen joints, stiffness, and fatigue seen in rheumatoid arthritis. When taken with methotrexate, Kevzara has been shown to relieve RA pain in as little as two weeks, while slowing the progression of the disease and protecting the joints from further damage.

Like other biologics, Kevzara works by impairing ability of the immune system to fight infections, which may result in the development of tuberculosis and/or viral, bacterial or fungal infections. Tell your doctor if you have current or recurrent infections, a weakened immune system, diabetes, HIV-1, or hepatitis B before taking Kevzara.

Kineret

Kineret (generic name, anakinra) is a biologic categorized as an interleukin-1 inhibitor that is used either by itself or with other medications to reduce the pain, swelling, and joint stiffness seen in rheumatoid arthritis. Kineret works by blocking the activity of interleukin-1, a substance that causes arthritis-related swelling and joint damage. Used only for those who haven't been helped by other RA medications, Kineret is given in the form of daily injections.

Some possible side effects include redness, pain, swelling, itching, or bruising at the injection site, and infections of the upper respiratory tract including serious infections like pneumonia. Tell your doctor if you currently have pneumonia or another infection, a history of serious infections, or asthma before taking Kineret.

Medrol

Medrol (generic name, methylprednisolone) is a steroid used to reduce the inflammation seen in rheumatoid arthritis, psoriatic arthritis, and lupus. It works by preventing the release of substances in the body that promote inflammation.

Some possible side effects include increased infections, diabetes, high blood pressure, skin thinning and easy bruising, increased weight, loss of muscle, osteoporosis, and glaucoma. This drug can also increase your susceptibility to infections and make them harder to treat and "hide" the presence of infections, making it difficult for your doctor to diagnose and treat them.

Miacalcin

Miacalcin (generic name, calcitonin salmon) is a synthetic hormone used to treat Paget's disease and osteoporosis (thinning and weakening of the bones). Also available as Fortical, Miacalcin helps regulate calcium levels in the bone and blood. It is given as an injection (either into the muscle or directly beneath the skin) or can be used as a nasal spray. Those using Miacalcin as a treatment for osteoporosis should also take a calcium and a vitamin D supplement.

Some possible side effects include diarrhea, upset stomach, flu-like symptoms, muscle aches, and fatigue.

Mobic

Mobic (generic name, meloxicam) is an NSAID used to reduce the joint pain, swelling, inflammation, and stiffness seen in osteoarthritis, rheumatoid arthritis, juvenile idiopathic arthritis, bursitis, ankylosing spondylitis, gout, and tendonitis. Taken once daily in tablet form, it is designed to ease pain by lowering levels of prostaglandin, a hormone-like substance that can cause inflammation.

Some possible side effects include difficulty breathing, drowsiness, skin eruptions, bleeding in general, stomach ulcers, itching, abdominal pain, bruising, and constipation. See your doctor regularly to monitor for possible internal bleeding, ulcers, and stomach ulcers.

Naprosyn

Naprosyn (generic name, naproxen) is an NSAID used to treat the joint pain, swelling, inflammation, and stiffness seen in osteoarthritis, rheumatoid arthritis, juvenile rheumatoid arthritis, bursitis, tendonitis, gout, and ankylosing spondylitis. It's also available under the brand names Aleve and EC-Naprosyn.

Some possible side effects include difficulty breathing, drowsiness, skin eruptions, bleeding in general, stomach ulcers, itching, abdominal pain, bruising, and constipation. See your doctor regularly to monitor for possible internal bleeding, ulcers, and stomach ulcers.

Olumiant

Olumiant (generic name, baricitinib) is part of a new group of immunosuppressant drugs called Janus kinase (JAK) inhibitors, that work much like the biologics. Used for people with moderate to severe rheumatoid arthritis who haven't found relief with methotrexate, Olumiant and other JAK inhibitors work by blocking the action of enzymes known as Janus kinases, which "turn on" a great many interleukins and cytokines. Blocking the action of Janus kinases, then, helps tamp down inflammation and decrease certain hyperactive functions in the immune cells. You can read more about the JAK inhibitors in Chapter 20.

The most common side effects seen with Olumiant are upper respiratory infections (colds or sinus infections), cold sores, nausea, and shingles, due to a lowering of immune function. More serious side effects include blood clots in the legs, tuberculosis, shingles, and bacterial, viral, or fungal infections. Tell your doctor if you have current or recurrent infections, a weakened immune system, diabetes, HIV-1, or hepatitis B before taking Olumiant.

WARNING

Since 2020, the FDA has required the JAK inhibitors Olumiant, Xeljanz/Xeljanz XR, and Rinvoq to include information about their risks of serious heart-related events, cancer, blood clots, and death. This is known as a *black box warning*, the most serious of the agency's safety advisories. While these may still be viable treatments for a lot of people, those who have history of clots, cancer, or certain kinds of heart disease may need to stay away from them.

Orencia

Orencia (generic name, abatacept) is an injectable biologic drug used to reduce pain and slow the joint damage seen in adults with moderately to severely active rheumatoid or psoriatic arthritis, and in children with one particular subtype of JIA. Orencia is usually prescribed after the failure of a DMARD like methotrexate.

Orencia works by suppressing T-cells, slowing the progress of rheumatoid arthritis and preventing joint damage. However it also increases the risk of developing infections or worsening existing infections. The most common side effects include upper respiratory tract infections, sore throat, headache, and nausea, with the more serious side effects including fever, flu symptoms, shortness of breath, serious infections, pain when urinating, and abdominal pain.

Orencia is sometimes prescribed in conjunction with certain DMARDs, but should not be used with other biologics or JAK inhibitors. For more on Orencia, see Chapter 20.

Pediapred

Pediapred (generic name, prednisolone sodium phosphate) is a steroid suspended in a raspberry flavored solution used to reduce the inflammation seen in rheumatoid arthritis, gout, psoriatic arthritis, lupus, dermatomyositis, and others. It decreases the immune system's response to these diseases and reduces inflammation, pain, and swelling.

Some possible side effects of Pediapred include increased infections, diabetes, high blood pressure, skin thinning and easy bruising, weight gain, loss of muscle, osteoporosis, and glaucoma. This drug can increase your susceptibility to infections and "hide" their presence, making it difficult for your doctor to diagnose and treat them.

Penicillin

Penicillin (generic name) is an antibiotic used to treat bacterial infections including Lyme disease. It works by killing or preventing the growth of bacteria. Penicillin is available under a variety of brand names including Amoxil, Bicillin L-A, Dynapen, Geocillin, Pfizerpen, and Staphcillin, and there are several kinds of penicillins, each designed to fight different kinds of infections. Penicillin can be taken as a tablet, capsule, solution, suspension, or injection.

Some possible side effects of penicillin include allergic reactions, such as rashes, tongue swelling, itching, nausea, diarrhea, and acute kidney failure.

Plaquenil

Plaquenil (generic name, hydroxychloroquine) is a DMARD and anti-malarial drug that is used to decrease the joint pain, swelling, and stiffness seen in rheumatoid arthritis, JIA, and lupus. It is a slow-acting drug given as an oral tablet with effects that may not be fully experienced for up to six months. Because it modulates the immune system rather than depressing it, Plaquenil does not increase infection risk.

Some possible side effects of Plaquenil include nausea, diarrhea, rash, changes in skin pigmentation decreased muscle coordination, and, rarely, vision changes. So long as you get regular eye examinations, it is generally it is safe to take Plaquenil, and it is important to do so, especially if you have lupus.

Relafen

Relafen (generic name, nabumetone) is an NSAID used to reduce the joint pain, swelling, inflammation and stiffness seen in osteoarthritis and rheumatoid arthritis. It works by reducing inflammation-producing hormones and usually starts working within a week of taking the first dose. Some possible side effects include itching, insomnia, nervousness, constipation, diarrhea, dizziness, ringing in the ears, and stomach inflammation.

Some possible side effects include difficulty breathing, drowsiness, skin eruptions, bleeding in general, stomach ulcers, itching, abdominal pain, bruising, and constipation. See your doctor regularly to monitor for possible internal bleeding, ulcers, and stomach ulcers.

Remicade

Remicade (generic name, infliximab) is a TNF inhibitor biologic that is used to block an inflammatory protein called TNF seen in excess in rheumatoid arthritis, psoriatic arthritis, JIA, and ankylosing spondylitis. By blocking excessive TNF, Remicade helps lower inflammation in the joints, skin, and GI tract, slowing the progression of joint damage, reducing pain and stiffness, and improving joint function. Remicade is infused intravenously every two months and is often used in conjunction with the drug methotrexate.

Side effects can include abdominal pain, cough, rash, muscle pain, lightheadedness, unusual fatigue, and shortness of breath. Infections have been reported with this treatment, so Remicade should not be used if a serious infection is present and should be discontinued if an infection develops.

TNF inhibitors such as Remicade lower the body's ability to fight infections, increasing your risk of developing serious infections like tuberculosis. Tell your doctor if you have ever had tuberculosis, recurrent infections, a nervous system disorder, diabetes, HIV-1, hepatitis B, a neurologic disorder such as multiple sclerosis, impaired heart function, or recent bouts of cancer, as TNF inhibitors can make these conditions worse.

Rheumatrex

Rheumatrex (generic name, methotrexate) is used for rheumatoid arthritis when drugs such as NSAIDs aren't effective. One of the most effective an most commonly prescribed medications for the treatment of autoimmune/inflammatory arthritis, whether used for RA, psoriatic arthritis, lups, scleroderma, or other conditions, methotrexate helps slow immune system reactions that cause many of the problems seen in these diseases.

Although it has a lesser infection risk than biologics or JAKs, it may lower your body's overall resistance. Because of this you should avoid getting any live vaccines while taking Rheumatrex, as you might end up contracting the same disease you're trying to avoid. It's important to note that Rheumatrex and other brands of methotrexate are taken once a *week,* not once a day.

Besides a greater susceptibility to infections, some possible side effects include liver toxicity, lung toxicity, bone marrow suppression, mouth ulcers, the blahs, hair loss, fatigue, and abdominal pain/GI upsets. It's important to get blood tests to check your liver and blood counts every two months and get immediate medical attention if a cough or shortness of breath develops.

Rinvoq

Rinvoq (generic name, upadacitinib) is a JAK (Janus kinase) inhibitor, which belongs to the larger group known as DMARDs. It is FDA-approved for use in adults with moderate to severe RA who haven't found relief with methotrexate. Rinvoq and other JAK inhibitors are immunosuppressants that work by blocking the action of enzymes known as Janus kinases. This helps tamp down inflammation and regulate an overactive immune system to help stop the attack on the joints. Rinvoq is taken once a day in pill form. Find out more about the JAK inhibitors in Chapter 20.

The most common side effects seen with Rinvoq are upper respiratory infections (colds or sinus infections), cold sores, nausea, and shingles, due to a lowering of immune function. More serious side effects include blood clots in the legs, tuberculosis, shingles, and bacterial, viral, or fungal infections. Lymphoma and other cancers can occur n those taking Rinvoq. Tell your doctor if you have any current infections) or have had recurrent infections), a weakened immune system, any type of cancer, diabetes, HIV-1, or hepatitis B or C before taking Rinvoq.

WARNING

Since 2020, the FDA has required the JAK inhibitors Rinvoq, Olumiant, and Xeljanz/Xeljanz XR to include information about their risks of serious heart-related events, cancer, blood clots, and death.

Rituxan

Rituxan (generic name, rituximab) is an anti-cancer medication that is also FDA-approved for the treatment of rheumatoid arthritis in adults. Rituxan zeroes in on a molecule on certain immune system cells called B cells, which are overactive in RA in many ways. Killing B cells helps modulate RA symptoms. Some studies have shown that over half of rheumatoid arthritis patients experienced improvement in symptoms when given Rituxan together with methotrexate, even though taking methotrexate alone was shown to be ineffective in all of the patients.

Rituxan is given through an infusion into a vein. Common side effects include low levels of white or red blood cells, nausea, diarrhea, painful urination, depression, and upper respiratory infections. Serious side effects include brain infection and other infections, heart problems, kidney failure, and intestinal blockage. If you have ever had hepatitis B, Rituxan use may reactivate or worsen the virus.

Simponi and Simponi Aria

Simponi (generic name, golimumab) is a TNF inhibitor biologic FDA approved to treat adults with moderate to severe RA in combination with methotrexate, active psoriatic arthritis in combination with methotrexate, and active ankylosing spondylitis. Given as a once-montly injection under the skin, it is often used in combination with methotrexate, Simponi Aria, which is given as an IV infusion, is also approved to treat these conditions, adding treatment of active polyarticular JIA in children age 2 or older, and expanding the treatment group for active psoriatic arthritis to include children age 2 older. Both work preventing TNF from binding to its receptors, which reduces inflammation in the joints, skin, and GI tract, decreases pain and irritation, and improves joint function.

Like all TNF inhibitors, Simponi and Simponi Aria lower the body's ability to fight infections, with side effects including an increased risk of developing a diseases like tuberculosis. Tell your doctor if you have ever had tuberculosis, recurrent infections, a nervous system disorder, a neurologic disorder such as multiple sclerosis, impaired heart function, diabetes, HIV-1, or hepatitis B or recent bouts of cancer, as TNF inhibitors like Simponi can make these conditions worse. For more on Simponi and Simponi aria, see Chapter 20.

Sulfinpyrazone

Sulfinpyrazone (generic name) is an antigout medication that works by increasing the levels of uric acid that are passed in the urine, which decreases the uric acid levels in the blood. It's available under the brand names Anturan and Apo-sulfinpyrazone. While it doesn't cure gout, sulfinpyrazone can help prevent attacks of the disease by removing extra uric acid from the body.

Some possible side effects include itching, redness, rash or other signs of skin irritation, difficulty urinating, nausea, and lower back pain. At the beginning of treatment, levels of uric acid in the kidneys greatly increase, which can produce kidney stones in some people. Drinking ten to twelve 8-ounce glasses of water each day will dilute the uric acid content of the urine and help prevent kidney stones.

Tacrolimus

Tacrolimus (brand name, Prograf) is an immunosuppressive drug used primarily to prevent the body from rejecting a transplanted organ. However, it has also been shown to be an effective and safe treatment for RA patients who have had an unsuccessful response to DMARDs when used alone or in combination with the DMARD methotrexate.

Tacrolimus is available in tablet or capsule form. Common side effects include infections, tremores, headache, diarrhea, constipation, nausea, tingling or swelling of the hands or feet, high blood sugar (diabetes), anemia, kidney problems, electrolyte imbalances, high blood pressure, bronchitis, heart problems, and an increased risk of cancer. Because tacrolimus makes you more likely to develop other diseases including cancer, it should not be taken with other immunosupressants.

Taltz

Taltz (generic name, ixekizumab) is a type of biologic that targets a different inflammation molecule than most other arthritis drugs: interleukin-17(IL-17). Used initially to stop the inflammation that causes psoriasis plaques, Taltz has since been found to be effective in treating psoriatic arthritis, ankylosing spondylitis, and certain other forms of spondyloarthritis. It works by binding to the IL-17 molecule, which helps block the release of pro-inflammatory substances. As inflammation decreases, so does joint damage.

Taltz is injected under the skin, usually every two to four weeks. Because it weakens the body's ability to fight infections, you can develop mild infections when taking the drug, with common side effects including upper respiratory symptoms (colds, sinus infections), nausea, fungal skin infections, and abnormally low levels of white blood cells. Less often, serious infections such as tuberculosis, pneumonia, and inflammatory bowel disease may occur. Your doctor may want to give you a medicine for tuberculosis before beginning your treatment with Taltz.

Tetracycline

Tetracyclines (generic name) are a class of antibiotics used to treat bacterial infections, including Lyme disease. They work by interfering with the building of proteins in the RNA of microorganisms like chlamydia, protozoa, and mycoplasma. Tetracyclines don't necessarily kill these organisms; mostly they keep them from multiplying. Thus, they are used to treat infections bodywide.

Many generic and brand name versions of the tetracyclines exist, including Broadspec, demeclocycline, doxycycline, minocycline, Panmycin, sarecycline, Tetracap, Vibramycin, and, of course, tetracyline.

Possible side effects include allergic reactions, tooth discoloration, diarrhea, pressure within the brain, drug rash, toxicity to a developing fetus, and skin sensitivity to sunlight.

Tremfya

Tremfya (generic name, guselkumab) is an FDA-approved biologic that blocks a substance called interleukin-23 (IL-23). Tremfya, which is used to treat adults with active psoriatic arthritis, works by suppressing the IL-23 cytokine, which plays a role in triggering inflammation. Fortunately, unlike some biologics, Tremfya has not been found to reactivate hepatitis B or worsen hepatitis C.

Tremfya comes in injection form that you can administer yourself. After two starter doses, injections are required every eight weeks. Some possible side effects include body aches, chills, infections, difficulty breathing, headache, nasal congestion and, in rare cases, burning or stinging of the skin, diarrhea, stomach pain, and tuberculosis.

Trilisate

Trilisate (generic name, choline magnesium trisalicylate) is an NSAID used to treat the joint pain, swelling, inflammation, and stiffness seen in osteoarthritis, rheumatoid arthritis, and juvenile rheumatoid arthritis. It's also used to treat fever in adults.

Trilisate may be linked to Reye's syndrome, a serious ailment. See your doctor regularly to monitor for this problem, as well as possible internal bleeding and stomach ulcers.

Some possible side effects include difficulty breathing, drowsiness, skin eruptions, bleeding in general, stomach ulcers, itching, abdominal pain, bruising, and constipation. See your doctor regularly to monitor for possible internal bleeding, ulcers, and stomach ulcers.

Tylenol

Tylenol (generic name, acetaminophen) is a fever- and pain-relieving analgesic used to treat aching joints and muscles. It is also available as Mapap and Panadol. It should not be used for more than ten days to relieve pain or three days to relieve fever.

Some common side effects of Tylenol include stomach pain, nausea, fatigue, loss of appetite, rash, and excessive sweating. Occasionally it can cause symptoms of an allergic reaction, such as hives, swelling, and difficulty breathing.

Voltaren

Voltaren (generic name, diclofenac sodium) is an NSAID found in the form of a standard or extended release oral tablet, a suppository, and an over-the-counter topical gel. All are used to treat the joint pain, swelling, inflammation, and stiffness seen in osteoarthritis, rheumatoid arthritis, and ankylosing spondylitis. While the tablets and suppository are only available with a prescription, the gel is purchased over the counter. Applied to the skin, the gel is most useful in easing osteoarthritis pain in the hands and knees.

Some possible side effects of diclofenac in oral form include stomach or intestinal bleeding and diarrhea, as well as itching, cramps, constipation, ringing in the ears, and increased risk of fatal heart attack or stroke when used long term or taken in high doses. The topical gel form has very few side effects, ranging from stomach upset to skin irritation where the gel was applied. Tell your doctor if you have kidney or heart problems or elevated blood pressure, and see your doctor regularly to monitor for these and other problems, including internal bleeding and stomach ulcers.

Xeljanz

Xeljanz (generic name, tofacitinib) is one of a new group of drugs called Janus kinase (JAK) inhibitors which are FDA-approved to treat adults with moderate to severe rheumatoid arthritis or active psoriatic arthritis, as well as children with a certain form of JIA. Xeljanz and other JAK inhibitors are immunosuppressants that work by blocking the action of pro-inflammatory enzymes known as Janus kinases, which tamps down inflammation and decreases certain overactive functions in the immune cells. Xeljanz is taken once a day in pill form.

The most common side effects seen with Xeljanz are upper respiratory infections (colds or sinus infections), cold sores, nausea, and shingles, due to a lowering of immune function. More serious side effects include blood clots in the legs, tuberculosis, shingles, and bacterial, viral, or fungal infections. Tell your doctor if you have current or recurrent infections, a weakened immune system, diabetes, HIV-1, or hepatitis B before taking Xeljanz.

WARNING

Since 2020, the FDA has required the JAK inhibitors Xeljanz/Xeljanz XR, Olumiant, and Rinvoq to include information about their risks of serious heart-related events, cancer, blood clots, and death.

Zyloprim

Zyloprim (generic name, allopurinol) is the first-line treatment for gout unless it's contraindicated by the patient's history or health status. People of certain ethnic backgrounds should be checked for the HLA B5801 gene before starting since this gene carries an increased risk of severe allergic reactions to the drug.It works Zyloprim works by reducing uric acid concentrations in the blood and urine. It does not stop gout attacks that have already begun; in fact, it can actually worsen acute attacks of gout. Instead, Zyloprim is used *after* an acute attack has subsided as a long-term treatment to prevent future attacks. The use of allopurinol (or Zyloprim) is a lifelong therapy. For it to work, the dose must be adjusted until uric acid levels are maintained at a certain level.

Some possible side effects include skin rash, chills, fever, diarrhea, nausea, itching, stomach pain and related problems, and headache. The most serious side effect is a life-threatening allergic reaction, which, although very rare, requires immediate medical attention because it is fatal about 25 percent of the time. Its symptoms include a skin rash, fever, and liver and kidney failure.

Chapter **9**

Cuts That Cure: Surgeries for Arthritis

he idea of having surgery is always a scary one. Any time you allow a surgeon to ply their trade on your body, you're taking certain risks, some great, and others small. But under the right conditions, surgery performed on a diseased joint can bring results that are nothing short of spectacular. Pain can be reduced or eliminated, range of motion restored, deformities corrected, and joint function vastly improved. Still, surgery isn't for everybody. Whether it's right for you depends on many factors. To help you weigh up the pros and cons of surgery, see the nearby sidebar "Finding out if you're (mentally) prepped for surgery."

If you're considering surgical treatment for your arthritis, you need to consult with an *orthopedic surgeon* or *orthopedist* (the kind of doctor who specializes in treating diseases of the muscles, bones, and joints). An orthopedic surgeon is trained in both surgical and nonsurgical methods. *Nonsurgical treatments* consist of casting, splinting, and joint injections. *Surgical treatments* include removal of the joint lining, cutting and resetting of the bone, bone fusion, and joint reconstruction. *Arthroscopic surgery* is a minimally invasive procedure in which a small tube containing a tiny video camera, lenses, and a light for viewing is inserted into a joint to allow the doctor to see what's going on and perform surgery, if necessary.

FINDING OUT IF YOU'RE (MENTALLY) PREPPED FOR SURGERY

Although your doctor can tell you all about what goes on inside your body, only *you* know what's going on inside your head. Do a little soul-searching to determine whether or not you really want and need the surgery by asking yourself the following questions:

- Is the pain interfering with my ability to lead a productive and satisfying life?

- Do I rely on pain relievers taken at the maximum allowable dosage to get through the day?

- Have I tried all other pain-relieving methods (physical therapy, exercise, pain management strategies, and so on) without success?

- Are my expectations of the results of the surgery realistic?

- Will I participate fully in my post-surgery rehabilitation?

If you can answer "yes" to all of these questions, you may be mentally and emotionally ready to undergo joint surgery.

Your family physician or internist may be able to refer you to a competent orthopedic surgeon, but don't automatically assume that this person is the right choice for you. Review the suggestions in Chapter 6 for finding a doctor; then apply them to your search.

Knowing What to Ask Your Doctor Before Undergoing Surgery

Because surgery is a drastic and at least somewhat risky option, you shouldn't even consider it until all other measures have been exhausted. First, you and your doctor should thoroughly investigate and make use of the many nonsurgical options, such as medication, diet, physical therapy, pain management strategies, exercise, and alternative methods. In truth, most people really don't need surgery to manage their arthritis.

In some cases, though, surgery can be a godsend. When rheumatic finger joints render your hands nearly useless, or when a painful, osteoarthritic hip makes walking out to the mailbox a major feat, certain surgical procedures may be able to give you a new lease on life. For more details on hip and knee replacements, check out the sidebars relating to these forms of surgery later in this chapter.

REMEMBER

The success of a surgery will depend mightily on two things: the disease itself and the body in question. Some disease states respond wonderfully to surgery, whereas others show little or no improvement. People are like that, too. One person may come through a surgical procedure with flying colors, zip through recovery, and be thrilled with the results. Another person, equally affected and undergoing an almost identical surgery, may be trapped in a long, drawn-out recovery period that garners less-than-optimal results. Putting it simply, surgery is a highly individualized matter and may or may not be the best option for you. To find out, begin by asking your orthopedic surgeon the following questions:

>> **Do my symptoms and my test results go hand-in-hand?** In other words, can your doctor confirm your diagnosis? You certainly don't want to undergo surgery for a problem that may not exist.

>> **Does my kind of arthritis respond well to surgery?** Surgery is most often performed on those with rheumatoid arthritis (Chapter 3) or incapacitating osteoarthritis (Chapter 2). In contrast, surgery is rarely the treatment-of-choice for gout (Chapter 4), scleroderma (Chapter 5), or lupus (Chapter 5). Those with ankylosing spondylitis (Chapter 4) are "iffy" candidates for surgery: sometimes it may be used to straighten their spines or replace certain joints, but excessive bone growth can complicate the recovery process.

>> **How do I know if I need surgery?** In most cases, surgery for arthritis is not an emergency — it doesn't absolutely have to be done at a certain time. The decision to undergo surgery and the timing of the operation is usually dictated by pain, overall health status, and the degree of disability. Although a few arthritis-related problems need surgery right away (for example, a ruptured tendon), most can wait. But delaying an "optional" surgery (for example, a hip replacement) for too long can be a bad idea, leading to a poor surgical outcome, the irreversible contraction of certain muscles supporting the joint, and increased postoperative pain. Ask your doctor about the possibility of irreversible damage or disability brought on by waiting too long.

>> **What results can I expect from this surgery?** In other words, what is the surgery going to do for you? How will it affect your pain, your range of motion, and the stability of your joint(s)? What kind of activities will you be able to participate in after you recover? What limitations will you have?

>> **What risks are involved?** Make sure the doctor explains all the complications that can result from the surgery (for example, infection, nerve damage, and so on), as well as the risks involved in undergoing the surgery itself (such as cardiac arrest).

>> **What is involved in the post-surgery rehabilitation?** Rehabilitation can be a long, sometimes painful process that usually requires hard work and your

utmost dedication. Be sure you know what lies ahead before you consent to surgery. If you're not willing to do the work, the outcome may very well be compromised.

>> **Am I physically able to withstand the surgery?** It is common practice to have a physical examination before surgery to make sure that your body is up to the procedure. The condition of your heart, respiratory system, blood, and overall health are taken into account when assessing whether or not you can withstand the rigors of surgery. Your habits and co-existing health problems are also taken into consideration. For example, most surgeons won't perform a knee or hip replacement if you smoke, your diabetes is uncontrolled, or you are severely overweight. These problems need to be solved before you can be a viable candidate for surgery.

>> **What does the future hold if I don't have surgery?** If you are already in great pain, finding out that it may get worse unless you have the surgery could tip the scales in favor of the procedure. In some cases, arthritis surgery can be put off indefinitely without compromising its effectiveness. But it can result in muscle wasting, decline in joint function, or permanent deformities, all of which can make future surgeries less likely to be successful.

Looking At Different Kinds of Joint Surgery

Because the joint is an intricate piece of "machinery" and many different things can go wrong with it, joint surgery is complex and wide-ranging. It can involve flushing the joint with water, resurfacing rough bone ends or cartilage, cutting away inflamed membranes, growing bone where it otherwise doesn't exist, and even removing the entire joint and replacing it with a new one.

Synovectomy: Removing a diseased joint lining

People who have inflammatory arthritis may benefit from a *synovectomy*, in which the surgeon removes an inflamed, overgrown joint lining (*synovium*).

In rheumatoid arthritis, the inflamed, thickened synovium can overgrow to the point that it invades the joint's supporting structures — the bones, cartilage, muscles, and ligaments. This growth can cause damage to the joint over time. At the same time, the synovium releases enzymes that cause both bone and cartilage to break down. Removing the offending lining stops the synovial invasion and reduces the amount of destructive enzymes released.

The surgeon may make a large incision that exposes the entire joint. Or, in the case of arthroscopic surgery, tiny incisions may be made that are just large enough to accommodate the insertion of an arthroscope. The *arthroscope* is a flexible tube about the diameter of a pencil that has a camera on the end. It's used for diagnostic and surgical purposes. In either procedure, the joint lining is cut away, leaving just enough behind to produce lubricating fluid. This type of surgery isn't a permanent cure, as the synovium will eventually grow back. However, pain relief and protection against joint destruction can last for a couple of years, allowing the postponement of more radical treatments, such as joint replacement.

Osteotomy: Cutting and resetting the bone

To perform an *osteotomy*, the surgeon removes a section of bone to correct joint alignment. (*Osteo* is the Greek word for *bone; tomy* means *to cut.*) Those suffering from osteoarthritis, especially of the knee (Chapter 2), and ankylosing spondylitis (Chapter 4) can benefit from this surgery. It's also helpful for joints that are wearing improperly but still have a healthy portion, as is the case with most bunions.

A misaligned joint can cause uneven wearing on the bones and cartilage as well as general joint pain. After proper alignment is restored, the force exerted on the joint is distributed more evenly. Excess pressure is released from cartilage and bone, "worn spots" have the chance to repair themselves, and pain is reduced.

If the patient is suffering from osteoarthritis, a slice or wedge of bone is surgically removed, allowing the joint to realign. The "raw edges" of the bone are connected with screws and eventually grow together again. If the patient has ankylosing spondylitis, the damaged tissue and bone that lock the spine into its unnatural, bent-over position are removed, allowing the spine can return to its natural, upright position.

Pain relief, improved joint function, increased range of motion, and greater joint stability are the benefits of this type of surgery.

Recovery may take anywhere from 6 to 12 months, and there is a possibility that joint function may not improve. Alterations in joint alignment can make future joint replacements difficult. And for many, the benefits last only a few years.

Arthrodesis: Fusing the bone

Folks who suffer from rheumatoid arthritis may benefit from having certain bones fused. The surgeon positions the joint into its most functional alignment and then "locks" it in place permanently.

In highly unsteady and painful joints, arthrodesis can provide stability and pain relief. It is primarily performed on the spine but can also be used on the thumb, hip, knee, and wrist when joint replacement is either not feasible or has already proved unsuccessful. Fusion of the hip joint may be required for those who need a total hip replacement but can't have one, either because their bones aren't healthy enough or because the person in question is too young or active. (Hip replacements typically last 15 to 20 years, and second replacements often don't work as well.) Fusion of the thumb joint can make grasping possible. Fusion of the knee is sometimes performed when a knee replacement becomes infected and won't "take." The wrist may be fused because it's a highly unstable joint and very difficult to replace.

The surgeon removes cartilage from the opposing bone ends and also removes a surface layer of bone. The joint is positioned in the way it can be of greatest use, and then the bone ends are joined using pins, rods, or screws. Splinting or casting helps keep the joint stable, while new bone growth fuses it permanently into place.

Arthrodesis helps to relieve pain and can increase the ability to use the joint (in a limited way). Although joint motion is forfeited, joint function improves. A person with a fused hip, for example, *can* walk, even if it is with a limp, which may be progress for one who is otherwise wheelchair-bound. Recovery from this surgery can take several months.

Arthroplasty: Replacing the joint

Sometimes a joint degenerates to the point where pain is severe or constant and function is seriously impaired. By surgically removing the old, diseased parts of the joint and replacing them with new, artificial ones, the pain can usually relieved with mobility restored. This procedure is called *arthroplasty,* or joint replacement surgery, and it has revolutionized the treatment of hip and knee arthritis over the past several decades.

In the past, hip and knee arthritis routinely sidelined people, especially the elderly. But today, replacing old worn-out joints with artificial parts can offer relief from excruciating pain, loss of mobility, and disability, with results that are nothing short of amazing.

Arthroplasty can help to stabilize a wobbly joint, realign a joint to improve its function and, in some cases, even make cosmetic improvements. After undergoing hip or knee replacements, many people feel they have a new lease on life. Suddenly they can walk, hike, cycle and just move around without pain! Hoping to experience similar benefits, and encouraged by the surgery's high rate of success (joint replacement surgery is successful in 9 out of 10 cases), more than 1 million Americans undergo joint replacement surgery every year. The hip and knee are the most commonly replaced joints (450,000 and 600,000 per year, respectively), but ankles, shoulders, elbows, and knuckles are also done routinely and successfully.

A better idea may be to get the surgery earlier, instead of waiting. A study of 222 OA patients undergoing total hip or knee replacement surgery found that those who delayed their surgeries until joint function had severely declined and pain was severe had the worst surgical outcomes. They were also more likely to need assistance with bathing, dressing, and other daily tasks.

Those with the best outcomes are usually older, have arthritis-related pain, loss of movement, or stiffness that hasn't responded to other forms of treatment, but are otherwise in good health. In addition, they're highly motivated to help themselves and willing and able to participate in an exercise regimen once they've received their new joint.

TIP

You have a much better chance of enjoying a successful hip or knee replacement if you exercise, stay away from high-impact sports and activities, and maintain your ideal body weight.

Joint replacement surgery involves the use of artificial parts as well as some existing natural tissues. With the patient under anesthesia, the surgeon opens the joint and detaches the tendons and ligaments from the bones,dislocates the joint, and cuts away the diseased or weakened parts of the bone. The surgeon then uses plastic and/or metal prostheses to replace the missing parts of the joint and may or may not cement them into place. Next, the joint parts are fitted together, and ligaments and tendons are reattached. Finally, the incision is closed. (See Figure 9-1 and the sidebar "Taking a look at the total hip replacement procedure" following this section.)

FIGURE 9-1:
The hip socket is replaced with a metal cup (usually made of titanium) lined with polyethylene (a kind of plastic), and the femur is replaced with a metal stem that has a ceramic ball (the new head of the femur) attached to the top.

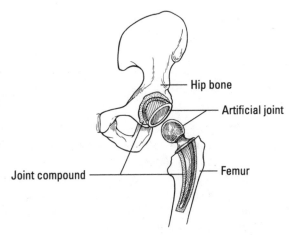

© John Wiley & Sons, Inc.

TECHNICAL STUFF

Although we call it "joint replacement surgery," a more accurate description is "joint rebuilding surgery." The surgeon tries to maintain the integrity of your natural joint as much as possible. Certain areas may simply be resurfaced and diseased tissue cut away. Just part of the joint may be replaced, for example the "socket" of the ball–and–socket joint in the hip, while leaving the "ball" intact. Or the entire joint may be reconstructed using artificial parts.

TAKING A LOOK AT THE TOTAL HIP REPLACEMENT PROCEDURE

The total hip replacement surgery gives you a good idea of how joint replacement (arthroplasty) surgeries are performed. As a ball-and-socket joint, the hip must provide a secure anchor between the pelvis and thigh bone (femur) to do its job properly. In a total hip replacement, the ball and the socket are separated, removed, and replaced with artificial structures. The surgery is completed in several stages:

- Through an incision made into the side, back, or front of the hip, the surgeon carefully detaches the tendons and ligaments connected to the femur's ball-shaped head.

- The femur head is cut away from the femur.

- A special tool is used to hollow out the hip socket to remove bone spurs and make it large enough to accommodate the new socket lining. The new lining, a cup-like structure typically made of titanium lined with polyethylene, is attached.

- The new socket lining will be held in place by your own bone which literally grows into it or by bone cement. Sometimes both methods are used. In an uncemented hip replacement, he upper end of the stem and the ceramic head are covered with a porous surface, through which your bone will grow, binding the implant to the bone.

- An opening is made at the top of the femur and the metal stem of the prosthesis is inserted. The ceraminc head of the prosthesis is attached to the top of the stem and the prosthesis is inserted into the shaft.

- The ligaments and tendons are repaired, and the wound is closed.

Recovery from a total hip replacement can take time. Patients usually stay in the hospital for a couple of days after surgery and may use a cane, a walker, or crutches during the first six weeks. After that, most normal activities can gradually be resumed — walking, bicycling, driving, golfing, and so on. Some doctors estimate that 80 percent of a patient's recovery occurs within the first 10 to 12 weeks after surgery, and the last 20 percent occurs during the following three to six months.

In the majority of cases, joint replacements provide pain relief, restored mobility, and improved joint stability. In the case of the weight-bearing joints, such as the hip or knee, this improved function can restore not only a patient's independence but also his or her overall outlook on life. Complications do exist, however. Infection at the site of the surgery may require removal of the implant; the prosthesis can loosen; or the joint may dislocate. Blood clots can occur (especially in the leg), the nerves surrounding the replacement can be damaged, and the surgery leg may not equal the other leg in length. Down the line, replacements of weight-bearing joints can wear out — hips typically last 15 to 20 years and knees may last 25 years (or even longer). When joint replacements do wear out, the surgery must be repeated.

There was a time when total joint replacement was thought of as a last resort because replacement parts tended to wear out or loosen with the passage of time. Those who might benefit from this kind of surgery were asked to hold out for as long as possible, because most implants had to be replaced within 10 to 20 years. But recent advances in the durability of implant materials have led to longer-lasting joint replacements, so earlier total joint replacement surgery is an option. As for the far end of the age spectrum, it seems that joint replacement surgery doesn't have a cutoff age. A study released by the Mayo Clinic found that even those aged 90 years and older may be able to undergo safe and effective hip replacements.

If you're planning to have a knee replacement, you may think it's a good idea to do both knees at once and save yourself some time and money. But studies show that those undergoing double knee replacements are more likely to suffer from serious complications like dislocation, inflammation, and nerve damage than those who take it one step (or one knee) at a time. Healing is typically easier when you have one "good" leg to put the bulk of your weight on, while giving your newly-replaced knee a break while it's healing.

Although the risk of developing infection in a joint replacement is relatively rare (1 in 100, or less), it's a complication that can require additional surgery and the removal of joint replacement parts. Any infection in your body can spread to the site of your joint replacement, so be scrupulous about taking the antibiotics prescribed for you before and after surgery. Also, your surgeon may recommend that during the months and years after surgery you take antibiotics if you develop a skin or bladder infection, undergo a dental treatment that's more than just a simple procedure, or have another surgery. (Yes, infection *can* occur years later!) All of these are high-risk times for infection because bacteria are more likely to enter the bloodstream and travel to the site of your joint replacement, where they can settle in and wreak havoc.

WITH CEMENT OR WITHOUT?

The majority of hip replacements performed in the U.S. today (up to 93 percent) are uncemented, which seems to be the preferred technique for patients less than 70 years old. In older patients, however, uncemented hip replacements are usually avoided because low quality bone and osteoporosis can prevent proper fusing of the bone to the prosthesis. For these patients, cemented replacements are often the better choice. However, cement can crack and break into little pieces over time, causing inflammation that can lead to the loosening of the implant. There is also a rare complication called *bone cement implantation syndrome* (BCIS) that happens when tiny pieces of cement travel through the bloodstream, leading to blood clots in the lung, cardiac arrest, and possible death. So which technique is best? Both cemented and uncemented replacements can provide excellent outcomes. Your surgeon will help you make the right decision. In the meantime, here's a quick rundown of advantages and disadvantages of each:

Advantages of uncemented replacements:

- There is no cement to crack and break away, leading to loosening of the implant.
- There is no risk of bone cement implantation syndrome.
- In younger patients, uncemented fixation survives better.
- Revision surgery can be easier.

Disadvantages of uncemented replacements:

- Recovery can take a long time, with activity limited for as much as three months while bone "grows into" the replacement part.
- Soft or porous bones may not be able to bond tightly enough to the prosethesis to allow a successful cementless hip replacement.
- It's hard to get a perfect fit — 10 to 20 percent of patients experience pain in the thigh that is sometimes severe.

Advantages of cemented replacements:

- There is a lower rate of implant-related bone fractures, compared to cementless replacements.
- The implant does not require bone to "grow into it" to achieve stability; therefore, lesser quality or osteoporotic bone is not an issue.

- In older patients, cemented fixation survives better.

- The positioning of the femoral stem is easier since it can be adjusted during cementing and stem insertion.

Disadvantages of cemented replacements:

- There is a possibility of developing bone cement implantation syndrome and cement-related destruction or disappearance of bone tissue.

- Cemented implants may loosen early on and continue to loosen.

- There is an increase in patient mortality from cemented hip replacements during the early postoperative stage.

TAKING A LOOK AT THE TOTAL KNEE REPLACEMENT PROCEDURE

If your knee is severely damaged by arthritis, and medications and/or assistive devices just aren't cutting it, you may be interested in getting a total knee replacement.

Total knee replacement surgery involves inserting a prosthesis made of metal and high-grade plastics that typically has three parts: the *tibial component* for the top of the shin-bone; the *femoral component* for the end (bottom) of the thighbone, and the *patellar component* for the bottom of the kneecap where it meets the thigh bone.

The surgery typically follows these procedures:

- The knee is placed in a bent position to expose all surfaces of the joint. The surgeon then makes an incision 6 to 10 inches long, and moves the kneecap aside.

- The damaged bone and cartilage is cut away from the shinbone (tibia) and thigh-bone (femor).

- The bone and cartilage that have been removed are replaced with metal implants on the tibia and femor to recreate these joint surfaces. The implants are attached to the bones using bone cement. (Uncemented prostheses are rarely used anymore, although in certain cases a combination of cemented and uncemented prostheses may work best.)

- The undersurface of the kneecap (patella) is cut and resurfaced with a plastic button, and a plastic spacer is inserted between the metal implants on the femur and tibia for a smooth, gliding movement.

(continued)

(continued)

- The ligaments and tendons are surgically repaired.

- The surgeon bends and rotates the knee, to make sure it works properly. Then the incision is closed.

Recovery/rehabilitation (the first 12 weeks after surgery) is a crucial stage in the total knee replacement procedure. Physical therapy begins the day after surgery if possible, with long-range goals of improving knee mobility and range of motion, andi increasing strength in the knee and supporting muscles. At two to three weeks post-surgery, most people can get around completely on their own or with the help of a cane. By week 12, there should be little to no pain during normal activities and full range of motion in the knee. However, it can take six months to a year before the knee regains its full strength and resiliency.

Autologous chondrocyte implantation: Cartilage transplants

Autologous chondrocyte implantation (ACI) is used to treat osteoarthritis of the knee in patients whose cartilage has worn away down to the bone. It's also used to treat defects in the knee cap and certain other joints in the body, including the thumb joint.

This is a two-part procedure that begins when the surgeon takes healthy cartilage cells (chondrocytes) from your knee (assuming that's where the problem lies) and sends the cells to the lab, where they are increased in number for six to eight weeks. During the second part of the procedure, the surgeon opens your afflicted joint and sews a small patch over the part of the cartilage that's defective. The healthy chondrocytes that have been growing in a lab are then injected underneath this patch, as a sort of "cartilage graft." The graft adheres to the problem area of your knee to form cartilage that resembles your natural cartilage in its healthy state.

Because the cells and fluid come from your own body, there is a much lesser chance of rejection. You will need to restrict weight-bearing activity on your affected knee for up to eight weeks in order to allow the cartilage graft to "take." Light sports activities may be allowed after about six months, but it may take up to a year before you can return to full sports activity.

The biggest advantage of the autologous chondrocyte implantation surgery is it helps relieve pain and restore mobility using a relatively noninvasive method with an overall success rate of 85 percent in the return to pain-free activities. The biggest disadvantage is that the cost of the surgery is very high (approximately $40,000). However some insurance companies will pay for the procedure if certain criteria are met.

Getting Ready for Surgery

TIP

If you decide to undergo surgery, you'll need to do a little planning that begins with getting yourself in to the best possible physical shape. Your doctor should review the medications, vitamins, minerals, herbs, and other supplements you're currently taking and tell you which ones to stop taking prior to surgery. (Certain drugs and supplements can increase the risk of bleeding.) You might need a pre-op clearance by your primary care physician or a cardiologist to make sure you're fit for surgery before you can be scheduled for it. You may also want to donate some of your own blood to the hospital or surgical center so you can receive it during or after surgery, if necessary. You should also make careful plans for your postoperative care, figure out the financial and insurance angles, and arrange for someone to handle your daily responsibilities while you're recovering. This ensures that you'll be able to relax while convalescing and concentrate on getting well!

Getting yourself into the best possible physical shape

Prepare for your surgery as if you were an athlete training for a competition. Eat highly nutritious meals, exercise regularly (if you're up to it), get plenty of sleep, and stay away from alcohol or unnecessary drugs. Surgery is performed carefully, utilizing every precaution, but it is still a major assault on the body. The better your health is going in, the better your body can withstand the trauma and the faster you'll recover.

Your doctor will undoubtedly give you several presurgical instructions. You may be asked to wash with a special soap or take a course of antibiotics. Most certainly, you'll need to avoid taking certain drugs and supplements that can thin the blood and increase bleeding time.

REMEMBER

If you take immunosuppressive drugs like DMARDs or biologics, you'll need to stop for a certain amount of time both pre- and post-op to decrease your risk of infection. Your surgeon should give you complete instructions about this.

Arranging adequate postoperative care

You'll need someone to take you home from the hospital, someone who can take care of you for the next several days, and someone who can help around the house for at least a week or two, depending upon the extent of your surgery. You may have an angel in your life who can play all three of these roles, or you may have to call on a variety of friends and family members to help fill the bill. One thing is sure: You can't recover alone.

Finding someone who can handle your responsibilities

If you are undergoing major surgery on a weight-bearing joint, you may be partially out of commission for months. Driving, shopping, taking care of children, doing housework, or going to work may be impossible during this time. You must arrange a solid support system. The last thing you need is to be forced into doing things that are beyond your capabilities.

Resolving financial and insurance matters

Before your surgery, find out exactly what your insurance company covers and how much of the tab you will have to pick up. The stress of unexpected medical expenses can be extremely disruptive mentally and emotionally and can be a major hindrance to your recovery.

Making a recovery plan with your doctor

Although no one can predict exactly when you'll pass certain milestones on the road to recovery, it may ease your mind and give you something to look forward to if you have a list of the progressive steps of healing. Ask your doctor to help you construct a recovery plan that maps out these steps. Studies show that people recover better and faster if they have a good idea of what to expect both during and after surgery.

Your recovery begins while you're still in the hospital, where you'll undergo physical therapy beginning the day after surgery. If you're doing well after two or three days, you'll go home. But if you need more help, you may need to go to a rehabilitation center for a short time for more in-depth therapy.

Once you're home, your doctor will set up an at-home therapy program for the first six weeks, during which you'll be visited by a physical therapist, who will prescribe an exercise program and help you follow it correctly. (This, of course, will depend upon your insurance program.)

After about three weeks, if all is going well, you'll begin an outpatient physical therapy program that lasts another five weeks, or longer if necessary.

The success of your joint replacement will depend heavily on your doing the required exercises regularly, and scrupulously following your treatment plan. It's a lot of work, but a successful surgical outcome is will worth it!

Chapter **10**

Overcoming the Ouch: Strategies for Pain Management

I t's hard to be happy when you hurt. Pain has a way of enveloping your mind, hijacking your brain, and making it difficult to concentrate on work, family, hobbies, or anything else. You desperately want to be fully involved in life, but the pain distracts, worries, irritates, and depresses you to the point where you can think of little else. The things that you used to do with ease can suddenly become difficult or even impossible to accomplish. Living with long-standing chronic pain can wear you down, exhaust you, discourage you, and make you feel that life isn't worth living. Fortunately, plenty of strategies (both physical and mental) can help you cope with pain, so even if your pain isn't completely banished, you can release its stranglehold on your life.

In this chapter, we focus on physical strategies for managing the pain. (See Chapter 14 for mental pain-management strategies.)

Understanding Arthritis Pain

Arthritis pain comes in many forms: stabbing, aching, twisting, burning, pressing, stretching, and crushing. Some people describe it as "a fire," "a knife that someone keeps jabbing into me," "a bowling ball knocking the pins down over and over," "a continual car wreck," and "something I wouldn't wish on my worst enemy."

Several things can cause the pain of arthritis. For example, it may result from something related to the disease process itself:

» **Inflammation:** Swollen, hot, inflamed joint tissues

» **Joint damage:** Bones grinding against each other, tendons that have slipped, joint misalignment or loosening, invasion of the bone by the synovium (joint lining), and so on

Arthritis pain may also be related to your body's response to the disease:

» **Muscle tension:** Tensing up as a reaction to your pain can spread pain to the muscles and make everything feel worse.

» **Strained muscles and supporting tissues:** When overcompensating for an injured area, you can unintentionally put excessive stress on a different area.

» **Fatigue:** Feeling dragged out due to illness can make your pain even more intense and difficult to cope with.

But when you're hurting, it doesn't matter much whether your pain is caused by or related to your arthritis. You just want it to stop! Yet for many people, the pain just seems to go on and on — and on.

Differentiating Between Acute Pain and Chronic Pain

The kind of pain you feel when you touch a hot stove, called *acute pain*, is absolutely vital to your well-being. Acute pain is a warning that you've injured yourself and you need to do something about it — now! Acute pain is episodic, meaning that it comes on quickly, builds rapidly to a crescendo, then tapers off and disappears. Suppose, for example, that you fall down and skin your knee: It really hurts! But, by the time you wash, disinfect, and bandage the area, your pain is already receding and soon disappears entirely. The acute pain has served its purpose — it got you to remove the source of the pain and attend to the damage that it caused. Although acute pain can be excruciating, at least it has a purpose and a definitive end.

Chronic pain, however, is another story. Like a barrage of telegrams repeating the same message over and over, chronic pain is not a useful warning, but an agonizing, debilitating tirade. More resistant to medical treatment than acute pain, chronic pain can become the constantly tormenting drumbeat underlying your every activity, day and night. Bam! Bam! Bam! It won't let up. Not surprisingly, one of the most common causes of chronic pain is arthritis, especially in older adults.

Breaking the pain cycle

Many arthritis sufferers become extremely frustrated and depressed by pain and the decline in their physical abilities. Unfortunately, stress and depression can, and do, make pain worse. The physical pain from arthritis causes stress and upset about the lost physical abilities. This stress, in turn, can trigger muscle tension that worsens the pain and further limits physical activities, causing even more stress and depression; thus, the cycle continues.

Fortunately, you can do many things to break the pain cycle and live more comfortably, even if your pain is chronic. The key is to block the pain signals moving through your nerves and spinal cord so they no longer register in your brain. The medicines discussed in Chapter 8 can eliminate a little or a lot of your hurting.

REMEMBER

With medication and the pain management methods we describe in this chapter and the next, you should be able to block many pain signals in your brain and manage your arthritis pain. But the key word is *manage.* Managing chronic pain means reducing its severity and decreasing it to the point where you can get on with your life, not eradicating it completely.

Dealing with chronic pain

You usually don't have to worry much about dealing with acute pain. It certainly hurts, but it often responds well to medicine and doesn't wear out its welcome. Getting rid of acute pain is typically your doctor's job. Dealing with chronic pain, however, is a different matter.

The goal in chronic pain management is to block pain messages *before* they reach the brain. You can try several natural approaches, apart from taking medication:

>> Exercise that's appropriate to your condition

>> Hot or cold treatments

>> Water therapy

>> Massage

>> Topical pain relievers

>> Relaxation

>> TENS (transcutaneous electrical nerve stimulation)

However, there are several "natural" things that can make your pain worse and also need to be addressed, all of which we discuss in Chapter 14:

>> Anxiety

>> Depression

>> Fatigue

>> Fixating on your pain

>> Physical overexertion

>> Progression of the disease

>> Stress

Assembling your treatment team

Chronic pain is a complex phenomenon that involves the original or ongoing disease process, the way your body deals with the problem mechanically, and your mental and emotional responses. A team of professionals, each with their own expertise, can best handle this multifaceted problem. Your treatment team may include these people who do the following:

>> **Your doctor** guides your treatment and prescribes medication, if necessary.

>> **A physical therapist** helps you build strength and restore range of motion. (See the sidebar "What does a physical therapist do?" later in this chapter.)

>> **An occupational therapist** teaches you how to place less strain on your joints when performing daily activities, overcome limitations, and prevent further damage.

- » **An exercise physiologist** helps you devise an exercise program that increases strength, flexibility, and endurance without putting undue strain on your joints. (This is also a function of the physical therapist, whose services may be paid for by insurance.)

- » **A psychologist, psychiatrist, or other mental health professional** helps you cope with depression, anger, and/or other emotional issues that may be increasing your pain.

- » **A pharmacist** offers advice on the proper use of medication.

- » **A social worker** recommends support groups or other special services.

You can also visit pain management clinics that have teams like these already assembled for you. Although some of these clinics specialize in treating specific types of pain, others treat all types. (Insurance coverage varies according to plan, and you may need a referral from your doctor.)

TECHNICAL STUFF

CONTROLLING PAIN THE NATURAL WAY

Your body makes certain substances that can decrease or even block pain sensations, as well as others that can increase your pain. The pain blockers include *endorphins* and *enkephalins*, substances that can slow or stop nerve cells from firing and sending pain messages to the brain. These chemicals are so powerful that their effects are often compared to those of morphine. Naturally, you want to produce more endorphins and enkephalins when you're in pain. You also want to have plenty of the brain hormone serotonin and other substances that play a role in manufacturing and releasing these internal painkillers.

Natural irritants — substances that increase the neurons' sensitivity to pain — are the flip side of the body's natural pain blockers. These irritants include *lactic acid, potassium ions, substance P,* and the stress hormones *noradrenaline* and *norepinephrine.* Most of the pain-control process revolves around increasing the production of the pain blockers while decreasing the production of the pain intensifiers. For example, massage can increase the production of endorphins while helping the body dispense with excessive amounts of lactic acid. Meditation, deep breathing, and a good belly laugh also can do much to increase endorphin levels, and transcutaneous electrical nerve stimulation (TENS — which is described later in this chapter) releases endorphins while decreasing substance P.

Relieving Pain with Noninvasive Therapies

Remember getting sick when you were a child? Your parents probably had a whole bag of tricks that could make you feel better: a cool cloth on your forehead, a warm bath, letting you lie inbed to watch television, chamomile tea, and so on. Their methods were just simple little things, but they really *did* make you feel better.

These methods were *noninvasive,* which means they didn't intrude on or cause harm to the body. Noninvasive methods may be physical or psychological, and they are the least traumatic approaches to pain management.

We discuss several noninvasive physical treatments below. Other techniques include psychotherapy, self-hypnosis, deep breathing, progressive relaxation, creative imagery, and biofeedback. (See Chapter 14 for more on these mental strategies for pain relief.)

At best, noninvasive approaches to pain management are very helpful; at worst they're probably harmless. With no side effects, incisions, blood loss, addiction potential, or other hazards, these techniques should be thoroughly explored by you and your doctor before you move on to harsher, more dangerous methods of pain relief.

You may be surprised at how much relief you can get from your arthritis pain by adopting the following simple physical strategies. Although these techniques don't *cure* your arthritis (the relief is temporary), any respite from the pain is always welcome! So, next time your arthritis pain flares, try some of the following methods.

Applying heat

Warmth encourages the blood vessels to expand, bringing more blood to the painful area and stimulating the healing process. It also helps your muscles relax, which may be just what you need if your pain makes you tighten up. You can use hot packs, heating pads, heat lamps with infrared bulbs, electric blankets, or hot paraffin wax treatments (see the nearby sidebar for more on these) to rev up your circulation, encourage overall relaxation, and make you feel better. However, sometimes heat increases swelling, so if swelling is a problem, try applying cold (see the next section).

TIP

Another way to apply heat is to wrap yourself in a flannel sheet or a throw blanket that you've just popped into the clothes dryer for a few minutes. Although the heat won't last long, it's very cozy!

HOT PARAFFIN WAX TREATMENTS

Hot paraffin wax treatments are a nice, comfortable way to warm up painful joints in your hands and feet. These treatments sustain their warmth because they use wax as insulation. A physical therapist usually applies hot paraffin wax treatments, but you can also do it yourself at home.

How do hot paraffin wax treatments work? Your painful hand or foot is repeatedly dipped into a blend of melted wax and mineral oil and allowed to cool in between immersions so that the wax can harden. When the build-up is thick enough, your hand/foot is wrapped in plastic and covered with towels to preserve the heat. The locked-in warmth can be very soothing to your stiff, painful fingers or toes, especially if you have osteoarthritis, rheumatoid arthritis, or fibromyalgia. After 20 minutes or so, the wrapping comes off, and the wax is peeled away.

As if pain relief weren't enough, hot paraffin wax treatments leave your skin wonderfully soft!

Don't use this treatment if your hands or feet show any signs of skin damage (excessive redness, blisters, and so on).

Ultrasound is a more high-tech way of accomplishing the same thing, and it can penetrate more deeply into the muscles and joints. High-frequency sound waves are aimed at the affected area, producing deep heating to soft tissues, which increases circulation and promotes muscle relaxation. Ultrasound is typically performed in your doctor's office or at a rehab center, although your physical therapist can bring along a portable machine for at-home visits. Ultrasound machines also are available for sale on the Internet, but they can be very expensive.

WARNING

Be careful not to damage your skin when applying heat from any source. Follow these rules to protect yourself:

>> Limit heat applications to no longer than 30 minutes in one area.

>> Wrap the hot pack or heating pad in towels to insulate it; don't place the source of heat directly on your skin.

>> To avoid steam burns or skin reactions, make sure that your skin is dry and that you haven't applied lotion or cream to it (particularly deep-heating creams).

>> Inspect the area every five minutes for purplish-red skin, hives, or blisters, which are signs of skin damage.

>> Allow your skin temperature to return to normal before reapplying heat.

Heat may make some conditions worse. Check with your doctor in advance to see if heat treatments are appropriate for you.

Applying cold

Cold packs are used to reduce inflammation, ease muscle spasms, and block pain signals by numbing the affected area. Although blood flow to the chilled area is temporarily reduced, cold applications eventually *increase* circulation, acting much like hot packs (perhaps because the body senses the need to warm up the area). Ice is the usual medium used to numb painful areas, but you may find it more convenient to use cold packs containing chemical mixtures that thaw slowly and don't drip.

A bag of frozen peas makes a good cold pack, because you can mold it around any shape, unlike a block of ice or bulky cubes. But make sure that you put the bag of peas inside an airtight plastic bag and wrap it in a towel, because it will drip.

Protect your skin and other tissues when using cold packs by following these steps:

>> Limit treatment to no longer than 20 minutes.

>> Remove the cold pack once the area becomes numb.

>> Be on the lookout for skin damage — redness, white patches, and so on.

>> Avoid cold packs if you have Raynaud's disease or phenomenon, poor circulation, sensitivity to cold, nerve damage, a lack of sensation, or heart problems.

In general, if inflammation is present, use cold; if not, use hot, although many doctors recommend that you use whatever feels good to you. The best advice, of course, is to consult with your doctor before using either method.

Washing away pain with water therapy

Ah, what feels better than easing your stiff, sore body into a nice warm bath? The ancient Romans evidently agreed, and built several health resorts throughout their wide-ranging empire for the express purpose of bathing. Most notable was their spa/bath retreat in the town of Bath, England, where people with arthritis came from far and wide to "take the waters." It makes perfect sense:

>> Warm showers, baths, and whirlpools can help ease your stiffness and make you feel better. Warm-water therapy is also a good way to warm up your

muscles before an exercise session, relaxing them and making movement easier.

>> Cool water can also help, especially when inflammation is present. Immersing a painful, swollen joint in cool water or using cool compresses is a milder, less jolting version of applying an ice pack.

Pool exercises are another extremely effective form of water therapy. Because water supports your body, exercising in a pool is like exercising in a weightless environment. With the tiresome pull of gravity greatly reduced in water, your joints can rest, even if your muscles go through a real workout. Because water provides resistance, your muscles have to work harder to perform a movement in water than they do on land. This combination adds up to more effective exercise, with less wear and tear on your joints. (See Chapter 12 for more on water exercise.)

Whether warm or cool, water can be used in a variety of ways to help ease your pain:

>> Cool hand or foot baths

>> Cool moist compresses

>> Warm tea to drink

>> Warm full-body baths

>> Warm hand or foot baths

>> Warm, moist compresses

>> Warm showers

>> Warm whirlpool baths

Trying topical pain relievers

Many topical creams, lotions, rubs, and sprays can help with chronic arthritis pain because they typically contain one or more of the following ingredients:

>> **Capsaicin** is a substance derived from chili peppers that decreases the nerves' concentration of substance P in the painful area, thus reducing pain. Earlier in this chapter, see the sidebar "Controlling pain the natural way" for more on substance P.

>> **Irritants** include menthol, camphor, and other substances that produce feelings of heat, cold, or itching. These can distract you from the sensation of pain.

>> **Lidocaine** in cream form (brand names BenGay, Aspercreme with Lidocaine, Xylocaine) are anesthetic creams available over the counter that promote a loss of feeling in the skin and surrounding tissues, which can help prevent and treat pain.

>> **Salicylates** are aspirin-like compounds that desensitize nerve endings.

>> **NSAIDs** in gel or spray form (generic name diclofenac topical; brand names Voltaren, Pennsaid) are over-the-counter preparations applied to the skin to treat the pain and swelling caused by osteoarthritis in the hands, wrists, elbows, feet, ankles, and knees. They work by inhibiting the production of prostaglandins, substances in the body that cause pain and inflammation.

Topical pain relievers are usually safe and at least somewhat effective. If you decide to use them, make sure you don't apply them to broken skin, and watch for signs of skin irritation.

Manipulating the joints

Joint manipulation is also known as *passive movement*, because something other than your own energy is moving your joints for you. That "something" is usually a physical therapist. During joint manipulation, the physical therapist uses their hands to move your joints through their range of motion. Then, by applying pressure (stretching) or simply moving the joint back and forth or around and around (depending upon the joint type), the therapist can help loosen up your joints. Joint manipulation must be done carefully, however, and never overdone. Otherwise, your joints may become even more irritated and painful.

WARNING

If you don't move your joints, you may lose the ability to do so. In most cases, some joint movement is *absolutely necessary*. People with arthritis have a tendency to guard their stiff, sore joints by moving them as little as possible. Unfortunately, this can be the worst thing for them. When the joints are held still, they aren't being lubricated or nourished. Their supporting muscles become weaker, circulation decreases, and ligaments and tendons tighten up, losing their resilience. Over time, an immobile joint can actually become frozen into position. That's why you must keep moving your joints, whether they hurt or not. Even splinted joints should be moved, at least a little, every day.

Helping the joints with splints and supports

Splints are designed to support and immobilize an injured or inflamed joint. A molded piece of metal or plastic is strapped to the affected area and then wrapped with elastic bandages. You can find splints for joint support in the wrists, fingers, hands, ankles, knees, back, and neck. Splints are widely available in off-the-rack varieties or can be custom-made by professionals who take an impression of your joint, then mold heat-sensitive material to replicate its shape. Splints help ease joint pain by doing the following:

>> Providing support, stability, protection, and rest for injured or inflamed joints

>> Immobilizing a joint after surgical fusion (arthrodesis), thereby allowing healing

>> Easing pain during arthritis flares

>> Keeping inflammation under control

>> Correcting or preventing deformities (in certain cases) by correctly positioning the joint

Supports (sometimes called *braces*) are strong, elasticized wraps designed to fit certain body parts such as your wrist, knee, ankle, and so on. Their tight fit lends stability to a joint, while their elasticity allows movement and blood circulation.

Supports are used in two ways: to support and stabilize an injured joint, or to protect a weakened joint from becoming injured. You should use supports in conjunction with a good exercise program, so the muscles and supporting structures themselves become strengthened and don't rely solely on the wrap for strength and stabilization.

WHAT DOES A PHYSICAL THERAPIST DO?

Described as a combination of buddy, drill sergeant, cheerleader, and workout partner, the physical therapist works with you to help increase your range of motion, reduce your pain, build strength, and decrease the disability associated with arthritis.

"The hardest part is getting the patients to do exercises that remind them they can't move like they used to," Kari, a physical therapist in San Diego, California, told us. "This seems to make them angrier and more depressed than feeling the pain does. But my job is to keep pushing, because that's the only way anybody gets better."

A physical therapist takes you through a series of exercises designed to get your joints lubed and to stretch your range of motion. Joint manipulation and massage are also important parts of the physical therapy session. Perhaps most importantly, the physical therapist will create a program of at-home exercises for you to do. Be aware that if you don't do these exercises regularly your progress will be slowed or stopped.

Transmitting a tingle with TENS

Transcutaneous electrical nerve stimulation (TENS) is a mild electrical buzz that overrides pain signals in tender areas. Studies have shown that TENS helps relieve osteoarthritis pain and decrease the need for pain medication. It may also be useful in relieving the pain of rheumatoid arthrhitis, fibromyalgia, tendinitis, and bursitis, although the jury is still out on these.

The TENS process may sound scary, but it really isn't, and it's easy to apply. Electrodes are affixed to your skin above and below (or parallel) to the painful joint with a small amount of gel. Then soothing pulses from a battery-powered unit connected to the electrodes) are transmitted to the area. Tthese electric currents override pain signals and trigger the release of endorphins, which are natural painkillers. TENS has also been found to ease inflammation.

The physiologic basis for TENS is the Gate Theory of Pain (discussed in Chapter 14). TENS helps to "close the gates," thus inhibiting pain impulses. It may offer welcome temporary relief for some people, but TENS isn't a cure.

You can purchase your own TENS unit and give yourself treatments at home. But if you decide to do so, knowing how to operate the TENS unit properly is important. Some people don't benefit from TENS simply because they use the equipment incorrectly.You should try TENS at your doctor's office or physical therapy clinic several times before purchasing your own unit to see if it seems like a worthy investment.

WARNING

Don't use TENS if you have a pacemaker, heart problems, epilepsy or you are pregnant. Also, don't use it on open wounds, rashes, inflamed skin, any part of the head, face or throat, or directly on your backbone.

Taking Pain Relief to the Next Level

When noninvasive techniques don't work and your pain is interfering with your ability to live a comfortable and productive life, you may want to look into medications or, in more serious cases, surgery.

Medicating the pain away

From the mildest aspirin to the powerful DMARDS or biologics, medicines can be beneficial but they are always risky. The most commonly prescribed painkillers for most forms of arthritis are NSAIDs (non-steroidal anti-inflammatory drugs, like ibuprofen) and analgesics (drugs that reduce pain without reducing consciousness, like acetaminophen).

If a joint is particularly painful and not responding to painkillers, your doctor may recommend injecting the afflicted areas with substances like steroids (high-powered anti-inflammatory agents). DMARDs (disease modifying antirheumatic drugs, like methotrexate) alter the way the immune system works and are reserved for autoimmune/inflammatory forms of arthritis including rheumatoid arthritis, psoriatic arthritis and ankylosing spondylitis. And biologics like etanercept and infliximab also target the immune system, but are used for those with autoimmune/inflammatory forms of arthritis that have not been relieved by one or more of the DMARDS.

REMEMBER

All medications, from aspirin to joint injections have side effects. Although they can be helpful initially, their long-term use can cause problems ranging from stomach upsets to drug dependence and death. Also, over time, their effectiveness can wane. It's vitally important that you take any medication exactly as it's prescribed and see your doctor regularly to monitor its effects on your body.

Chapter 8 tackles medication more fully.

Undergoing surgery

Surgery, which involves making incisions and manipulating the inner workings of the body, is always a risky and traumatic procedure.

Undergoing surgery to relieve pain can produce dramatic results in some cases, but always carries serious risks and side effects, ranging from infection to death. Consider surgery only as a last resort.

See Chapter 9 for a complete discussion of the surgeries for arthritis.

3

The Arthritis Lifestyle Strategy

Even though arthritis is a medical problem that continues to challenge even the top experts in the field, you can do a great deal to lessen your pain, improve your ability to perform everyday tasks, increase your enjoyment of life and, in some cases, even slow the progression of the disease.

In this part, we tell you how to ease arthritis pain through diet and supplements; how to keep your joints as healthy and mobile as possible through exercise; how to protect your joints from undue wear by walking, sitting, moving, and lifting loads correctly; and how to deal effectively with the stress, depression, and anger that may be getting your down. Plus, you'll get loads of tips on how to make day-to-day living with arthritis a lot easier!

Chapter **11**

Fighting the Pain with Foods and Supplements

The idea that food can cause or relieve arthritis isn't new. More than 200 years ago, English doctors prescribed cod-liver oil to treat gout and rheumatism. More recently, some health writers have insisted that people with arthritis should or should not eat certain foods. The debate is in full swing. Do certain foods cause arthritis? Is there an "Arthritis Begone" diet? While there is no miracle diet for arthritis, many foods have been found to fight inflammation and ease joint pain in certain people.

And what about supplements? Can they eliminate arthritis pain, unlock "frozen" joints, or prevent the immune system errors that lead to rheumatoid arthritis (RA)? Researchers have not yet come up with definitive answers, but some scientific studies suggest that various supplements may be helpful aids in the battle against arthritis. While much of the evidence is considered speculative, it may be worth your time to discover more about some of the foods, "food parts," and supplements that appear to help — and a few that might best be avoided.

Reviewing in detail all of the supplements that people take for various forms of arthritis is beyond the scope of this book, but this brief account will give you enough information to start a discussion with your doctor.

WARNING

Discuss *everything* you plan to take with your physician. There are subtle and sometimes hidden reactions caused by the combination of body chemistry, supplements, medications, and disease processes that may make your condition worse. For more on this, see the sidebar "Watch for food allergies" later in the chapter.

Finding Foods That Heal

Way back in the 1920s, researchers looked into treating osteoarthritis (OA) with the mineral sulfur. In 1963, a letter to the editor in the prestigious medical journal called *Lancet* described the use of a B vitamin called pantothenic acid in treating osteoarthritis. The idea that foods and the vitamins, minerals, and other substances they contain can aid in the battle against arthritis isn't new. What is new is that researchers are finding out why certain foods can be helpful — exactly *why* an apple a day may keep the doctor away.

Which fruits, vegetables, meat, or fish should you eat? There are no absolute rules, but the results of studies and case histories suggest that these foods may be helpful:

» **Anchovies:** Three-and-a-half ounces of anchovies contain almost a gram and a half of omega-3 fatty acids. The omega-3 fatty acids help regulate the prostaglandins, which play a role in inflammation and, hence, pain. Anchovies are extremely high in sodium, however, so if sodium-sensitivity or water retention is a problem for you, choose a different kind of fish. Because anchovies also are high in purines (nitrogen-containing compounds), you should probably avoid them if you have gout.

» **Apples:** Not only can an apple a day keep the doctor away, but it may also help to hold your arthritis at bay. Apples contain boron, a mineral that appears to reduce the risk of developing osteoarthritis. And when boron is given to people who have osteoarthritis, it helps relieve pain.

» **Broccoli:** This popular vegetable contains a powerful antioxidant and detoxifying agent called glutathione. Studies indicate that people with low amounts of glutathione are more likely to have arthritis. Other foods rich in glutathione include avocados, cabbage, cauliflower, grapefruit, oranges, potatoes, and tomatoes.

>> **Cantaloupe:** This sweet fruit contains large amounts of vitamin C and *beta-carotene,* the plant form of vitamin A. These two powerful vitamins help to control the oxidative and free radical damage that may contribute to arthritis. (For more on oxidative and free radical damage, see "Saving Your Joints with Supplements" in this chapter.)

>> **Curry:** A combination of spices that often includes turmeric, garlic, cumin, cinnamon, and so on, curry contains powerful antioxidants that may help relieve inflammation and reduce pain.

>> **Fish:** The omega-3 fatty acids in Norwegian sardines, Atlantic mackerel, sablefish, rainbow trout, striped bass, wild-caught salmon, and other fish may help reduce inflammation and pain. (See "Using omega-3s and omega-6s to fight arthritis pain and inflammation" in this chapter.)

>> **Garlic:** An ancient treatment for tuberculosis, lung problems, and other diseases, garlic also appears to relieve certain forms of arthritis pain, due to its anti-inflammatory effects. A study of 1,082 twins found that people who ate more garlic had a lesser risk of developing hip osteoarthritis. These helpful benefits may also be due to the fact that garlic contains sulfur, which plays an important role in manufacturing collagen and glucosamine, both of which are necessary for healthy joints.

>> **Grapefruit and other citrus fruits:** The skin, peel, and outer layers of citrus fruits are rich sources of bioflavonoids like quercetin, hesperidin, and rutin. Among other things, bioflavonoids help increase capillary strength and permeability, fight inflammation, inhibit viruses, and strengthen the collagen that's so important to joint health.

>> **Grapes:** This sweet, bite-sized fruit is a good source of the mineral boron, which is important for strong bones. The skin of the grape also contains resveratrol, a compound that can block the inflammation that causes arthritis pain.

>> **Mango:** A sweet treat, mangoes are packed with three powerful antioxidants. One medium-sized mango provides 90 percent of the vitamin C, 100 percent of the beta-carotene, and about 25 percent of the vitamin E that you need in an entire day.

>> **Nuts:** Almonds, peanuts, and hazelnuts are good sources of boron, a mineral that helps keep the bones strong and certain arthritis symptoms like inflammation at bay.

>> **Oysters:** Oysters are an excellent source of zinc: Six medium-sized oysters offer about 125 milligrams of the mineral, which is well over the RDA. This is important because RA patients often have low blood levels of zinc, and depleted zinc supplies have also been associated with the joint pain and stiffness of arthritis, in general.

Stay away from raw oysters, which are notorious for their high bacteria levels and are especially unhealthy for those who have compromised immune systems or liver disease. Either eat them well-cooked, or not at all.

>> **Papaya:** Long used as a folk medicine for diarrhea, hay fever, and other problems, a single papaya contains three times the RDA for the antioxidant vitamin C, plus more than half the daily allotment of beta-carotene. It also contains an anti-inflammatory compound called papain that has been proven to be effective at reducing joint pain and stiffness.

>> **Spinach and other leafy greens:** Unfortunately, eating spinach won't dispatch arthritis as quickly as Popeye does Brutus, but the vitamin E found in this vegetable can help reduce the pain of RA, inhibit the prostaglandins that help "stir up" inflammation, ease certain symptoms of fibromyalgia, and improve or stabilize lupus lesions.

>> **Water:** Drinking six to eight 8-ounce glasses of water per day can help prevent kidney stones in certain people who have gout. Eight glasses is also the amount recommended to keep your cartilage well-hydrated, thereby reducing the amount of friction between the bones.

>> **Whole grains:** Whole grains such as wheat, rye, and barley are good sources of B vitamins, which can be helpful in relieving some symptoms of arthritis. For example, vitamin B12 can help reduce the pain of both chronic and acute bursitis. Niacin can improve joint mobility in osteoarthritis patients, and may help lessen the skin lesions seen in lupus. Vitamin B6 reduced pain and improved performance in a study of patients with carpal tunnel syndrome. Because whole grains are an excellent source of B vitamins, eating at least four servings per day may help you battle arthritis.

Managing RA Mediterranean-style

Fat is considered a boogeyman by a lot of people because, in its saturated form, it can contribute to heart disease, obesity, cancer, and a host of other ills. We've all been told to cut the fat off of our meat and cut it out of our diets. But at least one diet that is high in fat (in unsaturated and monounsaturated fats, that is), is actually good for you — and may help ease rheumatoid arthritis (RA). And that's the Mediterranean diet.

The Mediterranean diet was first studied over 50 years ago, when researchers noticed that the people living on the Greek island of Crete had low rates of heart disease and certain types of cancer, plus a long life expectancy, even though they ate plenty of fat. Countless studies since that time found the same results in other areas of the Mediterranean region — Greece itself, Italy, southern France, and parts of Spain, Portugal, North Africa, and the Middle East. What were these people doing that the rest of us weren't? Part of the answer has to do with the kind of fat they ate.

Olive oil, which has long been linked to heart health, is the main fat used in the Mediterranean diet, replacing other oils, butter, and margarine. Olive oil can help lower harmful LDL cholesterol, and it contains antioxidants that discourage artery clogging and chronic diseases, including cancer. But it's only one part of this super-healthy style of eating. The bulk of the Mediterranean diet is made up of plenty of plant foods (vegetables, fruits, whole-grain breads, pasta and cereal, nuts, and legumes), eaten as fresh and as close to their natural state as possible. Cheese and yogurt are eaten every day, and small-to-moderate amounts of fish, poultry, and eggs are eaten a few times a week. Red meat is included just a few times a month, while a glass or two of red wine (it's loaded with antioxidants!) is taken just about every day, with meals. Sweets are limited, and fresh fruit is a favorite dessert. (See Figure 11-1 for the Mediterranean diet food pyramid.)

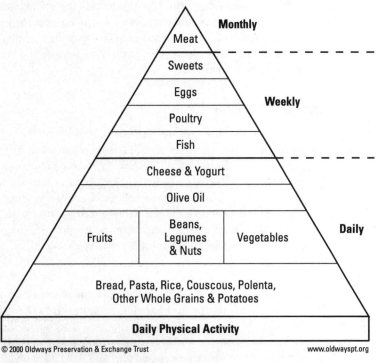

FIGURE 11-1: The Mediterranean diet provides a host of health benefits and helps ease the symptoms of RA.

Daily beverage recommendations: Drink six glasses of water. If you drink wine, do so in moderation.

If you have RA and you love hummus, tabbouleh, and baba ghanouj (traditional Greek foods), or you just like the idea of a fresh, plant-based diet, you're in luck: The Mediterranean diet may help ease your RA-related pain and swelling. When patients with active RA are placed on either a Mediterranean diet or a standard Western diet for three months, those who eat like the Greeks have much less inflammation and much greater physical function and vitality. The Mediterranean diet appears to suppress the activity of RA, at least for the short termand reduce inflammation in those with OA, and protect against weight gain, the risk of fracture, and disability.

Using omega-3s and omega-6s to fight arthritis pain and inflammation

Two other kinds of fat, the omega-3 and the omega-6 fatty acids, can also help fight arthritis. Omega-3s can be converted to natural anti-inflammatory substances called *prostaglandins* that help decrease the inflammation and pain that plague so many arthritis sufferers. And a certain type of omega-6 fatty acid (gamma linolenic acid, or GLA) can help lessen pain by calling off the disease-related invasion of white blood cells that trigger the joint swelling and tenderness seen in rheumatoid arthritis.

Omega-3 fatty acids

Studies have shown that the omega-3 fatty acids, which are found primarily in cold-water, fatty fish, can help reduce the pain and joint stiffness seen in RA by "dampening" the inflammation response. The results of at least 13 studies involving more than 500 RA patients found that those who took omega-3 fatty acid supplements had significant improvements in RA symptoms, including less joint pain, although joint damage did not decrease. In another study, patients with RA were able to ease pain and inflammation and reduce their use of NSAIDs (pain relievers such as aspirin and ibuprofen) just by eating a diet rich in antioxidants and omega-3s.

Good fish sources of omega-3 fatty acids include mackerel (Atlantic, Pacific, and Spanish), herring (Atlantic and Pacific), salmon (king, Chinook, and pink), and roe. Check out the sidebar "Sources of omega-3 fatty acids" for more. In general, the best sources of omega-3 fatty acids are fish that come from cold water. Fish from warmer waters and those raised on fish farms have smaller amounts. Some nonfish foods also contain omega-3 fatty acids, such as green soybeans, black walnuts, and flaxseed oil.

TECHNICAL STUFF

Omega-3 fatty acids have long, complicated names such as *alpha-linoleic acid*, *DHA (docosahexaenoic acid)*, and *EPA (eicosapentaenoic acid)*. But they're often referred to as omega-3s or *fish oil* (because that's where you typically find them in their most concentrated form), for short.

Taking high doses of omega-3 fatty acids (4 grams per day or more of EPA and DHA, combined) may help reduce inflammation due to RA. However, the average person must take the supplements for about three months before any improvement is seen.

REMEMBER

Take supplements only after discussing them with your physician. And make sure your doctor always knows what supplements you're taking, as they may interfere with certain aspects of treatment.

WARNING

According to the FDA, fish oil is likely safe when taken in daily doses of 3 grams or less. But since fish oil thins the blood, it can be dangerous if taken in larger amounts. Overly thin blood may not clot properly, causing bleeding to increase to dangerous levels. Consult your physician before taking fish oil supplements if you take blood-thinning medication, NSAIDs, supplements that contain ginger, or anything else that thins the blood. Fish oil should be avoided before undergoing surgical procedures to help ward off unnecessary bleeding.

WHAT DOES "OMEGA" MEAN?

A fatty acid is built around a line of carbon atoms. There may be a few, 6, 10, 12, or more carbons lined up, one behind the other, like a line of school children. Each of the carbons has a "left hand" and a "right hand," and can "hold" one hydrogen atom in each hand, off to either side. If each of the carbons in the line is holding two hydrogens, one in each hand, the fatty acid is saturated. Like a sponge that's full of water (saturated), the fatty acid can't possibly hold any more.

Often times, however, some of the carbons in the line "let go" of one of their hydrogens. Now they're each holding only one. When that happens, the fatty acid is either unsaturated or polyunsaturated (depending on how many carbons have let go of a hydrogen).

If the first carbon holding only one hydrogen happens to be the third in line, the fatty acid is called an omega-3 fatty acid. If the first carbon holding only a single hydrogen is sixth in line, it's called an omega-6 fatty acid, and so on. They're called "omega this" or "omega that" because the counting starts at the side of the fatty acid called the omega side.

SOURCES OF OMEGA-3 FATTY ACIDS

In general, the best sources of omega-3 fatty acids are fish that come from cold water. Fish from warmer waters and those raised on fish farms have less. The following statistics are calculated on 3½-ounce servings of fish.

Fish	Grams of Omega-3
Roe	2.3
Atlantic mackerel	2.3
Pacific herring	1.6
Atlantic herring	1.5
Pacific mackerel	1.4
King salmon	1.3
Spanish mackerel	1.3
Pink salmon	1.0

You'll also find omega-3 fatty acids in other foods, including butternuts, black walnuts, and green soybeans.

TIP Don't deep-fry your fish. Doing so destroys the omega-3s.

The good omega-6 fatty acid — GLA

Although most of the omega-6s are best avoided (see the section "Avoiding Foods That May Be Trouble," later in the chapter), one of them may give hope to people with RA: gamma-linolenic acid, or GLA for short, which is found in evening primrose oil, black current oil, and borage oil.

Your body converts GLA from another omega-6 fatty acid, linoleic acid, and oddly enough, although linoleic acid *promotes* inflammation, GLA actually helps *calm* it. Some studies have shown that GLA helps reduce the number of tender joints, pain, and inflammation in RA patients. In a study of 56 patients with active RA, taking 2.8 grams of GLA for six months significantly improved joint pain, stiffness, and grip strength. A 2014 study found that the daily use of borage oil reduced the need for disease-modifying antirheumatic drugs (DMARDs) in RA patients.

An often-suggested dose of GLA is 1.4 grams per day. However, you'll need to take a lot of borage or blackcurrant oil, and even more evening primrose oil to get

1.4 grams of GLA. Taking it as a GLA supplement in capsule form is easier and more convenient, although most of the research has been done using evening primrose oil or borage oil, instead of GLA supplements.

REMEMBER

If you do decide to take one of the oils rather than the supplement, make sure it lists the GLA content on the label so you know exactly how many spoonfuls provide the desired dose.

Getting a grip on arthritis with green tea

Green tea, that delicious drink sometimes referred to as a "cup of steaming medicine," has been linked to prevention of heart disease, strokes, and certain kinds of cancer. It may also protect against the cartilage breakdown seen in OA. That's because the unfermented green tea leaves contain large amounts of some potent health promoters called *catechins*, which are powerful antioxidants and disease fighters. Two of the most potent catechins, EGCG and ECG, may actually block cartilage-destroying enzymes. So when you drink green tea, your precious cartilage is better able to stave off the breakdown process and stay intact.

Green tea's EGCG can also put a damper on the inflammatory response. In a 2016 sutdy, people who had suffered from RA for at least ten years were given green tea (four to six cups/day), the RA medicine infliximab, or an aerobic exercise program, or a combination of any two for a period of six months. At the study's end, those treated with green tea, or green tea combined with either infliximab or exercise, showed significant signs of improvement in the disease. And those treated with green tea plus exercise *outperformed* those treated with infliximab plus exercise.

For best results, look for the higher grades of green tea, use loose-leaf tea, allow the tea to steep in just-boiled water for 3 minutes, and drink at least three cups of tea per day. Also, be sure to keep your tea in an airtight container as exposure to air or dampness lessens both the polyphenol content and the flavor.

Avoiding Foods That May Be Trouble

No foods actually *cause* arthritis, but some can exacerbate arthritis that already exists. For example, red meat, alcohol, and saturated fat can increase joint inflammation and pain. However, certain foods are known to give some people trouble, so you may want to consider cutting back or avoiding intake of the following:

>> **Nightshades:** Peppers, potatoes, eggplant, and tomatoes are some of the members of the nightshade family of vegetables. Some people feel that eating

nightshades aggravates their rheumatoid arthritis and other forms of the disease. Although it hasn't been proven, if you feel that eating nightshades worsens your symptoms, avoid them.

>> **Organ meats:** Liver, kidney, sweet breads, and other organ meats contain purines, which can trigger gout. If you have gout, avoid organ meats and other foods high in purines, including sardines, anchovies, and meat gravies.

>> **Processed meat:** Cold cuts, hot dogs, bacon, and other processed meats contain various chemicals that may trigger allergic reactions, bringing on arthritis-like symptoms. Or, they may cause flares of existing arthritis conditions.

It's not clear whether these substances actually trigger arthritis and allergies, or whether they tend to replace the vegetables, fruits, and whole grains that provide the nutrients needed to hold arthritis at bay.

>> **Foods containing linoleic/arachidonic acid:** The omega-3 fatty acids help reduce inflammation, but linoleic acid, an omega-6 fatty acid, tends to promote inflammation. Linoleic acid is found in salad or cooking oils, such as corn, safflower, and sunflower oils. It's found in many kinds of fast food, and large amounts of linoleic acid are fed to the cattle that eventually end up in the meat department of your grocery store. Linoleic acid is converted into arachidonic acid, which the body uses to build the substances that trigger inflammation and arthritic pain.

WATCH FOR FOOD ALLERGIES

If you've noticed that a food tends to make your arthritis worse, try eliminating it from your diet for a while. Reports abound (including some published in prestigious medical journals) of arthritis cases being "cured" when the sufferer stopped eating certain foods, including cheese, corn, milk, and various members of the nightshade vegetable family. Most likely, their arthritis-like symptoms were the result of simple food allergies. This diagnosis may not be true for you, but it can't hurt to check it out.

To test for a food allergy, eliminate all foods that contain the suspected culprit for at least two weeks and write down everything you eat and drink, plus your symptoms — especially any reactions or changes in the way you feel. After the two-week period, if there are no differences, gradually add the foods back into your diet, one at a time, in small amounts, recording everything you ate, symptoms, and any changes.

Remember: This is just a preliminary test, for your own information,. Only a health professional can conduct a scientifically valid elimination diet.

Naturally, the less linoleic acid you consume, the better for your arthritis! To avoid it, switch to olive, flaxseed, or canola oil for cooking, eat less meat and poultry, and avoid fast food. At the same time, increase your consumption of the fish and other foods that contain the helpful omega-3 fatty acids (see "Omega-3 fatty acids," earlier in this chapter).

Saving Your Joints with Supplements

Various studies have linked poor nutrition to rheumatoid arthritis, juvenile arthritis, and other forms of arthritis. However, the connection between nutrition and arthritis isn't yet fully understood. For example, researchers can't say that eating too few apples will cause arthritis or that drinking too much beer *always* triggers gout. However, good nutrition is an important part of the battle against arthritis, and evidence suggests that careful use of supplements can also be very helpful. It's not just the omega-3 and omega-6 fatty acids can help you out, though. Antioxidants and free radical scavengers, plus some regular vitamins and minerals, can also have beneficial effects.

REMEMBER

Take *all* supplements with care, because even helpful ones can interact with medicines or herbs that you may be taking and cause trouble. Supplements can increase the effect of blood-thinning medications (which makes you more likely to bleed unnecessarily), counteract the effectiveness of some immune system-suppressing drugs, increase the side effects of NSAIDs, make alcohol and sedatives more powerful, hinder the absorption of select nutrients, and so on. Always let your physician know about *all* the supplements, herbs, and other substances you're taking. Consult with them before beginning to take supplements, increasing or decreasing the dosage, or discontinuing their use.

What you need to know before taking supplements

WARNING

First of all, before you buy anything else, see your doctor, and bring a list of any medications, over-the-counter drugs, vitamins, minerals, herbs, or other supplements that you're currently taking. Be aware that supplements are not FDA approved and haven't been subjected to trials that confirm their safety. Some can interact with medications, change the results of medical tests, and cause side effects. Ask your doctor if the supplement combinations and amounts that you're taking are okay for your health and your body.

Then, tell your doctor about any supplement you're planning to take and ask these questions:

>> Will it interact with any medications I'm taking?

>> Will it interact with any other supplements I'm taking?

>> Will it have an effect on any of my medical conditions?

>> Are there side effects I should watch for?

>> Is there any good research that shows this supplement is safe?

>> Is there any good research that shows this supplement is worth taking?

>> What kind of results can I expect?

>> How much should I take?

>> How often should I take it?

>> How long should I take it?

>> How will I know when I should stop taking it?

Of course, your doctor may not know the answers to these questions. If that's the case, you might want to see a registered dietitian, or just do the research yourself online.

TIP

Your best bet is to find a supplement endorsed by the Arthritis Foundation, the American Dietetic Association, or the American Medical Association. The Arthritis Foundation puts out a special Supplement Guide each year that gives the latest information on supplements and other natural remedies for arthritis (find it at www.arthritis.org/health-wellness/treatment/complementary-therapies/supplements-and-vitamins/supplement-and-herb-guide-for-arthritis-symptoms). You can also contact the organizations listed in Appendix B for the latest nutrition and diet information. Don't turn yourself into a guinea pig. Get the facts first!

Fighting damaging oxidants and free radicals

Oxidants and free radicals are perfectly normal substances in the body; they're the result of normal metabolism. Unfortunately, if not properly controlled by the body, they can cause damage to cells, tissues, and organs, and have been linked to many ailments, including arthritis. Researchers can't absolutely say that oxidants and free radicals *cause* arthritis, but they're definitely implicated in actions that lay the groundwork for trouble — or make any current trouble worse. (For more information, check out the sidebar, "What oxidants and free radicals do.")

Fortunately, many oxidant quenching and free radical-corralling substances (known as *antioxidants* and *free radical quenchers*) can be found in foods and supplements. This section highlights some of the substances that may help you fight the cellular damage that can contribute to arthritis.

Vitamin C

This popular vitamin works together with vitamin E to scavenge free radicals or stabilize them so they're no longer dangerous. It also helps reactivate used vitamin E so it can charge back into the fray and protect your body. Researchers have reported that vitamin C may help ease the pain, reduce the inflammation and protect against the progression of cartilage damage seen in RA and OA.

Fresh fruits and vegetables, especially papaya, guava, red peppers, cantaloupe, sweet green peppers, oranges, broccoli, cauliflower, and asparagus are good sources of vitamin C. An often-suggested dose is 500 to 1,000 milligrams of vitamin C per day in supplement form.

Vitamin E

Vitamin E, like NSAIDs, slows the action of the prostaglandins that play a major role in producing pain. It also helps control the free radicals that promote inflammation and damage cells and tissues in and around the joint. And vitamin E may help by stabilizing the proteoglycans (the water-loving molecules in the cartilage), allowing the cartilage to stay moist and healthy. Individual reports have also suggested that vitamin E may reduce the risk of developing RA through its antioxidant effects.

Vitamin E is found in a variety of foods, including green leafy vegetables, broccoli, Brussels sprouts, seeds, nuts, green beans, and wheat germ oil. An often-suggested dose of vitamin E is 400 to 800 IU (international units) per day in supplement form.

Selenium

Selenium, an essential mineral with antioxidant properties, works together with *glutathione peroxidase* (one of the body's internal defenders) to control free radicals. Selenium also makes vitamin E more effective and plays an important part in regulating inflammation in the body. It also aids in the production of cartilage, a key component of the joints.

You can find selenium in whole grains, fish, poultry, and meat; smaller amounts are present in fruits and vegetables. Selenium levels in food vary, depending in part on how much of the mineral was in the ground where the food was grown. An often-suggested dose is 100 to 200 micrograms per day in supplement form.

WHAT OXIDANTS AND FREE RADICALS DO

Here's a short list of the damage that oxidants and/or free radicals can cause:

- They can attack the fatty membranes surrounding body cells. With repeated hits, the cell membrane may become damaged and unable to ferry water, oxygen, and nutrients into the cells while sending waste products out. In short, the cells can become unable to function properly.

- Sometimes they harm the outer wall of the cell, and parts of the cell will leak out. Besides damaging the cell itself, neighboring cells can also be negatively affected.

- They can severely damage the DNA that holds the genetic blueprints within your cells. When this happens, your cells may be unable to grow, function, and/or repair themselves properly.

- They can increase the inflammation response, which is the last thing you want in inflammatory conditions like arthritis.

- They can hamper the immune system, the same internal defense system that goes awry with certain forms of arthritis. (The immune system sometimes uses oxidants and free radicals to fight off certain germs. But these same "weapons" can harm the immune system: it's like a soldier being shot with his own gun.)

Warding off OA with boron

Low blood levels of boron have been shown people who have RA or OA, and those with OA have also been reported to have low stores of boron in their bones. Boron supplements, however, can help improve the body's absorption of calcium, magnesium, and phosphorus, and retention of calcium and magnesium in the bones. It also helps inhibit the inflammatory response, appears to be helpful in preventing OA, and combating JIA inflammation and pain.

Boron is found in a variety of foods, including apples, peaches, peas, beans, lentils, peanuts, almonds, and grapes. The World Health Organization estimates that an acceptable safe range of boron intakes is 3 to 13 milligrams per day in supplement form for adults.

Lowering homocysteine with vitamin B6 and folic acid

The combination of vitamin B6, folic acid, and vitamin B12 helps lower blood levels of *homocysteine*. High blood levels of this amino acid are linked to a higher risk of heart attack and stroke, and are also found in many people with lupus. Vitamin B6 alone may help relieve the pain and stiffness of carpal tunnel syndrome and, in some cases, can make surgery unnecessary.

You'll find vitamin B6 in brewer's yeast, sunflower seeds, and brown rice; folic acid in green leafy vegetables; and B12 in meat, fish, and dairy products. An often-suggested dose for reducing elevated homocysteine levels is 25 milligrams B6, 2.5 milligrams folic acid, and 0.4 milligrams B12 in supplement form.

Fighting OA and RA with vitamin D

Vitamin D helps build strong bones by aiding in the absorption of calcium, and it's also vital for preventing muscle weakness. But did you know that it may also play a part in warding off osteoarthritis and rheumatoid arthritis? Those who get adequate amounts of vitamin D appear to be less likely to develop OA of the hip, and if they do develop the disease, it progresses at a slower rate. Conversely, getting too little vitamin D may actually triple the rate of OA progression! Among those with RA, there is a high prevalence of vitamin D deficiency which is also link to RA disease severity.

An optimal daily dosage of vitamin D for fighting OA and RA hasn't been established, although a 2000 IU (international units) of vitamin D3 (the most easily absorbed kind) has been recommended for RA patients. Good food sources of the vitamin include fortified milk, egg yolks, butter, cheese, fish oil, and fortified cereals, although it's hard to get enough D from food alone.

Pumping up cartilage with hydrolyzed collagen

Also known as HC or collagen supplements, hydrolyzed collagen may help your cartilage absorb collagen, the "netting" that holds the proteoglycans (*water-loving molecules*) in place. Collagen gives cartilage its elasticity and ability to absorb shock. When collagen fibers weaken and thin, the cartilage dries out, cracks, and is more likely to show signs of wear.

Although HC is still in the experimental stage, recent studies have shown that it can help reduce OA related pain, stiffness, and impaired physical function. In a study of 250 people with OA of the knee who took 10 grams of HC every day for six months, significant improvement was experienced in knee joint comfort.

Hydrolyzed collagen is taken orally in tablet, capsule, or powder form, and can also be consumed in the form of bone broth or pork skin. The supplements are made from animal hides, bones or fish scales, or, more recently, genetically modified yeast and bacteria. Typical doses of HC range from 2.5 grams to 30 grams per day.

WARNING

Those who are allergic to fish or shellfish should avoid products containing these ingredients. Also note that HC supplements haven't been tested for safety, so consult with your physician before taking them.

Combating Raynaud's with niacin

Niacin, a member of the B-vitamin family, was first noted early in the twentieth century during a battle against *pellagra*, a disease that causes blotchy skin rashes, confusion, weakness, memory loss, and other problems. As pellagra is rarely seen today, doctors are primarily interested in niacin's ability to keep the skin, nerves, and intestines healthy, lower cholesterol, and possibly guard against cancer.

The Raynaud's Association suggests that those suffering from Raynaud's try taking niacin (vitamin B3) to dilate the blood vessels and increase blood flow. Inositol nicotinate, a compound made of niacin and inositol, has been used in Great Britain for years to improve the symptoms of poor circulation, including Raynaud's. Some research has shown that taking an oral inositol nicotinate product called Hexopal for several weeks modestly improved the symptoms of Raynaud's.

For health maintenance, a typical dose of niacin is 14 to 16 milligrams per day, but therapeutic doses in the form of inositol nicotinate are much larger and should be prescribed and monitored by your doctor.

WARNING

Niacin can produce liver damage when taken in large doses. Don't take more than the recommended dosage of niacin unless you're under a doctor's supervision.

Zapping RA and psoriatic arthritis with zinc

The mineral zinc is necessary for maintaining skin health and immune function. It also has anti-inflammatory properties. Zinc levels in the blood are significantly lower in those suffering from rheumatoid arthritis and/or psoriatic arthritis, and the lower the levels the more severe the symptoms.

The results of studies with zinc on arthritis have been mixed, some have shown that zinc sulfate improved RA symptoms, while others have found it eased symptoms of psoriasis. But others have shown that it has no significant benefit. This has led some researchers to suggest that zinc may not be helpful for everyone, but can be a great aid to carefully selected arthritis patients who have low levels of the mineral. And side effects don't seem to be an issue: Hundreds of thousands of people take it every day without a problem.

You can find zinc in oysters, seafood, eggs, meat, wheat germ, and plain yogurt. An often-suggested dose is 8 to 15 milligrams per day in the form of zinc sulfate, gluconate, or picolonate.

Relieving Arthritis Symptoms with Other Nutritional Substances

Omega-3 fatty acids, GLA (the "good" omega-6 fatty acid), antioxidants, free radical quenchers, vitamins, and minerals: The nutritional arsenal against arthritis is growing larger every year. And there's more. Here are a few of the nonvitamin, nonmineral, nonantioxidant substances that are gaining recognition.

Alleviating inflammation with aloe vera

Made from the leaves of the aloe plant, aloe vera juice is an ancient beauty aid, reportedly used by Cleopatra to keep her skin fresh and soft. It is also an all-purpose balm that was carried by Alexander the Great's soldiers as they conquered much of the ancient world. Today, aloe vera juice's popularity is partially due to its inflammation-relieving properties. Many people drink aloe juice as a laxative and health booster, and aloe vera creams or gels are used to treat sunburn, cuts, burns, and abrasions. Stabilized aloe vera juice contains numerous vitamins, minerals, and amino acids, which may explain its many beneficial effects.

There are reports that drinking aloe juice can help relieve symptoms of rheumatoid arthritis, as well as other inflammatory forms of arthritis. A few animal studies back up these claims, and many arthritis sufferers are eagerly awaiting human studies that will show that aloe can help knock down arthritis symptoms. Meanwhile, many people insist that moderate amounts of aloe juice relieve swelling.

You can find aloe vera in juice, cream, gel, and capsule form. An often-suggested dose is up to 200 milligrams or more per day in capsule form.

Supporting your joints with SAMe

SAMe (short for S-adenosyl-L-methione and pronounced *sammy*) is naturally produced by the body which, among other things, helps the body manufacture a hormone called melatonin, vital to sleep, and protects DNA.

Since at least the late 1980s, SAMe has also strutted its stuff as an anti-inflammatory and painkiller that may be particularly effective for those with osteoarthritis. In Europe, where SAMe is sold as a drug, it has been used to treat OA for many years. And no wonder. It has been shown to be as effective at easing OA pain as the prescription drugs celecoxib (Celebrex) and the NSAID nabumetone. Clinical trials involving thousands of people suffering from OA have shown that SAMe helps improve the health of joints, most likely by repairing and rebuilding the cartilage. It's also been shown to counteract fibromyalgia better than a placebo, and fight depression just as well as a standard antidepressant, with few side effects. Results have been experienced after just one week, although they may take more than a month.

An oft-suggested dose of SAMe for OA is up to 400 milligrams, three times a day. For fibromyalgia, 200 to 400 milligrams twice daily is recommended. Make sure you get plenty of vitamins B-12, B-6 and folate while taking this supplement, because SAMe works closely with them and can use them up quickly. SAMe is available without a prescription online and in many health food and vitamin stores.

WARNING

High doses of SAMe can cause headache, nausea, vomiting, diarrhea, and flatulence. SAMe can worsen bipolar disorder and Parkinson's disease, and may interact with antidepressants, especially monamine oxidase inhibitors (MAOIs).

Battling inflammation with bromelain

An enzyme found in pineapple, bromelain is often used as a digestive aid because it can help break down protein. But bromelain also has anti-inflammatory properties that may help reduce the swelling and pain of arthritis. In one study of 73 people with OA of the knee, bromelain, combined with rutin (a citrus flavonoid) and trypsin (a pancreatic enzyme), relieved pain and improved function as well as an NSAID. However, as yet there is no evidence that bromelain alone is effective.

Bromelain comes in capsule form, and an often-suggested dose is 80 to 300 milligrams of extract taken two to three times per day, or one or two 200 milligram tablets.

WARNING

Bromelain can increase the effects of medications that thin the blood. Large doses can cause stomach upset or cramps. Avoid bromelain if you're allergic to pineapple.

Curtailing the pain with capsaicin

Chili peppers have long been used to treat numerous ills, including (surprisingly enough) indigestion! Today, researchers know that *capsaicin*, the ingredient that gives chilies their bite, can help relieve pain. Applying cream that contains capsaicin stimulates the pain impulse (it feels hot!) and then blocks it. It works by depleting the nerves' supply of substance P, a messenger that carries the pain message to the brain. Substance P also revs up the inflammation process, so decreasing your substance P stores can translate to less pain *and* less swelling. A 2018 study found that capsaicin cream was just as effective as topically applied NSAIDs in relieving the pain of knee OA.

Creams containing capsaicin are available online and in many drugstores without a prescription. Apply the cream to the painful area, following the instructions on the label.

WARNING

Some people find capsaicin irritating, so if you decide to try it, start with a very small trial dose and work your way up.

Guarding your joints with grapeseed extract

Medical researchers haven't yet discovered all the ins and outs of grapeseed extract, a potent antioxidant made from the ground-up seeds of red wine grapes, but it appears to help vitamin C cross into certain body cells. With a good supply of vitamin C safely tucked inside, these cells are better able to prevent and/or repair oxidative damage. Grapeseed extract, a great source of powerful antioxidants, may also help combat the inflammation associated with many forms of arthritis by slowing the body's release of inflammation-producing enzymes. Animal studies show that it reduces the tissue destruction seen in RA and OA, strengthens bones, and reduces joint pain.

Grapeseed extract is available as a supplement. Dosages of 75 to 300 milligrams per day for three weeks in capsule form,settlng at 40 to 80 milligrams per day for maintenance.

WARNING

Don't use grapeseed extract if you're currently taking blood-thinning medication, as it increases the risk of bleeding.

Fighting disease with flaxseed oil

Many people swear by flaxseed oil, which contains many "parts" that the body can turn into the helpful omega-3 fatty acids known as EPA and DHA. Although there aren't any good studies showing that flaxseed can actually ease the symptomsRA, flaxseed does increase levels of EPA, while decreasing swelling, which is why some people use it for RA. One study found that flaxseed oil put the kibosh on autoimmune reactions just as effectively as EPA. It's also believed to improve kidney function in those with lupus by decreasing the thickness of the blood, lowering cholesterol levels, and reducing swelling.

Plus, taking flaxseed oil brings some hefty side benefits: It helps inhibit tumor growth, balance your hormones, ward off heart disease, and reduce high blood pressure

Flaxseed comes in oil or capsule form, and as flour or meal. Whole seeds need to be ground into meal, or your body will just pass them right through without absorbing the helpful linolenic acid. The oil spoils easily and shouldn't be heated to high temperatures (as in frying), although you can cook with it and bake with the flour or meal. An often-suggested daily dose is 1 to 3 tablespoons of the oil, the equivalent in capsule form, or up to a third cup of the flour or meal.

Jettisoning OA pain with ginger

Ginger has been used for more than 2,000 years by the Chinese to treat coughing, diarrhea, vomiting, and fever. Today we know that it contains ingredients that can ease nausea, alleviate motion sickness, and prevent heart attacks by thinning the blood. But it also may help ease the hurt of osteoarthritis, thanks to its pain-relieving and anti-inflammatory properties. A 2015 review study involving 593 people with OA found that those who used ginger had 30 percent less OA pain than those given a placebo. A 2019 study found that ginger powder decreased two major inflammatory markers (CRP and IL-1B) in people with active RA, and improved inflammation.

As for how much to take, one double-blind study found that 225 milligrams of highly purified ginger extract, taken twice daily, reduced OA knee pain.

WARNING

Don't take ginger if you have gallstones or are on medications for blood pressure, heart problems, blood thinning, or diabetes. Ginger can cause heartburn, diarrhea, or stomach discomfort in sensitive people.

Glucosamine sulfate and chondroitin sulfate: Cures for osteoarthritis?

In 1997, two supplements burst onto the arthritis scene: glucosamine sulfate and chondroitin sulfate, touted to be the "arthritis cure" due to their ability to relieve arthritis pain and prevent joint disease. Glucosamine, which is derived from shrimp, crab, or lobster shells, was believed to provide the building blocks for cartilage growth, maintenance, and repair. Chondroitin, which comes from pork byproducts or the tracheas of cattle, was thought to attract water to the cartilage, thus improving its shock-absorbing properties, while slowing the action of certain enzymes that prematurely destroy cartilage.

Now, more than two decades after the debut of these two supplements, multiple studies have found that they don't appear to deliver as promised. A 2010 meta-analysis involving more than 3,800 people with OA found that glucosamine, chondroitin, or a combination of the two weren't any better at relieving OA symptoms than a placebo. A 2016 study involving 164 people with knee OA that compared glucosamine and chondroitin to a placebo had to be stopped early because OA symptoms in those taking the supplements actually got worse compared to those taking the placebo. And, according to the National Institutes of Health (NIH), the results of large, high-quality studies showed that chondroitin wasn't helpful for easing OA pain of the knee or hip, and it was unclear whether glucosamine could ease OA knee pain.

However, there were also some positive study results. A 2018 meta-analysis of 30 studies on the effects of glucosamine and chondroitin on OA found that chondroitin could alleviate pain and improve joint function, while glucosamine showed improvement in joint stiffness. And severals studies of people with OA have shown that glucosamine helps slow knee joint degeneration, improve joint function, reduce joint swelling and stiffness, and provide pain relief.

So what's the takeaway message? Study results on the effectiveness of glucosamine and/or chondroitin on OA are inconclusive and additional research is needed. But since side effects are minimal to nonexistent, it probably wouldn't hurt to experiment with these supplements if you're so inclined. There are many different brands online, in pharmacies, health food stores and big box stores. An often-suggested dose is 500 milligrams of glucosamine three times a day and 400 milligrams of chondroitin three times a day.

There are several forms of glucosamine, including glucosamine sulfate, glucosamine hydrochloride and n-acetyl glucosamine. Although most of the studies have been conducted with the sulfate form, the hydrochloride form is believed to be better absorbed. Some researchers feel that the n-acetyl form is weaker than the other two.

If you're allergic to sulfates, avoid glucosamine sulfate and chondroitin sulfate. Glucosamine may also cause a reaction in those allergic to shellfish and reduce the effectiveness of acetaminophen. Chondroitin, when taken with medications that thin the blood (like NSAIDs or warfarin), can increase the risk of bleeding.

Chapter **12**

Oiling Your Joints with Exercise

O ur local gym has a sign that says, "Warning: *Not* Exercising Is Hazardous to Your Health!" This goes double for arthritis sufferers, because a lack of exercise can really do a number on your joints, making them stiffer, less mobile, and more likely to degenerate. The old saying, "Use it or lose it!" is an appropriate one for those who live with arthritis. In this chapter, we discuss the elements of a good fitness program and give you tips on setting up a plan that can help strengthen your joints without disrupting your lifestyle.

WARNING

Before you start on any kind of exercise program, consult your physician to determine whether or not your body can accommodate the stresses of exercise. This is especially critical when you haven't exercised in a while, you're over 40, or you have heart disease or high blood pressure.

Achieving Different Goals with Different Exercises

Every good fitness plan, no matter how simple or complex, includes three basic kinds of exercise: *cardiovascular endurance, strength training,* and *flexibility.* Together, these three types of exercise can build a strong, toned, and healthy body better able to withstand physical, mental, and emotional stresses. Your initial goal should be to follow a short, easy fitness plan that includes all three of these. Then you can slowly increase the length and intensity of the exercises as you become more physically fit.

WARNING

A physical therapist or exercise physiologist experienced in working with people who have arthritis is the ideal person to design and supervise your fitness program. Any kind of exercise, whether cardiovascular endurance, strength training, or flexibility, can cause injury if done improperly, especially over time.

Building cardiovascular endurance

Countless studies have shown that people who regularly perform cardiovascular endurance exercises have less heart disease, more energy, less body fat, lower blood pressure and cholesterol levels, faster metabolisms, higher self-esteem, and a greater sense of well-being. So be sure to included plenty of these!

After you've warmed up with some moderately paced walking or calisthenics, you can safely move on to cardiovascular endurance exercises, which will rev up your body's motor. You'll have to become a heavy breather, however, because cardio-vascular endurance exercises done properly will make your breath come faster and your heart beat more quickly.

You can choose from a host of invigorating activities: walking, swimming, cycling, ballroom dancing, and so on. If you enjoy the outdoors, try a brisk walk or hike, or maybe some tennis. If you prefer climate-controlled conditions, why not dance or ride a stationary bike? You might also try a water aerobics class held in a heated pool.

Take advantage of the great variety of fun and exciting cardio-endurance exercises, and mix them up within your individual fitness plan. For example, you may swim during one session, ride a bike in the next, and take a jitterbug class in the third. Doing different kinds of exercise that work different parts of your body is important. You'll increase your overall fitness without putting too much stress on any one area.

Most people with arthritis tend to gravitate toward three kinds of cardio-endurance exercises — walking, cycling, and water exercises — because they're easy on the joints. You may want to start with these, then investigate other activities as you get stronger and more adventurous.

TIP

Start small, even if it's just five minutes a day. Then slowly add a couple of minutes of exercise each week until you reach the recommended 30 minutes per day at least five days a week.

WALKING

Unless you have severe trouble with your feet, ankles, knees, or hips, walking can be an ideal exercise. It's easy, inexpensive (all you really need is a good, supportive pair of shoes and some absorbent socks), and can be done just about anywhere. It also provides the weight-bearing exercise you need to keep your bones in shape without exerting the heavy impact of running or jogging.

In order to get cardio benefits, though, you'll need to work your way up to *brisk* walking. Strolling is certainly pleasant and beneficial, but you'll have to pick up the pace if you want walking to qualify as a true cardiovascular endurance exercise. That means walking fast enough to make you somewhat winded, but not gasping for breath.

CYCLING

Whether you do it by flying through the park on an autumn day or pumping away in the comfort of your own bedroom, cycling can be a great way to get your heart racing without putting much strain on your joints. Start on flat ground. Then after several sessions (if your joints permit it), raise the level of incline on your stationary bike or find a road that slopes upward slightly as you ride your outdoor bike. Take it easy, though. Strenuous uphill cycling is not recommended for those with osteoarthritis of the knees or hips.

As with walking, you'll need to pick up the pace. Coasting along is certainly pleasant but doesn't count for much if you're trying to give your heart and lungs a workout. If you're riding outdoors, look for a place free of traffic lights, pedestrians, and other impediments, because you'll have a hard time raising your heart rate and keeping it there if you're forced to stop every two minutes.

EXERCISING IN WATER

Exercising in the water is just what the doctor ordered for most arthritis sufferers. It offers overall physical conditioning and great cardio-endurance with little or no pressure on the joints. With water to buoy you, you can say goodbye to gravity's woes and get your heart pumping without feeling that nagging pain in your knees or hips.

Swimming is one of the best exercises you can do to increase your head-to-toe fitness. When you swim, more than two-thirds of the muscles in your body go into action, giving you a good total workout in a short time. It's an efficient and enjoyable way to increase your overall strength, endurance, and flexibility — and even improve your posture!

For those who like the water but aren't keen on swimming, water aerobics can be a good choice. Offered by many local YMCAs and approved by the Arthritis Foundation, these classes are held in warm water pools. Those with arthritis or other joint problems are led by a qualified instructor through a series of gentle range-of-motion, cardio-endurance, and flexibility exercises. Many people find that not only is their pain reduced during the time they're in the water, but their mobility and relief from pain are increased for hours (or even days) after a workout.

For more on the amazing benefits of exercise in general, see the nearby sidebar "Positive side effects of exercise."

Strength training

Strength-training exercises improve the ability of your muscles to do work by increasing the force they can exert (*strength*) plus the length of time they can exert that force (*endurance*). If you have arthritis, strength training is particularly important because strong, well-toned muscles and other supporting structures can help absorb the stress and strain placed on your joints during weight-bearing movement. Weak muscles force your joints to bear the brunt of impact, which encourages joint misalignment or slippage. Your weight-bearing joints (those in your spine, hips, knees, and ankles) and their supporting structures (tendons, ligaments, muscles, and so on) also need to be sturdy and strong enough to take on an additional load as your body tries to protect an injured or diseased area by shifting the weight elsewhere. Performed regularly, strength-training exercises can help fight weakness, frailty, falls, and disability.

Weight and repetition are the basis of strength training. You can build your strength by gradually increasing the amount of weight that your muscles must lift, which will make those muscles bigger and bulkier. And by increasing the number of times your muscles perform a certain movement (repetitions or reps), you can increase your endurance, which is even more important. Bulkier muscles are less flexible, more likely to be injured, and less likely to improve joint range of motion than muscles conditioned for endurance.

REMEMBER

Don't be fooled into believing that you can only do strength training with a set of barbells. When a dancer slowly lifts their leg and holds it in position, they is lifting weight — the weight of their leg as gravity pulls against it. When a swimmer pulls their arms through the water, they is working against the resistance of the water. With exercises like dancing and swimming, you don't need additional weights!

You can (and should) do different strength-enhancing exercises to vary your workouts and keep your exercise routines fresh and interesting, while toning different muscle groups. Strength-enhancing exercises include the following:

>> Isometric exercises

>> Sit-ups

>> Push-ups

>> Leg lifts

>> Weight training

>> Swimming

>> Stair climbing

>> Cross-country skiing

>> Dance or yoga (sustained poses)

>> Running

You can do two kinds of strength-training exercises — *isotonic* and *isometric*. When performing *isotonic* exercises, your muscles move against the resistance of gravity, water, light weights, or your own body weight, and your joints bend and straighten. Weight lifting and swimming are two examples.

Isometric exercises, on the other hand, are done *without* moving your joints. Muscles are contracted and released, but the joint stays in a static position. Often, your body itself provides the resistance. For example, clasping your hands in front of you and pushing them together is an isometric exercise for your arms and pectoral muscles. These exercises are great for toning your muscles and supporting structures on days when your joints are just too painful to move.

Increasing flexibility

Flexibility exercises (stretching) increase your ability to bend, reach, twist, and stretch. They help you maintain or increase your *range of motion* — the amount of movement your joints allow in various directions. Flexibility exercises also improve the elasticity of your muscles, which makes them more resistant to injury. If you have arthritis, flexibility exercises are crucial, because pain, stiffness, and restricted range of motion tend to make you move your joints less, which only increases pain, stiffness, and movement limitation over time. For more on the effect of exercise on pain and physical function, see the sidebar "What you may *not* know about exercise and arthritis," later in the chapter.

POSITIVE SIDE EFFECTS OF EXERCISE

If you don't already have enough reasons to exercise, here are a few more that don't directly relate to joint fitness but certainly boost your health in other ways. By getting regular exercise you can:

- Reduce stress
- Improve the quality of your sleep
- Increase your physical abilities
- Regain or maintain your independence
- Reduce body fat while increasing muscle mass
- Improve your balance
- Increase the activity of your immune system
- Promote relaxation
- Improve your sexual function
- Enhance your emotional health

You may think that you already bend and stretch enough while doing housework or gardening, and that you can just skip flexibility exercises. But because everyday activities don't move your joints through their full range of motion, you need to make flexibility exercises a regular part of your daily program. Try to do them every day if possible.

Easing Joint Pain with Exercise

Countless exercises can help make you stronger, more fit, more flexible, and better able to fight arthritis. Those that you choose should depend upon what you and your physical therapist feel are best for your particular condition. Having said that, we include the following exercises as good ones for stretching or strengthening the indicated areas.

TIP

For some of the exercises in this section, you'll need to use an exercise mat to protect your weight-bearing joints from excessive pressure whenever they're in contact with the floor.

Stretching your neck

Use this exercise to stretch and relieve tension in your neck muscles:

1. Sit cross-legged on your exercise mat, hands resting comfortably on your knees or thighs.

2. While facing to the front, drop your head to the right side, as if trying to touch your right ear to your right shoulder.

   Don't scrunch up your shoulders!

3. Put your right hand over the top of your head, and your left hand on top of your left shoulder.

4. Exert gentle pressure with each hand, stretching your neck.

5. Repeat on the other side.

Stretching your hand and wrist

This stretches and strengthens your fingers and wrists:

1. Make a fist.

2. Fling your fingers out to their straightened position, fingers spread.

3. Return to the fist position.

4. Repeat five times for each hand.

The following exercise increases finger and hand flexibility:

1. Open your hand flat.

2. Touch the tip of your thumb to the tip of each of your fingers, one at a time.

3. Repeat ten times per hand.

Extending the shoulder and arm

Use this exercise to strengthen your upper back and shoulder muscles:

1. Get on your hands and knees on an exercise mat.

   Make sure your neck is straight and parallel to the floor.

2. **Slowly reach your right arm out in front of you, keeping your arm straight, parallel to the floor and about the height of your ear.**

   Your fingers should point at the wall on the opposite side of the room. (See Figure 12-1.)

3. **Hold for five seconds, if possible, and then slowly return your arm to its starting position.**

4. **Repeat with your other arm, and then alternate, doing as many reps as you can manage.**

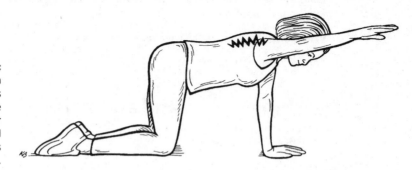

FIGURE 12-1: Shoulder arm extension. This exercise strengthens your upper back and improves posture.

© John Wiley & Sons, Inc.

Stretching your side

This exercise tones your side and back muscles and helps prevent sudden back spasms that can result from turning or twisting the wrong way.

1. **Stand straight with your feet about 18 inches apart.**

2. **Bend your left elbow, placing your left hand at your waist.**

3. **Straighten your right arm above your head while trying to keep your right shoulder level with the left one.**

4. **Bend slowly toward the left (toward your bent elbow), keeping your right arm above your head, as shown in Figure 12-2.**

5. **Hold this position for a count of five.**

   You should feel a pull in your right side. Be careful not to push your right hip to the side as your bend — that's cheating, and it can put stress on your knees.

6. **Slowly return to an upright position.**

7. **Repeat on the other side.**

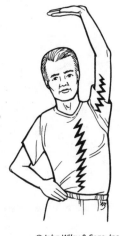

FIGURE 12-2: Side stretch. You should feel a nice pull in the muscles running from your upper arm all the way down to your hip.

Lifting your lower back and pelvis

This exercise tightens your rear-end muscles and stretches your lower back.

1. **Lie on your back on your exercise mat, knees bent and a couple of inches apart, with the soles of your feet flat on the mat.**

   Your arms should be straight and about 3 inches away from your sides, with your palms flat against the mat.

2. **Tighten your buttock muscles and slowly raise your pelvis, supporting your weight with your feet and your lower arms.**

   Try to keep your spine straight — don't arch up — but don't let your rear-end sag, either. You should have a nice straight line from your shoulders to your knees. (See Figure 12-3.)

3. **Hold this raised position for five seconds.**

4. **Slowly ease your back down, vertebrae by vertebrae, beginning with your upper back and ending with your tailbone.**

5. **Repeat slowly at least five times.**

Stretching your hamstring

Use this stretch to help you loosen up your lower back and back of your thighs (hamstrings), as well as to improve your ability to bend over.

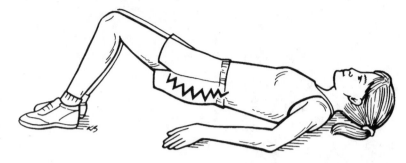

© John Wiley & Sons, Inc.

FIGURE 12-3:
Lower back and pelvic lift. A good exercise for tightening the buttocks and releasing tension in the lower back.

1. **Lie on your back on your exercise mat with your knees flexed and arms at your sides.**

2. **Bend your right knee and grab the back of your thigh with both hands.**

3. **Pull your knee toward your chest, keeping your foot pointed rather than flexed.** (Flexing stretches the sciatic nerve.)

4. **While holding onto your thigh, extend the lower part of your leg until your leg is completely straight, as shown in Figure 12-4.**

   If you can't straighten your leg in that position, lower your leg until you can straighten it. Hold for a count of five.

5. **Bend your knee and move your leg back to the mat.**

6. **Repeat with the other leg.**

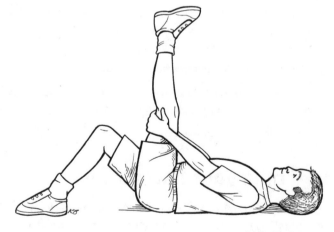

FIGURE 12-4:
Hamstring stretch. This loosens up the hip joint and stretches the back of the thigh.

© John Wiley & Sons, Inc.

TIP

If your arms aren't long enough to hold your leg while it's straightening, slide a towel or a belt around the back of your thigh and hold on to the ends of it. To benefit from this exercise, you need to keep your working leg as straight as possible, your supporting leg bent, and your back flat on the ground.

Doing mini-sit-ups

This exercise is great for tightening the abdominal muscles, which support your lower back. The mini-sit-up causes your abdominals to contract and hold at the point of maximum resistance, without putting too much strain on your back and neck muscles.

1. **Lying flat on your back on your exercise mat, bend your knees, keeping your feet flat on the floor.**

   Your knees shouldn't be more than an inch or two apart.

2. **Fold your arms across your chest and raise your head, neck, and shoulders off the floor, as shown in Figure 12-5.**

   Your head and neck will curl forward, but they shouldn't curl so far forward that your chin is on your chest.

3. **Hold this position for a count of five.**

   Try not to let your stomach muscles pop out; instead, suck them in.

4. **Slowly release and roll back down to your starting position.**

5. **Repeat this exercise five times, if possible.**

FIGURE 12-5: Mini-sit-up. This exercise tightens the abdominal muscles without putting a lot of stress and strain on the back and neck.

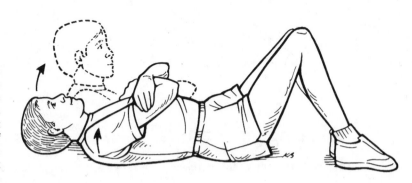

© John Wiley & Sons, Inc.

TIP

If you can't get your shoulders completely off the floor at first, don't worry. Do the best you can and work toward that goal in the long run.

Extending your hip and back leg

The buttock muscles are important in maintaining good posture. When they are contracted and "tucked under," the stomach muscles automatically contract, too. This contraction helps you support your lower back, while avoiding the sway back, stomach out, knees locked position that is so detrimental to your joints. Use this exercise to tighten up your rear-end muscles:

1. **Get on your hands and knees on an exercise mat.**

    Make sure your neck is parallel to the floor.

2. **When you feel comfortable and balanced, flex the toes of your right foot.**

3. **Slide your right leg out behind you until it's straight and supported only by your toes.**

4. **Slowly lift your right leg up until it's parallel with the floor, as shown in Figure 12-6.**

5. **Hold the position for five seconds.**

6. **Lower your leg slowly, bend it, and bring it back to its original position.**

7. **Repeat exercise with your left leg.**

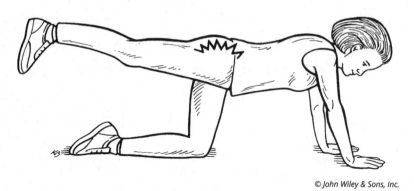

FIGURE 12-6: Hip and back leg extension. This exercise helps support your lower back by strengthening the buttock muscles.

© John Wiley & Sons, Inc.

Rotating your ankle

This exercise is great for increasing the range of motion in your ankle.

1. **Lie on your back on your exercise mat, legs bent and arms at your sides.**

2. **Raise your right leg into the air, keeping it bent, and hold onto your right thigh for support.**

3. **Rotate your foot slowly in a circle to the right, as if drawing a circle in the air with your big toe.**

4. **Rotate four times to the right and four times to the left.**

5. **Repeat the exercise with your left foot.**

Using Yoga to Ease Arthritis Pain

Yoga is an ancient practice for bringing your physical, mental, and spiritual "selves" into balance and harmony, thus achieving the highest form of good health. All of the many kinds of yoga involve assuming various sitting, standing, or lying-down postures called *asanas*. The postures are held for anywhere from seconds to minutes and are accompanied by deep breathing.

The benefits of yoga for arthritis sufferers are many, including relaxation, stress reduction, increased energy, improved flexibility, increased strength, and improved circulation. As an added bonus, many people find that regularly practicing yoga helps to relieve depression, increase alertness, and improve overall well-being.

The snake

Use this posture, or *asana*, to stretch your chest, stomach, and upper back muscles while strengthening your arms and upper body.

1. **On your exercise mat, lie face down on your stomach with your arms bent and hands palm down resting on either side of your neck, as shown in Figure 12-7a.**

2. **Pressing your hands and lower arms into the mat, slowly raise your head and upper chest until they're completely off the floor. See Figure 12-7b.**

3. **Gradually straighten your arms as you push your head, chest, and torso as far up as you can, as shown in Figure 12-7c.**

   Be sure to keep your pelvis flat on the floor and your legs extended.

4. **Hold the position for a count of five.**

5. **Slowly bend your arms as you ease your torso down to the mat.**

6. **Gradually return to the starting position with your face on the mat.**

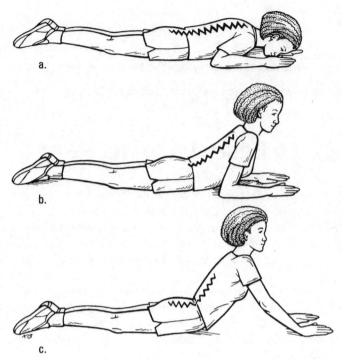

FIGURE 12-7: The snake is a great stretch for the upper back, chest, and stomach muscles.

The cat

This exercise helps increase spinal flexibility.

1. Get on your hands and knees on an exercise mat.

Make sure your neck is parallel to the floor. Your knees should be about 12 inches apart, with your arms straight down and your fingers pointing forward. See Figure 12-8a.

2. Contract your stomach muscles and roll your head forward until your chin touches your chest as you round your back upward toward the ceiling.

Your entire torso should be contracted, forming a hollow. See Figure 12-8b.

3. Gradually release the contraction and roll your head back to its original position.

4. Arch your back slightly, creating a curve going the opposite way.

Don't stick your rear-end out, let your stomach muscles relax, or sway your back to accomplish this position; these things can put too much pressure on the disks between your vertebrae. See Figure 12-8c.

5. Repeat, slowly forming the hump, and then ease into a slight arch.

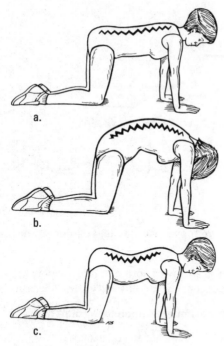

FIGURE 12-8:
The cat.
Contracting your
stomach muscles
then arching your
back helps
increase spinal
flexibility.

The pretzel

Use this exercise to stretch your inner thigh and hip.

1. Lie on your back on your exercise mat, legs bent and arms at your sides.

2. Cross your right leg over your left leg, with your right foot just clearing your left knee.

3. Grab your left thigh with both hands and pull it toward you while keeping your legs in the crossed position, as shown in Figure 12-9.

4. Hold this position for at least five seconds.

5. Slowly release, and then repeat with the opposite leg.

Knee-to-chest stretch

This exercise loosens up the hip joint while stretching your lower back and buttock muscles:

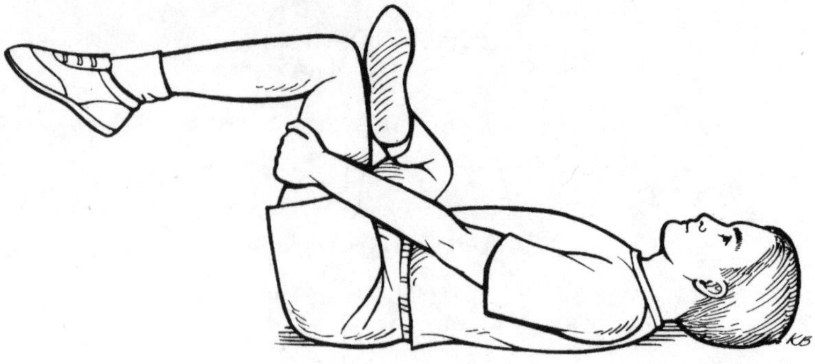

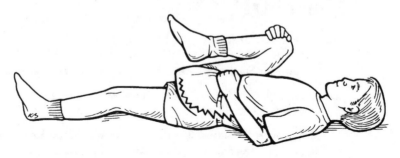

FIGURE 12-9:
The pretzel. A nice relaxing stretch that loosens the hip and increases the flexibility of the inner thigh.

© John Wiley & Sons, Inc.

1. **Lie on your back on your exercise mat, legs extended and arms at your sides.**

2. **Bend your right leg, grab it with both hands just below the knee, and pull it gently toward your chest as far as it will go, as shown in Figure 12-10.**

3. **Hold your leg at its maximum position for a count of five.**

   Make sure your other leg is straight and on the floor.

4. **Slowly release and repeat with your left leg.**

FIGURE 12-10:
Knee-to-chest stretch. This stretch is great for your lower back, buttock, muscles, and hip joint.

© John Wiley & Sons, Inc.

The spinal twist

Exercises that twist the spine are good for maintaining the flexibility of the spine and the oblique muscles — muscles that run diagonally along your side and allow you to reach for something in back of you without completely turning around.

1. Lie on your back on your exercise mat, legs extended and arms at your sides.

2. Bend your right knee and bring it toward your chest, grabbing hold of it with both hands behind the thigh.

3. Extend your right arm straight out to the side, keeping it flat on the floor to make a 90-degree angle to your body.

4. Using your left hand, pull your right knee across your body, as if to touch it to the floor beside your left hip.

    Your right foot should stay in contact with your left knee, and your right shoulder should stay flat on the floor. Your left leg should stay straight.

5. Turn your head to the right, as if looking at the right wall.

6. Hold this pose for a count of ten, and then slowly return to your original position.

7. Repeat, bending your left knee this time.

    One time on each side is sufficient.

The child's pose

This posture stretches your entire back, your buttock muscles, and your upper arms, while putting you into a dreamy state of relaxation.

1. Sit on your mat with your legs tucked under you, heels directly under the buttocks.

    Your knees should be about 12 inches apart.

2. Roll your upper body head first toward the floor, until you can place your forehead on the floor in front of your knees.

3. Place your palms on the floor on either side of your head.

4. Slowly extend your arms in front of you as far as possible.

    Your buttocks should stay in contact with your heels, and your feet should stay on the floor.

5. Hold this position for a count of ten, then slowly return to the sitting position.

6. Repeat five times.

Using Chair Exercises to Save Your Joints

If you like the idea of exercising without putting weight on your joints, consider *chair exercises,* which are performed while sitting in a straight-back chair. The following subsections give instructions for some simple chair exercises that can be used for warm-ups (or for aerobic exericses, if performed more vigorously).

Chair marching

This is a good one to do with music — try a Souza march! But be careful not to slam your feet on the ground in your enthusiasm.

1. **Sit up tall in your chair with feet planted on the ground and pointing straight ahead.**

2. **March your feet in place, beginning slowly then gradually picking up the pace.**

   Be sure to lift your thighs as far off the chair seat as possible.

Chair running

Follow the directions for chair marching, but move at a much faster pace. It's fair to "run" on your toes (it's too fast a pace to put your whole foot down), and you won't be able to lift your thigh off the chair as high as you do during chair marching. But a couple of minutes of chair running are guaranteed to make you "glow" and start shedding your sweater.

Chair dancing

You can do the hora, the heel-toe polka, or the shuffle-off-to-Buffalo all while sitting in a chair. Not only will it warm you up, it's fun!

In addition to the following, many more dance steps can be performed while in a chair; it only takes a little imagination. Try out some of your favorites. You may be surprised by how enjoyable this kind of exercise can be.

The hora

As with all dancing, the right music can make you forget you're exercising and imagine you're just kicking up your heels. Music for the hora can be found under "Jewish folk music" online.

1. **Starting with your right foot, step to the side.**
2. **Cross behind your right foot with your left.**
3. **Step to the side with your right.**
4. **Do a small kick with your left foot.**
5. **Then kick with your right foot.**
6. **Reverse it: step side with your left, back with your right, side with your left, kick right, kick left.**

Heel-toe polka

The count should go: heel, toe, step-together-step, or 1, 2, 1-2-3.

1. **Start with your right foot. Touch your right heel to the floor, and then touch your right toe to the floor.**
2. **Step to your right side with your right foot, then bring your left to meet it.**
3. **Step to the right again with your right foot.**
4. **Reverse: Left heel touches, then left toe, step side with left, bring right to meet it, step left.**

Shuffle-off-to-Buffalo

The sequence goes hop-step, cross, step, cross, step, cross, step, with a count of "and one and two and three and four."

1. **Begin with both feet all the way to the left of your chair. Lift your right foot slightly off the floor and "hop" on your left foot.**
2. **Step to the side with your right foot.**
3. **Cross your left behind the right.**
4. **Step right again, cross left behind.**
5. **Step right again, cross left behind.**
6. **Step right.**
7. **Reverse, starting with your left foot.**

Chair fencing

Although true fencing is a real strain on the knees — all that deep lunging! — chair fencing spares your knees while giving your arms a good workout.

1. Sitting up straight, extend your right leg forward as far as you can while keeping your foot flat on the floor, toes pointing straight ahead.

2. Extend your right arm forward, in a thrusting position, with left arm against your side, elbow bent and fist curled against the front of your shoulder.

3. Reverse, extending your left leg and left arm. Continue to change positions, as if you were "fencing."

WHAT YOU MAY *NOT* KNOW ABOUT EXERCISE AND ARTHRITIS

If you have arthritis, getting up and moving around may be the last thing you want to do, especially when you're in pain. But studies have shown that exercise may actually be an arthritis sufferer's best friend because it can lessen pain, improve joint function, and even protect against the development of certain kinds of arthritis. Here are a few fascinating facts about exercise and arthritis:

- Those with OA of the knee often experience less pain if they use free weights or machines with fixed weights to strengthen their knees *before* exercising.

- A team of Dutch researchers found that moderate-to-high intensity exercise (75 minutes, twice a week) performed over a two-year period helped increase functional ability in RA patients, with no additional damage to the large joints. This finding was surprising because RA patients are often told that strenuous activity can increase joint inflammation.

- Kids who engage in vigorous physical activity may enjoy some protection against OA later on. This is partly due to the fact that exercise stimulates the production of cartilage. An Australian study found that inactive children had 22 to 25 percent less cartilage than those who were just mildly active. But cartilage volume in the knee in children who were very active increased up to 15 percent per year in boys and 10 percent per year in girls. However, too much high-impact exercise, or sports that contribute to joint injuries, can lead to premature OA.

- Both high-intensity *and* low-intensity aerobic exercise seem to be equally effective in improving joint function, gait, pain, and aerobic capacity for people who have OA of the knee.

- T'ai chi, the ancient Chinese form of exercise that involves slow, fluid movements, helps improve physical functioning and ease the symptoms of OA. Those who participate in t'ai chi exercise programs (one-hour sessions at least twice a week) can expect to see improved walking speed, bending ability, arm function, balance, management of arthritis symptoms, control of fatigue, and ability to do household tasks. One study found that this was true even for those with severe limitations, including obesity or the use of a walker or oxygen tank.

Maximizing the Healing Effects of Exercise

Performing the proper exercises on a regular basis is a vital part of almost any arthritis treatment program. But to gain maximum benefits, you'll also need to be aware of proper exercise techniques, and always make sure that you're completely warmed up before exercising. A warm bath or shower can help, but you should also do some light cardio or strengthening exercises until you break a sweat. If you have painful, inflamed joints, you may find that icing them before your warm-up helps keep the pain at a minimum.

As for exercising when you're in the midst of an arthritis flare, begin with a warm shower or bath, and add some gentle stretching to get a little circulation going. Take it easy, though. If stretching causes too much pain, stop. You can always try again later.

Warming up your muscles through light exercise or a warm shower is just one idea for making the most of your exercise sessions. Some other helpful tips include:

>> Start slowly with a program you can do fairly easily.

>> If you feel dizzy, nauseated, faint, or there is a tightness in your chest, stop exercising and call your doctor.

>> Pick a cardio-endurance activity that you can do continuously for ten minutes, if possible. (If not, try five minutes or even one minute, and gradually increase your time.)

>> Make your cardiovascular-endurance exercises vigorous enough so that you sweat, your heart beats faster, and your breath comes more rapidly. Find a pace at which you feel slightly short of breath but can still maintain a conversation.

>> Do your cardiovascular endurance exercises three days a week (every other day, with one day off per week) for at least 10 minutes, working your way up to 30 minutes.

>> Exercise at a slower pace to cool down after doing cardio-endurance exercises. For example, you can walk slowly until your heart rate returns to normal.

>> Do your strength-training exercises three days a week, on the days you don't do cardiovascular endurance exercises. Leave one day a week free for rest.

>> Do some flexibility exercises (stretching) before your strengthening routine, and then again afterwards. This will help decrease the likelihood of injury to your muscles.

>> Ask your physical therapist to supervise your stretching sessions, at least in the beginning. Incorrect stretching can cause more harm than good. Stretching sessions should last from 10 to 20 minutes, with each stretch held at least five seconds. As you become more flexible, gradually increase the holding time to 10, 20, or even 30 seconds. Stretch every day, if possible.

>> Always stretch slowly and carefully — don't bounce. Move your body to its maximum position, hold it in place for at least 30 seconds, then ease into your stretch just a little more before releasing.

>> Don't hold your breath while stretching — breathe slowly and deeply and try to relax into the stretch.

One of the most important things you can do to help make exercise a permanent part of your life is to keep a positive attitude toward yourself, your body, and your program. Remember, the more you exercise, the easier it gets.

Although we've said that exercise may help ease your current joint pain and lessen tomorrow's pain, we don't suggest that you go for a jog when your arthritic knee is acting up or do push-ups when your wrist aches. If an exercise or activity hurts, or causes your joints to become inflamed, *stop immediately*. Pain is a message from your body telling you that tissue is being damaged. Respect the pain. Engage in a different kind of exercise, or call it a day and try again tomorrow.

Designing Your Workout Program

In this section, we tell you how to make your exercise program everything it needs to be to improve your health, keep you safe, and maximize the benefits of exercise.

What you discover by reading this book isn't a substitute for professional advice. Doing the wrong exercises, or even the right exercises in the wrong way, can make your condition worse. Enlist professionals to help you design your exercise program, then supervise you as you exercise so you do the right exercises in the right way.

Your doctor can advise you as to which kinds of exercise are helpful for your condition, how much is too much, and when to stop. A physical therapist can also be extremely helpful by suggesting appropriate exercises, teaching you correct techniques and positioning, and urging you on when it's time to increase the length and/or intensity of your workout. (An *exercise physiologist* can do much of what a physical therapist does, but make sure that he or she has experience working with arthritis patients.) And an occupational therapist can teach you how to use your joints in the least stressful ways.

Considering the basic game plan

With the help of your healthcare professionals, you can begin to devised and carry out an exercise plan. Ideally, you'll do some kind of exercise six days a week, taking one day off to rest. A good exercise session contains each of the following elements:

WARNING

>> **Warm-up:** A good warm-up lasts at least ten minutes and should make you break a sweat. If your joints can handle it, calisthenics (jumping jacks, jogging in place, and so on) make ideal warm-up exercises. If not, try doing the slow version of the activity you plan to do next — slow walking or relaxed cycling, for example — before beginning a brisk walk or bike trip.

Don't begin your warm-up with big stretches (for example, the hamstring stretch). Stretching a cold muscle invites injury. Save your flexibility exercises until after the bulk of your exercise session has been completed. (A small amount of gentle stretching is okay during the warm-up, but be careful.)

>> **Cardiovascular endurance exercises:** According to the American College of Sports Medicine, you should do at least 20 minutes of continuous cardiovascular endurance exercises at least three times a week. This means doing 20 minutes of walking, cycling, or water exercises (or something similar) every other day. However, if you haven't exercised in a while or you're experiencing a lot of joint pain, this may not be possible. The best idea is to start wherever you are right now. If you can do only five minutes worth of aerobic exercises, then so be it. Perhaps by next week you'll be able to increase it to six minutes. The point is to get moving and gradually improve.

If you find that you're doing great at your present level and aren't experiencing any physical problems, you can increase the length of your cardio workout and/or the number of sessions you do per week. Just make sure you don't do so much that you exhaust yourself or cause injuries. See the earlier section, "Building cardiovascular endurance" to find out more.

>> **Strength-training exercises:** On the days that you don't do cardio exercises, do about 20 minutes of strength training, in the form of weight training, swimming, stair climbing, or other exercises that involve pitting your muscles against some form of resistance. Check out the earlier section, "Strength training" to find out more.

>> **Flexibility exercises:** You should do exercises that involve stretching, bending, twisting, and reaching six or seven days a week for at least 10 minutes. To avoid muscle strains and sprains, flexibility exercises should be performed only after your body is well warmed-up. The safest strategy is to stretch at the end of an exercise session.

>> **Cool-down:** At the end of your exercise session, it's important to cool down for five to ten minutes to help your heart rate, breathing, and blood pressure return to normal. Begin by tapering off your activity; for example, slow your brisk walking down to an easy stroll. When your breathing has become easy again, you may want to do some gentle stretches, which will not only improve your flexibility, but reduce your risk of future injury, remove waste products from your muscle tissue, and lower the amount of muscle soreness you'll feel later on.

Figuring out if you're working hard enough

First of all, as long as you're doing some form of exercise, you should be congratulated! A whopping 33 percent of American adults, many with no excuses for their idleness, get no exercise at all. If you're at least making an effort, especially on a daily basis, you're definitely on your way to better fitness and better health.

But to get the most out of your cardiovascular endurance exercises without running the risk of exhaustion, you need to remember two things while exercising:

>> Your breath should be coming faster and harder, but not to the point where you're panting.

>> Your heart should be beating faster, but not pounding in your ears!

So how do you figure out if you're doing enough, but not too much? Try using the Target Heart Rate system.

1. **First, subtract your age from 220.** (Example: 220 – 60 = 160)

2. **Then, multiply the answer by .9 and by .6** (example: 160 x .9 = 144; 160 x .6 = 99).

Your two answers indicate the upper and lower ends of your target heart rate zone. That means that for maximum cardio–endurance benefits, your heart rate should fall somewhere between these two numbers while you're exercising — in this case somewhere between 144 and 99 beats per minute.

To figure your current heart rate, all you need is a watch or clock with a second hand and your own fingers:

1. **Place your index and second fingers across the inside of your opposite wrist.** There's a little "well" on the thumb-side of the tendon that runs up the middle of your wrist. Your two fingers should easily slide over that tendon and into this "well," where it should be easy to feel your pulse.

2. With an eye on the second-hand of your watch or clock, count the number of pulse beats you feel in 15 seconds.

3. Multiply by four, and you have the number of times your heart beats in a minute.

If you do this either during or immediately after your cardio-endurance session, you should be able to figure out whether you're "in the zone" or not.

TIP

Here's an easy way to find out if you're working hard enough (or too hard) while exercising. You should be breathing too heavily to be able to sing, but not so heavily that you can't talk. If you can sing while you're exercising, you may want to step up the intensity a bit. But if you find you can't catch your breath enough to talk during exercise, you're probably overdoing it.

Taking it easy!

REMEMBER

Whenever you start a new exercise program, add a new activity, or increase the frequency or duration of your workout, the number one rule is this: Start slowly. Many would-be exercise enthusiasts are sidelined by doing too much too soon, winding up either injured or just plain burned out! Your exercise sessions should emphasize enjoyment. They should require some effort but should never be grueling. If you're more than just a little bit sore a day or two after the workout, you've done too much.

Finding a good class

After you've done some initial training with a physical therapist or exercise physiologist, you may feel ready to join a class. You can enjoy several advantages by working out in groups — it's a lot less expensive than private instruction, classes usually have more space and a greater variety of equipment, and the friendships formed among classmates can make exercise more fun. But where can you find a class suited to the special needs of those with arthritis? The best bet is to contact your local chapter of the YMCA and ask about its Aquatics Program for people with arthritis. At YMCA's that offer this program, the pool is typically kept at about 83 degrees, and soft music is often played in the background. A specially trained instructor takes the class through a variety of stretching, strengthening, and aerobic exercises, and the buoyancy of the water allows participants to increase overall fitness without putting excessive strain on their joints

TIP

The Arthritis Foundation also offers a few exercise DVDs for those with moderate to severe arthritis. See Appendix B for more information.

Chapter **13**

The Right Stride and Other Ways to Protect Your Joints

Y ou may not realize that how you sit, stand, and walk can help determine how healthy or hurtful your joints are today and how well they'll fare tomorrow.

You probably think that sitting in a chair or walking down the street is a natural behavior that you instinctively perform correctly. After all, you've been doing these things all of your life. But believe it or not, almost everybody misuses their joints by doing some of these things incorrectly. And over time, repeated abuse of your joints can cause permanent tissue damage and a lot of unnecessary pain. Luckily, by using certain joint-saving techniques, you can take undue pressure off your joints today, thereby helping to prevent tomorrow's problems. In this chapter, we tell you how you can take a load off your joints while doing everyday things that you probably don't realize can be harmful.

Believing in Biomechanics

Biomechanics is the study of how your body handles the impact of its own weight against gravity. When your body is in a "biomechanically correct" position, the force of the impact created by movement is spread out over a large area. During correct walking, for example, when your heel strikes the ground, the impact travels up your entire leg and is absorbed along the way by your foot, ankle, knee, and hip, and all of their supporting tissues. But during incorrect walking, the brunt of the impact may be taken by the ankle and knee alone. By distributing the load as widely as possible and positioning the joints for maximum impact absorption, joint stress and damage can be reduced considerably.

Everybody should use correct biomechanical (joint-saving) techniques. But for those who already have joint problems, observing correct biomechanics is absolutely essential. Still, most people have a hard time analyzing their own posture or the ways they move, which means they also have a hard time figuring out how they may be overstressing their joints. So you may want to be evaluated by a practitioner who specializes in biomechanics, such as a physical therapist or a physician trained in sports medicine or osteopathy.

In addition, you may want to consider a practitioner trained in one of the following areas to help you with overall body alignment (Appendix B tells you where to find more information about each):

>> **The Alexander Technique:** Developed by F. Mathias Alexander, an actor who couldn't shake a lengthy case of laryngitis, the basis of this technique is that faulty posture and poor movement habits contribute to problems in both the physical and emotional realms. (Alexander found that his laryngitis was the result of tension and moving improperly.) Students are taught to stand, walk, and sit in ways that are less stressful to the body through the use of movement, touch, and awareness.

>> **The Feldenkrais Method:** Moshe Feldenkrais, a physicist, martial arts expert, and engineer, devised this method to heal a sports-related knee injury without resorting to surgery. By changing unhealthy movement habits, breathing deeply, and improving the self-image, patients begin to ease their pain. Classes are held in which patients are taken through exercises that increase flexibility, range of motion, and body awareness.

>> **Trager Approach:** Milton Trager, MD, believed that stress and pain originate in the mind and that bodywork can change the mental and physical habits that lead to them. Although the Trager Approach is more like a massage (you lie on a table and the practitioner manipulates your body), the gentle moving of your body (rocking, stretching, and so on) can help you relax and increase your mind-body awareness.

Although no bona fide studies prove that any of these methods work for arthritis, many physical therapists extol their benefits for rheumatoid arthritis, osteoarthritis, and fibromyalgia. In the end, you'll have to decide for yourself whether or not one or more of these methods is worthwhile. (Remember that it may take several sessions and a significant investment of time and money before you can come to a well-founded decision.) But if one of these methods does make you feel better, great! Just make sure you find a certified therapist (see Appendix B), listen to your body, and don't do anything that causes you pain.

Waxing Ergonomic at Your Workstation

With so many of us permanently wed to the computer, the incidence of neck, back, wrist, and hand problems has risen phenomenally, giving birth to a field of study called ergonomics. *Ergonomics* involves the design of equipment that "fits" the body and allows it to function in its least stressful positions. As a result, bodily stress, strain, fatigue, and repetitive motion injuries can be reduced.

TIP

When sitting at the computer, think 90-degree angles. Your head and torso should be erect, as if a piece of string attached to the top of your head is pulling you toward the ceiling. Your chin, arms, thighs, and feet should make 90-degree angles to your body as you type. See Figure 13-1 for an example.

Remember that angling your neck and head downward to read is stressful to your neck. A bookstand or a document holder that attaches to the side of your computer can help you maintain the proper position of your head and neck while reading printed material. When you're sitting at your desk and working at your computer, your body should be aligned as shown in Figure 13-1.

Take a look at your workstations (at work and at home) and see if they meet the following requirements. If not, start making ergonomically correct changes today!

>> The top of your computer screen should be just below eye level.

>> Your eyes should be 18 to 28 inches away from the screen.

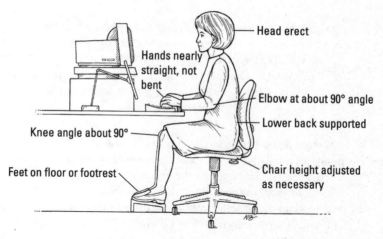

FIGURE 13-1:
Proper sitting
position at the
computer.

Head erect

Hands nearly straight, not bent

Elbow at about 90° angle

Lower back supported

Knee angle about 90°

Feet on floor or footrest

Chair height adjusted as necessary

© John Wiley & Sons, Inc.

>> Your chin should be at a 90-degree angle to your neck when you look at the screen.

>> Shoulders should be relaxed but not hunched over as you type. Forearms should be at a 90-degree angle to your body, and your wrists and hands should be flat (not bent, flexed, or curled) on the keyboard.

>> The chair should have adjustable armrests that support both your forearms and elbows at a 90-degree angle. This eliminates neck strain and positions the wrists properly.

>> The chair's built-in lumbar support, a rolled-up towel, or a cylinder-shaped pillow should support your lower back.

>> Knees should be bent, creating a 90-degree angle between your upper and lower legs.

>> Feet should be flat on the floor.

TIP

Save your own neck! Don't hold your phone with your shoulder as you talk. Either hold it with your hand or get a headset.

REMEMBER

Even if your workstation is ergonomically perfect, sitting in one position for too long can wreak havoc on your body. Every 15 minutes or so, get up, stretch, and move around a little to get your circulation going and relieve muscular stress and strain. Do some head rolls, shoulder rolls, and neck stretches. Gently stretch your fingers toward the back of each wrist. Shake your arms and hands and let them dangle loose at your side. Your body will thank you for it!

Standing Tall: Body Alignment

You can start improving your posture right now, just by becoming aware of certain general principles. Correct posture doesn't just mean a straight back; it's a group effort involving many parts of the body.

Focusing on feet

As you might imagine, standing up straight starts at the ground level. The way you position and use your feet determines how the rest of your body functions.

You should stand with your feet slightly apart and toes pointing forward or just a little turned out. *Turnout* means the toes are pointed away from the center of the body. If you think of your feet as the hands of a clock, pointing at 12 when they're straight forward, a slight turnout would put your left foot at 11 o'clock and your right foot at 1 o'clock.

Distribute your weight evenly across your heel, along the inner edge of the outside of your foot, and up to the ball of your foot. (Don't walk on the outside "rim" of your foot, but don't transfer your weight inward toward your arch, either.) The weight should also be borne by your big toe, second and third toes, and on the ball of the foot directly under the big toe. Figure 13-2 shows an example of the proper distribution of weight on the foot.

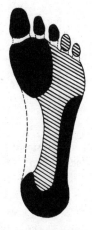

FIGURE 13-2: Proper distribution of weight on the sole of the foot.

© John Wiley & Sons, Inc.

WARNING

Many people carry their weight primarily on the inner edge of their feet, in a line that runs directly from the big toe down to the arch side of the heels. This causes the arches to collapse and the ankles to roll inward or *pronate*. Because the feet and ankles make up the base of the body, pronation throws the alignment out of whack all the way up. (Can you imagine the result if the Eiffel Tower had pronated ankles?) Pronation is a major cause of poor posture, and if you pronate, simply trying to stand up straighter won't solve your posture problem. You need to correct the pronation first. (You may need to see a physical therapist to help you correct this problem.)

If you're a pronator, try rolling your weight more toward the outer edge of your feet, but not so far that your big toe is no longer bearing weight. See Figure 13-3 for the correct and incorrect position of the ankles.

A. Correct

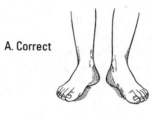

B. Incorrect

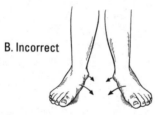

© John Wiley & Sons, Inc.

Bending your knees – just a bit!

Another cause of misalignment is *locked knees*, in which the front of the knee is completely straight (with no give to it at all) and the back of the knee is swayed backwards or *hyperextended.*

Many people adopt the locked knees position, because standing this way requires less muscular effort: Your leg and rear-end muscles aren't really holding you up; it's your leg bones locked into an unbending position. It's as if your upper body is perched on two stilts. The locked knee position is tough on knee joints, because it forces them into misalignment. But it's even worse for the lower back, which automatically sways in response (called *lordosis* or *swayback*), which leads to excess pressure on the spine that can cause pain, discomfort, and decreased mobility.

The locked-knees habit is a hard one to break, because most people are completely unaware that they're doing it. If you have this habit, remind yourself to keep your knees slightly bent whenever you're standing, especially for long periods of time. Specifically, this means when you're standing in line at the grocery store or bank, when you're ironing, doing dishes, waiting for a streetlight to change, or when you're standing over your child while she does homework. Standing with slightly bent knees takes a little more effort, but you'll be building up your "good posture muscles" while you work on healthier joint alignment.

TIP

If you're standing in line at the movies, you can also ease the pressure on your knees by shifting your weight subtly back and forth from foot to foot. Don't put all of your weight on one foot; just transfer the bulk of the burden. If you find yourself standing for a long time (for instance, while ironing), you might try putting one foot up on a stool, which helps to flatten your back and keep you from slouching.

"Unswaying" your lower back

Your pelvic bones should face straight forward like headlights on the front of a car. If yours point slightly downward, you may have a swayback — a lower back with an excessive curve. Swaying your back often results from locked knees and relaxed stomach muscles. A major cause of back pain, swaying puts extra pressure on the ligaments, muscles, and joints in your spine.

TIP

If you're wondering whether you have a swayback, try this test:

1. **Stand with your back to a wall and assume your typical relaxed posture.**

2. **Slide your hand behind your lower back into the space between your back and the wall.**

3. **Your hand should almost be able to touch both your back and the wall at the same time.**

   If you have extra room between your hand and your back, you're probably swaying your back. Try contracting your buttock muscles and tucking them under a bit in order to flatten your lower back. Contracting your stomach muscles will also help.

TIP

Surprisingly, one of the best ways to protect your lower back is to keep your stomach muscles firm and toned. If the stomach muscles are weak, your center of gravity will be thrown off, your posture distorted, your back muscles and ligaments strained, and the discs in your lower back overly stressed. So, rather than just "letting it all hang out" when your'e sitting or standing, contract your stomach muscles and tuck your rear-end under a bit. Your posture will automatically improve, the pressure on your lower back will ease, and you'll give these your stomach and gluteal muscles a mini-workout.

Relaxing your shoulders

Your shoulders should line up with your ears — not pushed forward or pinned back behind you. Rounding the shoulders is a common bad habit that lengthens the upper back muscles and exaggerates the upper back curve while causing the chest cavity to cave in. Not only is this hard on your back and neck, but it's also a very low-energy position. Your lungs can't fill themselves to capacity when your chest is sunken.

Pull your shoulders back to a *midline position* (pulling too far back will throw off your alignment), and press down the area between your neck and the shoulders, lengthening your neck. Raised shoulders are full of tension that will eventually express itself as neck or back pain.

Holding your head high

The average human head weighs around 11 pounds, so no wonder your neck sometimes bows under the strain of holding it up! The back of your neck should have a gentle forward curve to it that's similar to the shape of a banana. But many people jut their heads forward (known as a *forward head*), which distorts the natural shape of the neck and puts excessive pressure on the vertebrae in the lower part of the neck, just above the shoulders.

A forward head is the natural result of the round-shoulders, caved-in-chest position that so many of us assume. To correct this, first pull your shoulders back until they line up with your ears, and open up your chest. Then gently pull your chin in toward your neck — not to the point of making a double chin, but a little more than what feels natural to you. Your eyes should look straight ahead and your chin should be parallel to the floor as you do this.

Putting the posture points together

From stem-to-stern, here are the elements that make up the most efficient and least stressful ways to position your body:

>> Head erect, with chin slightly pulled in

>> Neck long

>> Shoulders relaxed and slightly pulled back so they line up with your ears

>> Buttock muscles slightly tightened and tucked under to counteract a swayback

>> Stomach muscles contracted

>> Knees slightly bent

>> Ankles directly over the feet (not pronated)

>> Feet apart, with weight evenly distributed across the heels, the first three toes, and the ball of the foot directly under the big toe

Now that you know how to stand correctly, you'll be able to alleviate plenty of uneven wear and tear on your joints. Of course, you don't just stand around all day — you move, too! Fortunately, just as you can save your joints by standing correctly, you can also save them by moving in the proper ways.

Reducing Joint Stress with the Right Stride

Our Aunt Bessie used to say, "My mother never taught me how to walk correctly which is why I have bad ankles today." We all pooh-poohed this idea (although not to her face). How ridiculous, we thought. Walking is just putting one foot in front of another! What was Bessie's mother supposed to do, other than get her up on her feet and let her go?

Today we know that dear old Aunt Bessie was right — there's a correct way to walk, as well as plenty of incorrect ways. And no matter how natural it may feel to you, walking incorrectly will throw off your body's alignment. The end result can be pain, uneven wear and tear on your joints, and even permanent joint damage. Think of a car that's out of alignment: Eventually some areas of the tires will wear smooth while others still have plenty of traction. If this goes on long enough, the tires will become worthless, and you'll have to buy a whole new set. The same is true of your joints — although buying a whole new set isn't usually an option! See Figures 13-4 and 13-5 for the correct position of the feet and the proper angle of the body when walking.

Correct walking is based on the principles of good posture with just a few additions:

>> Turn your feet out slightly, just 15 or 20 degrees (see Figure 13-4). Feet that are turned out more than about 20 degrees (think ballet dancer), or pointed straight ahead, or turned slightly inward (think pigeon-toed) will throw off your body alignment.

>> Make sure your heel is centered as it strikes the ground. (Remember: Avoid "rocking in" on your ankles, otherwise known as pronating.)

>> Your feet should be about 8 to 10 inches apart as you walk. (Don't cross one foot over the other as you step, unless you're a super-model on the runway.)

>> Keep your knees in an ever-so-slightly flexed position at all times (no "locking").

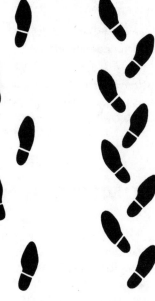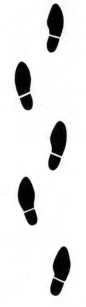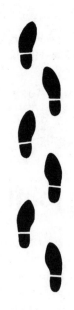

FIGURE 13-4:
Which way do
your toes point?

A. Proper position of
feet when walking

B. Too much
turnout

C. Not enough
turnout

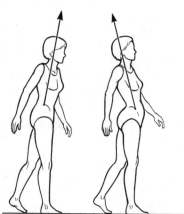

FIGURE 13-5:
Proper angle of
the body
when walking.

A. Proper-Upper
body angled forward

B. Improper-Upper
body angled backward

>> Swing your arms naturally as you walk, moving them in a straight line forward and back, not around your body. Palms should face inward toward your thighs.

>> Keep your head erect, with your eyes and chin just slightly lower than horizontal level.

>> Tilt your body slightly forward, keeping your weight mostly on the balls of your feet. This will bring your center of gravity forward and help stamp out the old locked-knees, swayback, stomach-out alignment. See Figure 13-5 for an example.

Saving Your Joints When Hitting the Hay

Remember when you were a kid and one of the most fun things in the world was to fly through the air and belly flop on your parents' bed? This approach is the exact opposite of the way you should lie down today.

The best way to go from upright to lying flat is to follow these steps:

1. **Sit on the edge of the bed.**

2. **Support your body weight by placing your hands flat on the mattress to one side of your body.**

   You may need to bend one of your arms and lean on your elbow.

3. **Draw your legs up, knees bent, until you can lie on your side.**

4. **Adjust your arms, legs, and pillows until you are in a comfortable position.**

Although most people arise by sitting straight up in bed and then throwing their legs over the side, it's much easier on your joints if you follow these steps:

1. **Scoot over to the edge of the bed while lying on your side, facing the edge of the mattress.**

2. **Place your hands flat on the mattress and push yourself up while you simultaneously swing your legs down to the floor.**

   The weight of your legs counterbalances the weight of your upper body and helps pull you to a sitting position.

TIP

If you're lying on the floor during an exercise session and you want to sit up, don't just throw your body up like you're doing a sit-up. Roll to your side and push off with your hands. You'll help save both your back and your neck in the long run.

Painful joints can make it hard to sleep, and your pain can get worse when you're tired. You can also increase joint pain if you sleep in the wrong position. It's best to sleep on your side or your back, rather than your stomach, which forces your neck to take a twisted position. For less pain and joint stress during sleep, try to keep your head, neck, spine and hips in a straight line.

>> If you're a side sleeper, use a pillow that keeps your neck in line with your spine; not propped up too high or drooping toward your supporting shoulder. A small pillow between your knees will help your hips stay in alignment.

>> If you're a back sleeper, use a fairly flat pillow that won't make your neck jut forward, and place a pillow under your knees to help maintain the normal curve of your lower back. You might also want to put a small pillow or rolled towel under the small of your back for additional support.

Just changing your sleeping position can do a lot to decrease arthritis pain and help you get some much-needed rest!

Lifting Without Losing It

By now, everybody should know that you don't just bend over to pick up a heavy load. This position puts great stress and strain on your back muscles, especially those in the lower back. But if you think about how most people pick up small children, you'll realize that improper lifting goes on all the time.

Lifting any size load (even baby-sized ones) should always be done this way:

1. **Make sure the load is as close to your body as possible before lifting it.**

   The farther away an object is, the greater the strain on your lower back.

2. **Keeping your back straight and your neck in line with your spine, bend your knees until you can get your hands under the load.**

   Use two hands for lifting instead of one.

3. **After you have a good grasp, rise by straightening your legs, while keeping your back straight at all times.**

Setting down a load should be done in the same way; just reverse the process. And whenever possible, slide the load along the floor instead of lifting it.

WARNING

If you feel pain while lifting, you're overdoing it. Stop immediately and find another way to get the job done.

Chapter **14**

Controlling Your Stress, Aggression, and Depression

W e used to believe that pain was simply a matter of an uncomfortable impulse traveling from the "ouch point," through the nerves, and to the brain. For example, say the bones in your right knee were rubbing together. The nerves would send a pain message up to your brain, and you'd feel a throbbing, grinding, burning sensation in your knee.

But in 1965, two doctors decided that it wasn't quite that simple. They introduced the "Gate Theory of Pain," which suggests that "gates" exist along the nerve pathways. Like the locks on a canal, these gates can raise or lower to either let pain messages through or block them. This means they *don't* automatically have to open wide in response to every pain message.

Several factors influence the opening and closing of the gates — including your feelings about pain and your experiences with it. Here are some of the things that can get those gates swinging one way or the other:

>> **The way you think about the pain.** Not only what kind of pain, when it arises, and where it occurs, but also your perception of its intensity, duration, and quality.

>> **The way you feel about the pain.** Emotions that accompany your pain, such as fear, depression, anger, and despair . . . or acceptance and the belief that you don't need to worry about it.

>> **Your tendency to take action in response to the pain.** For example, whether you tend to isolate yourself from others when you're hurt, immediately take pain pills, or engage in positive self-help measures.

>> **Your prior experience with pain.** Memories, comparison of this pain to others, your perception of your own coping ability, and so on.

In other words, pain is more than a physical problem at the "ouch point." Your thoughts will help determine whether the pain messages race through the gates to the brain, move at a more leisurely pace, or crawl slowly along.

Understanding Why We Hurt More Than We Have To

The bad news is that many of us hurt more than we have to, because we're quick to think the unhappy thoughts that open the gates to pain messages. The good news is that positive thoughts and feelings can close those gates — a little or a lot — and make it harder for the pain messages to get through. Of course, pain is pain, and a brick dropped on your toe is going to hurt. No amount of positive thinking can close the gate on that kind of pain message! But good thoughts can act as healing balms for a fair amount of the chronic pain that comes with arthritis.

Switching from one set of thoughts to another will definitely help reduce your pain, but which thoughts are "good" and which are "bad"? The good thoughts will be discussed later in this chapter. But in this section, we'll focus on the thoughts and feelings you need to clear out of your mind to help reduce your pain, namely a trio of notorious gate openers: stress, aggression (or what is called *Type A* behavior), and depression.

Ratcheting up the pain with stress

Flares of rheumatoid arthritis and certain other forms of arthritis are often associated with stressBut any kind of pain, brought about by any ailment, can be worsened by stress. Reducing and managing your stress, then, can be a very helpful technique for managing pain.

In simple terms, stress is your body's response to *stressors,* which can be anything that causes you stress; that is, anything that frightens, angers, annoys, scares, challenges, or forces you to change or respond to a change. Cars about to ram into you are stressors, as is a nasty boss who's giving you a rough time. Other stressors include illness, the loss of a loved one, and failed relationships. Even good things, like getting married or having a baby, can be stressors because they force you to respond to major challenges and change. Stress, on the other hand, is your response, physical, mental and emotional, to one or more stressors. You may feel tense, angry, frustrated, helpless or hopeless in response to a stressor — in other words, you're stressed. Or you may simply ignore the stressors, laugh them off, or find a calm way to deal with them, and you don't get stressed. The facts are the same; it's your reaction that differs.

Stress can make the "pain gates" swing wide open. If you respond to stressors by getting riled up, there's a very good chance that whatever is already hurting your will hurt even more.

This is not to say that eliminating stress (even if it were possible) will magically make your pain disappear. But controlling your stress can ensure that you don't hurt any more than you absolutely have to — and that's a big change for most of us.

REMEMBER

You're always going to face stressors, many of which you can't do anything about. What you *can* do is change your attitude toward them. Reshaping your view of events and taking a more positive approach that calms your reaction (check out the section "Discovering the Healing Power of Positive Thinking" later in this chapter) can help reduce your stress and close the pain gates.

Increasing pain the "A" way

People often equate the hectic pace of modern life with stress: We wake up early to get the kids ready for school, then hurry to work, race through errands during lunch, drive the kids around, run more errands in the evening, then scramble to throw dinner together with our cell phones glued to our ears. It's no wonder so many of us are stressed out. Or is it? Several studies suggest that feeling harassed and under pressure aren't to blame. The real culprits are anger and hostility.

You may have heard about the Type A personality — the often angry, hostile, hard-driving, competition-loving person who seems to relish going into battle. Unfortunately, anger, hostility, and aggression can trigger stress and open the pain gates wide.

Are you a Type A personality? Do you

>> Hate to waste any time?

>> Feel like you always have to be accomplishing something?

>> Love to compete with others, just for the fun of winning?

>> Often think about your life and accomplishments in terms of dollars earned, cases won, opponents defeated?

>> Feel somewhat unsatisfied after each success and immediately begin working for the next?

>> Anger easily?

>> Always feel like you're behind or that you're racing against the clock?

>> Leave little time for hobbies and relaxation, often taking work with you on vacation?

>> Generally dominate conversations, finding it boring to listen to other people talk about themselves or their interests?

>> Make snap decisions that you "know" are right?

>> Often feel like other people are in your way?

>> Often find yourself locking horns with others?

>> Feel threatened when someone questions your achievements?

If you answered yes to more than a few of the questions, you may be a Type A personality, and this may be increasing your pain.

If you're a Type A, the odds are that you can't simply stop acting that way. You can, however, do quite a bit to reduce your hostility and calm yourself physically, mentally, and emotionally. Try integrating the following behaviors into your busy life:

>> Slow down!

>> Make it a point to find someone or something to admire every day.

>> Take time each day to relax — really relax, not just move your work to a nicer, seemingly more relaxed environment.

>> Make loved ones and friends a top-of-the-list priority.

>> Go easy on others.

>> Go easy on yourself.

>> Have some fun!

>> Accept the things you can't change.

Heightening pain when you're feeling low

Depression, a common companion to lingering and painful arthritis conditions, can make your pain feel worse because it affects both your body and your mind.

On the physical front, depression leads to inactivity — at times you may not even want to get out of bed. Inactivity, in turn, leads to a general de-conditioning of the body, joint stiffness, decreased flexibility, and weak muscles, all of which can increase arthritis pain. Depression can also raise your sensitivity to pain because it causes insomnia, fatigue, irritability, stress, and anxiety.

On the emotional front, depression is associated with a low level of endorphins, the body's natural painkillers. Too few endorphins can translate to increased pain. Your perception of pain also increases when you focus on it. Depressed people typically withdraw from life and become inactive, which increases their self-awareness and focuses their attention on themselves and their pain. In short, depression may be the result of pain, but it can cause pain, as well.

As many as 80 percent of those suffering from chronic arthritis pain become depressed about it from time to time. That's not surprising, given that doctors are unable to cure the disease.

The good news is that when depression is recognized and treated, pain tends to lessen as well. A study reported in the *Journal of the American Medical Association* found that when 1,001 older adults with arthritis received normal or enhanced depression care, more than half of them enjoyed a 50 percent drop in pain intensity, along with significant improvements in their quality of life and ability to function.

Identifying the symptoms of depression

Many people don't realize that they're depressed, because the signs of depression aren't always obvious. Besides sadness and feeling low, other possible emotional symptoms of depression include:

>> Anxiety

>> Brooding

>> Difficulty concentrating

- Disturbed sleeping patterns

- Excessive or inappropriate crying

- Fatigue

- Feelings of worthlessness or hopelessness

- Irritability

- Loss of interest in formerly pleasurable activities

- Loss of sexual desire or pleasure

- Not laughing as much as usual

- Thinking and speaking slowly

- Withdrawal

- Weight gain or loss

And in some people, depression can show up as physical symptoms that can lead to expensive and unnecessary testing and treatment. These symptoms include:

- Abdominal pain

- Back pain

- Headaches

- Worsening of joint pain

Any of these emotional or physical symptoms can and do strike from time to time; we all get the blues. But when several of these symptoms linger day after day for a couple weeks or more, it's considered depression. See your doctor or a mental health professional to help you get through this difficult period.

Seeking medical treatment for depression

REMEMBER

Depression should be taken seriously. If you recognized the symptoms of depression in yourself, feel unable to help yourself, or find yourself becoming suicidal, see your doctor or a mental health professional immediately. Although many of the milder forms of depression respond well to the self-help approaches discussed in this chapter, more severe depression can require medication, face-to-face psychotherapy, and careful monitoring by a mental health professional.

Lifting your mood to ease your pain

If you have arthritis or any other painful condition, you need to guard against depression and look for ways to take control of your situation and your life.

Thinking good thoughts acts like a medicine for the body. It can increase your body's production of natural painkillers, help boost your immune system, and speed healing.

Depression, on the other hand, can increase the sensation of pain, weaken the immune system, and interfere with your ability to participate in effective treatment and rehabilitation.

Although we can't offer you an instant cure for depression, we can suggest several steps that can help lift your mood:

>> **Express your feelings.** Don't pretend everything is all right to please others. If you're frustrated or angry because you're stuck with arthritis and its resultant pain, say so. This doesn't mean that you should misbehave, throw temper tantrums, or break things. Look instead for the middle ground between bottling up your feelings and blowing your top.

In other words, express yourself in an assertive, yet moderate and positive way. Tell your doctor what hurts and ask for help. If a certain pill or procedure doesn't help, say so and ask for another approach. Tell your family if your pain is preventing you from performing your normal activities and ask for help and understanding. It can also be very helpful to join a support group and express your feelings there. (See Chapter 15 for more information about online support groups.)

>> **Don't get caught in the "Love Me Because I Hurt Syndrome."** Some depressed people may subconsciously enjoy what they consider the "good" parts of being depressed. (For example, you get lots of sympathy, you're excused from certain chores, you're allowed to act out, you may be given extra treats, and so on.) Don't get attached to these secondary gains. Remember, depression can breed more depression, so you'll need to break this cycle as soon as it appears.

>> **Exercise regularly, even when you don't feel like it.** Take brisk walks, ride a bicycle, or otherwise rev up your body and body chemistry to increase the production of *endorphins,* which are the natural feel-good hormones.

>> **Try to avoid seeing yourself as a victim.** Some forms of arthritis are still mysterious to us, but they're physical diseases, not the results of curses or black magic. New breakthroughs are constantly happening and new therapies and drugs are constantly being developed. At the very least, you can manage your disease. And you can always hope that someone will discover a cure in the near future.

>> **Walk, talk, and act positively!** Even if you don't feel good, approach life with a positive attitude. If possible, don't shuffle. Instead, walk tall and with vigor. Don't mumble; speak clearly and enthusiastically. Don't look down at your

feet; look up. Don't avoid other people's gazes; look them straight in the eye. Even if you're only pretending, always walk, talk, and act positively. You may be surprised to find that soon you're not acting any more — you really *are* feeling better.

To find some great tips for dealing with unwanted advice, see the sidebar "Dealing with 'helpful' loved ones" at the end of this chapter.

Discovering the Healing Power of Positive Thinking

Stress, type A behavior, and depression can change your perception of pain, shoving the pain gates wide open and making you hurt more than you have to. That's one of the reasons why doctors have trouble dealing with pain: They can see how much of your cartilage has been worn away and guess how much it *should* hurt, but they can't gauge whether your attitude is making the pain better or worse.

Just thinking positively may help you close the pain gates, a little or a lot. For example, researchers have found that people who had positive expectations before going into hip replacement surgery were more satisfied with their results than those who doubted that they'd benefit. And those who imagined that they would enjoy complete relief from pain actually *did* experience significantly less pain and better physical function than those who weren't so optimistic. So maybe you really *can* make good things happen just by expecting them.

REMEMBER

Thinking positively doesn't mean you have to love everyone you meet and everything that happens to you. You can be a positive thinker and still get upset now and then, and it's fine to avoid people or situations you don't like. In fact, letting off a little steam once in a while or staying away from annoying people can be a good idea.

The next few sections present a few of the many techniques you can use to better equip yourself emotionally to deal with physical pain, and keep that pain from being worse than necessary. Which approach is the best one for you? It's the one that works. Give them all a try; the ones that help you control your stress and your pain most effectively are the ones you should use.

Relaxing the pain away through biofeedback

Although the body usually runs things as it sees fit, you *can* override some of its instructions. Biofeedback operates on the premise that "seeing" what's happening inside your body may help you control it. During biofeedback sessions, you're hooked up to sensitive electrical equipment that monitors the physical signs and symptoms of stress, including increased blood pressure, heart rate, muscle tension, body temperature, and so on. A continuous display shows fluctuations in these levels, and these numbers, displays, lights, and beeps give you something tangible to work with as you learn to control the physical and psychological effects of stress. By using certain relaxation and visualization techniques, you'll find that you can alter these bodily functions for the better and see the results on the monitors. With practice, many people can lower their blood pressure, heart rates, and muscle tension, and otherwise calm themselves during periods of stress.

Biofeedback is a wonderful teaching tool that gives immediate reinforcement as you practice relaxation techniques. Eventually, you should be able to apply these techniques in your daily life without using the equipment.

You can find a biofeedback practitioner in the yellow pages or by contacting the Association for Applied Psychophysiology and Biofeedback. (See Appendix B.) The best plan, however, is to get a referral to a biofeedback technician from your physician. Or your insurance company may have a list of biofeedback technicians who are covered under your plan.

Quieting your mind with meditation and programmed relaxation

Practiced in many different forms, meditation is designed to help quiet both your body and your mind. Some forms of meditation are exotic, using chants, incense, and foreign terms, but others are plain and simple. However, all of them have one thing in common: a strong, deliberate focus on something outside the self. Meditation reduces stress by giving you a break from your thoughts and problems, and the stressors in your life.

In basic meditation, you focus strongly on your breath or a *mantra,* a special word that is believed to have mystical powers. Practicing slow, deep breathing or repeating your mantra over and over again in your mind are ways of keeping your mind still. As thoughts and images drift into your mind, you simply ignore them and concentrate on your breath or your mantra. Soon, the thoughts and images will just drift away.

During programmed relaxation, also known as the relaxation response, you tune in to your muscles, feeling them tighten and relax in a prescribed manner. Programmed relaxation can help relieve the stress that accompanies chronic pain, reduce your overall pain load, and promote better sleep.

You can find out more about meditation and programmed relaxation from many sources, including psychologists, mental health experts, and meditation centers. Some HMOs and hospitals offer courses in meditation, and certain large companies offer them for their employees. You can also find a meditation or programmed relaxation practitioner by contacting the organizations listed in Appendix B.

Moving to a stress-free place through guided imagery and hypnosis

Although no hard scientific data proves that guided imagery can dramatically change body chemistry and functioning, many people have benefited from learning to transport themselves to a better place by imagining happy scenarios. For example, you may imagine yourself relaxing on a beautiful tropical beach when you're actually caught in bumper-to-bumper, rush-hour traffic. By doing this, you may manage to remain calm, at ease, and even happy while everyone around you seems ready to scream with frustration.

The same effect can be accomplished with hypnotherapy. Hypnosis doesn't cure arthritis, but it can help you handle emotional upsets caused by pain, which can ease the sensation of pain. Besides helping you relax in the face of pain and stress, hypnosis can reduce your levels of stress and anxiety, and make you feel as if you're no longer a prisoner to your pain.

You can ask your doctor or psychologist for a referral to an expert in hypnosis and guided imagery. (Many psychologists are, themselves, experts in both of these areas.) Or you can contact the organizations listed in Appendix B.

Controlling your breathing

Think about your breathing when you're stressed: You probably take short, shallow breaths. But when you breathe in the opposite manner, with long, deep breaths, your body naturally moves toward a relaxed state. By making a point of breathing slowly and deeply when you feel stressed, you can help short-circuit the stress cycle. And by focusing on your breath rather than your fear, frustration, anger, or pain, you can help derail your negative feelings.

Using cognitive behavioral therapy

Cognitive behavioral therapy (CBT) is a form of psychotherapy that helps you discover how certain thinking patterns exacerbate your problems. It also teaches you how to change your habitual reactions to these problems, and think more positively and rationally about them.

One study of 53 RA patients (reported in the journal *Rheumatology* in 2003) found that CBT not only helped the patients deal with their anxiety and depression, but also decreased their disability and significantly improved their joint function. A 2016 review study published in the *Journal of Pain Research* found that psychological therapy was definitely helpful for managing pain in RA patients, with CBT being the most effective kind. CBT fostered more positive attitudes in the patients toward the illness and challenged erroneous beliefs (such as, "I'm going to end up in a wheelchair, so why should I make things worse by exercising?") that tended to drag them down. Patients found out how to couple optimism with realism and manage their conditions more effectively.

In addition, a 2014 clinical review published in the *Journal of the American Medical Association* found high-quality evidence that supported the use of CBT for managing fibromyalgia symptoms.

TIP

Many (but not all) psychologists use cognitive behavioral therapy in their practices. To find one in your area, contact the National Register of Health Service Psychologists (https://www.nationalregister.org).

Laughing your way to relaxation

Undoubtedly, the most enjoyable stress reliever is laughter. A good, hard laugh is believed to lower the levels of cortisol, one of the stress hormones. It also helps you relax all over. Laughing takes your thoughts away from whatever is going wrong in your life, so you can't stew in your own negativity. In fact, many health experts believe that a good sense of humor is like a vitamin for body and soul. And laughter heightens the activity of the body's natural defenses. So the more time you spend laughing, the better your health should be!

Spend time with friends who make you laugh and, most importantly, look for the funny side of whatever life throws you. If you can laugh at your problems, they can't control you. There's almost always something funny in a situation — if you look hard enough. To find out more, contact the Association for Applied and Therapeutic Humor (https://www.aath.org/).

Forgetting all about it

Even something as simple as distracting yourself from your problems can be helpful. Instead of focusing on your pain, which will only increase your stress, try going for a walk with a friend, getting involved in an arts and crafts project, volunteering, going to a singalong, taking a fun dance class, watching an interesting movie or television show, reading an engrossing book, or listening to some great music. Distraction won't cure arthritis, but it will help prevent the stress caused by focusing on the pain.

Easing Depression and Anxiety with Prayer and Spirituality

Several studies have shown that people who belong to religious groups and regularly attend services are less depressed and anxious than those who don't.

Studies with hospitalized patients support the notion that religion is an antidepressant. We can't be certain why this is so, but it may be because being religious makes you feel that:

>> Someone very important (a higher power) is looking out for you.

>> You belong to something large and wonderful.

>> You have a role to play in life.

>> You're loved.

>> You belong to a community of people who can help support you.

You can also find plenty of opportunities to help others through your church, temple, or mosque. There's nothing like reaching out to others to help you forget about your own pain and feel better about yourself.

Prayer goes hand-in-hand with religion, and can also be an antidote to stress. The simple act of praying can relieve anxiety, and the thoughts expressed in many prayers can have a calming effect. Of course, you don't have to be religious to be spiritual. Spirituality is the quest for a connection with a higher power, however you may define it. You can also think of spirituality as a search for meaning in life and an attempt to understand the world and your place in it. You can express your spirituality through religion or find your own path. Some people find spirituality via meditation or yoga. Others commune with nature, write poetry, or do charitable deeds. The road to spirituality is yours to choose; you may even define a new one that's all your own. However you approach it, you may find spirituality a helpful balm for your pain.

DEALING WITH "HELPFUL" LOVED ONES

As if you didn't have enough in your life to make your blood pressure rise, well-meaning friends and relatives can make you crazy by "helping" you deal with your arthritis.

Mary Dunkin (writing in *Arthritis Today*) describes the types of helpful loved ones who may be driving you nuts with their well-meaning advice. Beware of the following types:

- **The caretaker:** This person hates to see you suffering and tries desperately to get you to try one treatment after another. That's because they need to see you well again; what *you* want takes second place in their mind. You gotta love them, but they can drive you crazy.

- **The blamer:** This one insists that things would be much better if you would just stop doing things a certain way, or thinking certain "silly" thoughts. This may be their way to get out of having to help you. After all, if you'd just shape up, everything would be fine (according to them).

- **The evangelist:** This exceedingly "helpful" person absolutely, irrevocably, and unshakably knows exactly what will cure you — and insists that you try it. Maybe they were cured by the same thing, is making money off the therapy they're pushing, knows someone who was cured this way, or just believes in it wholeheartedly. Whatever the reason, they never let up about it. This is the loved one who's most likely to make you run and hide when you see them coming.

- **The minimizer:** This person has a very simple cure, even though you have a very complex problem. "No sweat!" they say. They know exactly how to set things right in one fell swoop. Naturally, it doesn't wipe out your arthritis, but they continue to insist that it will, if you'll just give it a fair try.

What do you say to the caretaker, the blamer, the evangelist, the minimizer and everyone else who offers you unwanted advice? Gently but firmly tell them you appreciate their concern, but you're following your doctor's advice.

If they're really annoying, you can say, "Thanks for your ideas; you're a sweetheart to care so much! But I've got my own thoughts about my illness." That ought to do it!

Chapter **15**

Day-to-Day Living with Arthritis

A rthritis or not, you have a life to live! Like everybody else, you probably have a lot on your plate — a job, family responsibilities, household and gardening chores, a social life, a romantic life, pets, hobbies, and maybe more. But some days, those twin demons, pain and fatigue, may make you wonder if you can even make it to the next room. On those days, you need to find the most efficient, least stressful ways of accomplishing your goals. But don't wait until you're having a rough day before beginning to think about how to simplify your life. Start today by making a list of the things you typically need to accomplish each day. Then read this chapter to find ways to take on those tasks with greater ease and efficiency. Jot down ideas as you read and start to make a plan.

Studies have shown that people who take an active part in managing their arthritis and finding new ways to cope with physical disabilities do better and feel less pain and fatigue. Don't let yourself be sidelined as life's parade marches by!

In this chapter, we show you how to wrest control of your life from arthritis by applying these three watchwords to your daily activities: *organizing*, *planning*, and *prioritizing*. When you do, you may be surprised at how much you can accomplish and how good you can feel about yourself, even on a bad day.

Taking Care of You

When you've got arthritis, everyday stresses and activities can become twice as hard to handle. But you can help yourself by visiting an occupational therapist to learn the easiest, most efficient ways to get through the day, figuring out how to make the best use of your precious energy, and getting a good night's sleep. Another important part of taking care of yourself is taking care of your sex life, which can still be a fun, healthy, and fulfilling part of life.

If you're pregnant, we've included a section especially for you; see the sidebar "Coping with arthritis when you're pregnant," later in the chapter.

Working with an occupational therapist

The occupational therapist (OT), a vital member of your treatment team, helps you get through your everyday activities despite your arthritis. A licensed health care professional, the OT interviews and examines you to determine how your arthritis affects the things you do on a daily basis, such as getting into and out of bed, dressing, grooming, eating, drinking, cooking, getting around, shopping, doing housework, and working.

After the OT gets a sense of where and when you may be having trouble, they come up with ideas and recommendations. An OT can design splints or supports that conform to your affected body parts, recommend and locate a wealth of assistive devices, and come up with plans to help you get through the day with greater ease and efficiency. The OT can also show you joint protection techniques that reduce joint strain and help prevent further damage.

Many people are tempted to skip occupational therapy, thinking it's not really necessary. But those who do will cheat themselves of a great opportunity to solve the practical problems posed by arthritis. Even though medical attention and physical therapy are vital parts of the treatment program, they can't help you figure out how to change a light bulb in the ceiling when you can't raise your arm, or how to put together a decent meal when you can barely shuffle around the kitchen. Occupational therapy helps you discover easier, more efficient ways of getting through the day. But possibly the most important thing it can show you is how to conserve your energy.

Conserving your energy

Even if you're the most organized person in the world and you follow absolutely every principle of arthritis management, you only have so much energy. After it runs out, you're like a car that's out of gas — you have to pull over and stop. Don't waste your precious energy; conserve it so you have the "gas" to get through the day's most important tasks.

TIP

The Arthritis Foundation suggests the following ideas for conserving your energy:

>> **Balance activity with rest.** Don't try to do everything at once; work in some breaks between activities. When tackling chores, don't do two difficult ones in a row. Alternate heavy chores with light ones. In the long run, you'll accomplish more tasks and experience less fatigue by pacing yourself.

>> **Plan ahead.** Find shortcuts, combine activities that can be done simultaneously, figure out what you can skip, and organize the execution of tasks for maximum efficiency.

>> **Do the most important things first.** If something absolutely *has* to be done, do it first to make sure it doesn't fall by the wayside as your energy wanes.

Getting a good night's sleep

The best fatigue fighter in the world is a good night's sleep. If you sleep well, you find yourself better able to handle pain, less stressed, less depressed, and more energetic. Unfortunately, many people develop trouble sleeping as they grow older, especially if they're suffering from pain.

TIP

To give your body the best possible chance of a good night's sleep, follow these sleeping guidelines:

>> **Go to bed and get up at the same time every day (even on weekends).** Getting up at 7:00 a.m. Monday through Friday and then at 10:00 a.m. on Saturday and Sunday throws off your body's internal clock and makes it harder to fall asleep and stay asleep.

>> **Keep your sleeping area as dark and quiet as possible.** Block the light with heavy drapes or blackout shades. Get a white noise machine or turn on a fan to cover up noises that may disturb your sleep.

>> **Make sure your mattress and pillow are comfortable.** A mattress that is either too hard or too soft and a pillow that doesn't support your head and neck comfortably can interfere with your sleep more than you realize. If you think you need to make a change, you have loads of options. Begin by asking your OT for recommendations.

>> **Use your bed for sleep and sex only.** Some people use their beds as the Grand Central Station of their lives — they eat, watch TV and videos, pay bills, read, play with the kids, do office work, and perform beauty routines while

firmly ensconced between the sheets. Then they wonder why they can't fall asleep there, too. Your bed should be associated with just two activities — sex and sleeping. It should be the place you go to relax, not to handle the business of living.

>> **Get some exercise every day, but not in the latter part of the evening.** Exercising after dinner tends to rev up your body, making it harder for you to fall asleep. Finish your heavy exercise by about 6:00 p.m. Light exercise, however, like a stroll or some yoga before bedtime, is fine.

>> **Relax for about an hour before bedtime.** Doing yoga, meditating, reading, taking a warm bath, or listening to soft music or a relaxation tape are all good, calming activities that can help you wind down before going to sleep. Don't try to do 101 chores before falling into bed. You may end up exhausted, but your mind will be racing and unable to relax.

>> **Stay away from caffeine in the evening (this includes coffee, tea, soft drinks, and cocoa).** Caffeine is a stimulant that can keep you awake, even if you ingest it hours before bedtime. Try to avoid caffeine after 6:00 p.m.

For tips on the best sleeping positions for those with arthritis, see Chapter 13.

Holding on to your sex life

Having arthritis doesn't mean you can't have a romantic relationship. Nonetheless, you may find that sex takes a back seat when you're trying to manage pain, medication, emotional issues, and physical limitations. Arthritis may have made you more dependent on your partner, which can change the nature of your relationship. Perhaps physical limitations and/or deformities caused by arthritis have altered your self-image. And medications may put a damper on sexual desire or performance.

You may also be worried that physical lovemaking will be painful: This fear alone can cause a lack of lubrication and/or orgasm in women, and problems getting and maintaining an erection in men. Both partners may be acutely aware of the "pain factor," and even when everything seems to be going along okay, as soon as one partner winces, the other immediately becomes concerned rather than desirous. Lubrication stops, erections disappear, and the thought of sexual relations goes out the window.

Fortunately, satisfying and pleasurable sex can still be yours. The most important thing is to focus on the intimacy and closeness that it can bring, rather than on some preordained standard of performance. Gentle stroking, kissing, caressing, and massage are wonderful ways of expressing sexuality and nurturing one another at the same time. In most cases, intercourse is also possible, although it may require careful positioning and gentle technique.

To make sex easier and more pleasurable, try the following suggestions:

>> Take a warm bath beforehand to relax your joints and muscles and ease pain. This can also help increase circulation in your fingers and toes, which is particularly important for those with Raynaud's. Light exercise and stretching may help, too.

>> Take your pain medication in time for it to kick in before your session.

>> Some medications can bring on chemical imbalances that cause yeast infections, which can be annoying at best. If you get one of these infections, ask your doctor to prescribe treatment.

>> Talk to your partner about what feels good and what doesn't. Explore various methods of achieving mutual satisfaction. Good communication is an important part of any sexual relationship, but it's absolutely vital when physical difficulties exist.

If you have sexual problems that you and your partner can't seem to resolve by yourselves, seek help from a counselor, doctor, or nurse experienced in dealing with the problems of living with arthritis.

COPING WITH ARTHRITIS WHEN YOU'RE PREGNANT

Becoming pregnant when you've got arthritis can affect your body in several ways. You may find that your joints become less stable and "looser." The additional weight may increase symptoms of osteoarthritis to the knee. Your back will tend to sway in response to the additional weight of the baby, so back pain, muscle spasms, or numbness and tingling in your legs can occur. An increase in water weight can intensify stiffness in the hips, knees, and ankles (the weight-bearing joints) and worsen carpal tunnel syndrome.

On the bright side, some forms of arthritis actually seem to improve during pregnancy. Approximately 50 to 60 percent of women with rheumatoid arthritis notice a decrease in disease activity and an improvement in the signs and symptoms of RA, beginning in the first trimester and lasting through delivery,. However, some 90 percent of women with RA experience a flare soon after the birth of the baby.

It's important for you to see an obstetrician *and* a rheumatologist during the course of your pregnancy. You should also continue to take your arthritis medicines (if advised to do so by your doctors); exercise to keep your weight under control, your joints flexible, and your muscles strong; follow a nutritious eating plan; observe the rules of joint protection; and use stress management techniques to control mood swings and encourage relaxation.

Finding an Easier Way to Get Through the Day

For many people, one of the most frustrating things about arthritis is that it can get in the way of going about their daily activities, making it hard or even impossible to do certain things that used to come easily to them. When arthritis pain strikes, it can be a big effort to get something off a high shelf or to bend over to make a bed, and just getting dressed can be very tiring. That's why it's important to learn how to simplify everyday tasks to conserve your energy.

Simplifying your household

You can take steps to make various areas of your home easier to manipulate and deal with on a daily basis. Try the following:

» If you have trouble closing the door behind you, install two cup hooks — one in the door, near the doorknob, and one in the door frame, just outside the hinge area. (Position the cup hooks so they're level with each other.) Run a string or an elastic cord between the cup hooks. You now have an easy-to-grab cord that pulls the door shut behind you.

» Wrap rubber bands around a doorknob that is difficult to turn. This will give you a better grip.

» Try using a beaded seat cover on your car seats. The beads roll and make it easier for you to slide in and out of your car and adjust yourself after you settle in.

» Instead of the traditional lace-up style tennis shoes, try the kind with Velcro closures.

TIP

Personalize your kitchen to help make your daily tasks easier to perform. A few ideas include:

» Screw a cup hook underneath one of your cupboards and use it to pry open pull-tab cans. (In order to get the pull-tab started before the hook can grab it, slide a dinner knife or spoon under the tab and push the tab up slightly.)

» Put Lazy Susans (turntables) on your refrigerator shelves in your cupboards and any other storage areas that can accommodate them. This eliminates reaching, straining, and shuffling things around when you need to get an item that's at the back.

>> If dialing a phone is difficult, get one with an extra-large keypad or use a pencil to push the buttons. Most phones offer an automatic dial feature that lets you call frequently dialed numbers at the touch of a button.

>> Single-arm faucets (the type that lets you control the temperature and amount of water with just one lever) are the easiest kind to use and don't require two hands. Consider getting your kitchen and bathroom faucets converted to this style. If you want to keep your double-arm faucets, try getting wing-type handles that can be operated with your hand, wrist, or forearm.

>> Use the pointed tip of a can opener to open boxes of rice, cereal, or mixes with a "press here" type of opening, or to get the metal spouts started on boxes of nonfat milk powder.

>> Buy kitchen utensils (carrot peelers, can openers, stirring spoons, and so on) that have extra large, rubber-covered handles for easier gripping.

Making household cleaning easier

Back in the 1960s, a popular household cleaner claimed it was so fast and versatile that it could whip through your house like a "white tornado," cleaning everything in sight in no time at all. Although the tips that follow won't exactly make a "white tornado" out of you, they may reduce the time and effort you spend on household chores.

Remember to spread out your chores; don't try to get the whole house clean in one day!

TIP

If bending over while doing chores is difficult for you, use these tips to make cleaning easier:

>> Try sitting down while sweeping, using a broom with a handle that has been cut in half to make it shorter. Or you can use a child's broom. If you spray the bristles with water or furniture polish before using, the broom will do a better job of collecting dust and dirt.

>> For a dirty bathtub, mix together 1/2 cup of automatic dishwashing detergent and 2 cups of hot water. Plug the tub, add the mixture, and swirl it around with a long-handled mop. Let it stand for 20 minutes, then rinse thoroughly with cold water.

>> Instead of constantly bending over to plug and unplug your vacuum cleaner, add a 30-foot extension cord. You'll plug and unplug a lot less!

TIP

If you have arthritis in your hands, try to eliminate any chores that involve scrubbing with "elbow grease" or using intricate movements. Here are a few suggestions:

» Cleaning the fireplace is a dirty, unpleasant job, but you can make it easier if you line the fireplace with aluminum foil before you put in the grate and add the wood. After the ashes have cooled, spritz them with water (to keep ashes from flying), remove the grate, carefully pull the foil toward you. Then put the whole mess in the trash!

» Instead of scrubbing a pot that has burned-on food, sprinkle 1/2 cup baking soda in the pot, add a cup or two of water, and put it on the stove to simmer for 20 minutes. Then turn off the heat and allow to mixture to stay in the pot for two hours. The burned stuff should wipe right off.

» If clutching a dusting rag hurts your hands, try putting old socks on both hands, spraying the socks with a small amount of furniture polish, then wiping off tabletops and counters with ease.

» Foam pipe insulation is great for covering the handles of tools to make them easier to grasp. You can find it in the hardware store in several sizes and slip it on the handles of your knives, carrot peelers, screwdrivers, mops, or anything else that has a tendency to slip out of your hand.

Using assistive devices

One of the best ways to conserve your energy and keep from putting undue stress and strain on your joints is to use assistive devices — that is, equipment that can make performing a task easier, safer, and more comfortable.

Assistive devices run the gamut from long-handled shoehorns to hydraulic seat lifts that boost you out of a chair; from bathtub benches to computerized wheel-chairs. Some of these devices may require professional installation, while others are ready to use upon purchase. You can find many assistive devices online or at medical supply houses. Your occupational therapist can steer you to reputable sources. Most likely, the hardest part will be deciding which devices are right for you. Your OT can also help you with that task.

Here's a partial list of what's currently available:

» **Bathing and grooming:** Bath and shower grab bars, toilet safety frames, bathtub benches, foam tubing for handles (for example, toothbrush, hair brush, and so on), raised toilet seats, toothpaste tube squeezers, long-handled bath sponges, and makeup and razor holders are just a few items that can make bathing and grooming much easier.

- **Dressing:** Button hooks, zipper pulls, sock aids, long-handled shoe horns, shoe removers, cuff extenders, stretch shoe laces, and watch winders can help simplify getting dressed and undressed.

- **Food preparation and eating:** Large grip utensils (knives, carrot peelers, silverware, and so on), jar openers, can openers, pull-tab can openers, plastic bag openers, nonslip grips for plates and cups, easy-hold cups, and glass holders (with two handles) can aid in meal preparation and eating.

- **General household:** Doorknob turners, key turners, car door openers, faucet turners, voice-activated telephones or speaker phones, telephone headsets, voice-activated computer programs, reachers (long-handled devices that grab items), grips for phone receivers, and long-handled sponges and dusters for cleaning can make the handling of household tasks and communication much easier.

- **Cleaning the house:** A long-handled mop can be used to clean the bathtub or shower, while a long-handled feather duster can get those cobwebs out of the corner, and floor cleaner can be applied evenly with a long-handled paint roller.

- **Getting around:** Canes, crutches, stair walkers, walkers, portable stools, scooters, and wheelchairs can help you become more mobile.

For a list of online retailers featuring assistive devices, see Appendix B.

Getting help from other people

If you live alone and don't have the luxury of assistance from family and friends, you can handle personal care, household chores, gardening, and transportation in several ways, without having to do everything yourself. Home health care workers can come to your home and help you dress, bathe, do housework, prepare meals, get to the doctor's office, or do just about anything else you can imagine. House-keepers and gardeners can take care of cleaning, laundry, and yard work. But if these kinds of help are too pricey, look to the less expensive sources of assistance:

- Teenagers (either from your own family or your neighbor's) are often willing to do yard work or other chores for a small fee.

- A stay-at-home parent in your neighborhood may be willing to make some extra money by preparing meals and/or taking you to the doctor.

- Your church, mosque, or synagogue may have volunteers who are willing to help you out for free.

> » Your doctor, social worker, or another health care worker may be able to refer you to various nonprofit organizations that can offer either inexpensive or free services. Just ask!

Joining an Arthritis Support Group

Support groups are as individual as the people who join them. Some are quite structured, emphasizing education, but others stress emotional support and the sharing of experiences. Some may be designed for those with a particular kind of arthritis, such as osteoarthritis or rheumatoid arthritis, while others are all inclusive.

Support groups generally have a leader, who may be either a medical professional (for example, a doctor, nurse, psychologist, or social worker) or simply a member of the group. Groups that are run by their members are often called self-help or peer groups.

If you think you'd like to try a support or self-help group, keep in mind that it may take some detective work and a sizable investment of time before you find the one you really like. Visit several groups (either in person or online) and try each one at least twice. If you drop in for just one meeting, it may be an off night for an otherwise dynamic and helpful group. Or a good night for an otherwise disorganized and not-very-helpful group.

One of the great things about support groups is they remind you that you're not alone! There are thousands of experts out there just waiting to help you. Who are these experts? Other people who have arthritis, just like you.

Finding help and hope through the group

Joining an arthritis or pain support group can be both educational and comforting. Within these groups, you can find the following:

> » A chance to talk about your feelings

> » A good reason to interact with other people

> » Encouragement

> » Information

> » People who can tell you what to expect from a certain test or treatment, because they've already been through it

>> People who understand exactly what you're feeling

>> Great role models — people who are much more "advanced" in their arthritis than you are and are living happy, productive, and wonderful lives

Locating a support group

To find a support group, ask the members of your health care team for referrals. You can also contact the Arthritis Foundation at 800-283-7800, or contact any of the Support Groups Online listed in Appendix B.

For information on how to start your own arthritis support group, contact the National Mental Health Consumers' Self-Help Clearinghouse, 1211 Chestnut Street, Suite 1100, Philadelphia, PA 19107; phone (800) 553-4539 or (215) 751-1810; email info@mhselfhelp.org; web site: https://www.mhselfhelp.org.

Dealing with Arthritis in the Workplace

When you have arthritis, you have some days when you just don't feel like going to work. But you may not have the luxury of staying home every time you experience a flare, especially if they occur often. That's why it's important to simplify your tasks at work, just like you did at home, to make them as easy on your joints and as energy-efficient as possible.

REMEMBER

If your pain seriously interferes with your ability to do your job and you've done all you can to control it, you may want to consider leaving work behind and applying for disability insurance benefits.

Easing the pain when you work

Many of us spend our workdays sitting in an office, whether at home or in a workplace. It sounds easy, but working on a computer, handling correspondence, and doing other paperwork can be difficult if your hands hurt or you can't sit comfortably in a chair.

TIP

Consider these ideas for streamlining paperwork and making desk duties easier:

>> Large scissors with well-padded handles can make cutting easier.

>> A rubber grip that fits around the barrel of a pen or pencil makes it easier to hold and less likely to slip.

>> Rubber fingers (which look like a thimble made of rubber) can help you turn pages or thumb through a sheaf of papers without fumbling. You can twist a rubber band around the end of your finger for the same effect.

>> If you have trouble handling scissors, seam rippers make a good substitute.

>> Tape dispensers with some weight and a rubberized bottom make it easier to grab a piece of tape using just one hand, because they don't slide around.

Applying for disability benefits

According to the Social Security Administration, if you can no longer do the kind of work you're accustomed to doing, *and* you can't engage in any other kind of "substantial gainful activity" because of your age, education, and/or work experience, you may be eligible for disability insurance benefits.

To qualify, you must be a U.S. citizen or have a Permanent Resident card number, and have a Social Security number.

TIP

To apply online, do the following:

1. **Go to** www.ssa.gov/benefits/disability **and select "Apply for Disability."**

2. **Fill out the Disability Benefit Application.**

3. **Answer the disability questions.**

4. **Mail or take the documents you're asked for to your Social Security office.**

Be aware that receiving disability benefits doesn't mean that you can't continue to work. If you don't relish the idea of sitting at home, look into a special program run by the Social Security Administration called Ticket to Work that can help you find a job suited to your abilities while you continue to collect your disability benefits. You can contact the help line for Ticket to Work at https://choosework. ssa.gov/mycall, or by phone at 1-866-968-7842 or 1-866-833-2967 (TTY).

4

Is Alternative Medicine for You?

If the treatment of arthritis were as straightforward and effective as, say, getting rid of a mild headache (that is, take two aspirin and forget it), alternative therapies might not be so popular. But because medical doctors don't offer a real "cure" for arthritis, many people turn to alternative medicine. Some feel that traditional methods just aren't working, others want help with pain relief and additional symptoms, while still others believe that they really *can* find a cure if they just look hard enough.

In this part, we discuss the most popular alternative therapies for arthritis, from herbs and homeopathy to "hands on" healing methods, and everything in between.

Chapter **16**

Exploring Alternative Medicine

A lternative therapies have become increasingly popular, with half the population worldwide using some form of non-traditional medicine. There have also been major changes in the way people firmly entrenched in traditional Western medicine now view these therapies. In the early decades of the 20th century, Western medical doctors positively vilified other therapies and crusaded to make practicing other approaches illegal!

Fortunately, the attitude that everything Western medical doctors do is great while other therapies are just plain evil, has definitely fallen by the wayside. As a society, we've realized that our medical doctors don't have the cures for all of our ills, while other approaches may have a lot to offer. Yet, alternative approaches aren't perfect, either. Many alternative theories and practices aren't backed by enough scientific proof to be declared valid, and may have even been proven dangerous. Regardless of the debates surrounding these therapies, alternative medicine is close to becoming mainstream. Countless testimonials exist about the effectiveness of nearly all types of alternative therapies, and a fair number of studies indicate that some of these approaches work as well as standard medicines — or even better.

For a look at who uses complementary and althernative therapies and why, see the nearby sidebar, "CAM you dig it?"

Understanding the Many Faces of Alternative Medicine

Alternative, complementary, holistic, unorthodox, integrative, and preventive medicine: All of these terms are used to describe non-traditional approaches in medicine. But what do they mean?

Defining modern Western medicine (the drugs-and-surgery approach traditionally used by medical doctors) as *conventional medicine* is the first step in deciphering the many names used for alternative medicine. Anything that's not conventional is considered *unorthodox medicine*. *Alternative medicine* is an approach used in place of conventional medicine, while *complementary medicine* works with conventional therapies. The concepts of *holistic* and *integrative medicine* are related to each other: Instead of focusing only on the symptoms or the damaged part of the body, holistic and integrative medicine examines and treats the entire person, including the body, mind, emotions, and spirit. With *preventive medicine*, the goal is to keep disease from striking in the first place. Education, lifestyle changes, and improving the body, mind, emotions, and/or spirit are parts of this preemptive campaign.

CAM YOU DIG IT?

According to the Center for Disease Control (CDC), 36 percent of U.S. adults over age 18 currently use some form of complementary medicine. Several studies have estimated that some 30 to 40 percent of U.S. adults with arthritis use CAM. This may not be surprising since Americans pay more visits to complementary and alternative healers than to their primary medical doctors. The most popular treatments for arthritis include dietary supplements (including glucosamine and chondroitin sulfate), massage therapy, herbal medicine, acupuncture, and meditative therapies such as yoga and tai chi.

Who sees CAM healers? Middle-aged people make up the largest chunk of patients, especially women, and those who have graduated from college. CAM users usually have more than one health condition. In addition those with arthritis, approximately half of cancer patients have used some form of CAM at some point during their illness, while half of asthma patients use it to manage their symptoms. Those with HIV/AIDS are also very likely to use CAM, in spite of a lack of evidence that these therapies can actually help them.

The most recent term used to describe this wide variety of treatments is *complementary and alternative medicine*, or CAM for short. According to the National Center for Complementary and Integrative Health (NCCIH), which is a part of the National Institutes of Health, complementary health approaches can be classified by the way they are taken in or delivered: nutritional, psychological, physical, or a combination of any of these three. The mere fact that the National Institutes of Health has a division dedicated to CAM means that acupuncture, massage, nutritional healing, herbology, and other non-traditional therapies have gained both popularity and recognition. Establishing the NCCIH has also helped legitimize many of these therapies by defining their usefulness and safety through rigorous scientific investigation. Another indication of the acceptance of CAM is the fact that more than two-thirds of United States medical schools offer at least one course in these subjects.

Easing Arthritis Through Alternative Approaches

Look into the medicine cabinet of just about anybody who has arthritis and you're bound to find at least a few bottles of herbs, vitamins, or other supplements that promise to relieve arthritis symptoms. Because there is no real cure for arthritis, alternative approaches to treating this disease are wildly popular and run the gamut from bee venom to prayer. And in most cases, they work — at least to some extent.

In Chapters 17, 18, and 19, we discuss some of the most popular alternative approaches to treating arthritis-related pain, inflammation, and joint dysfunction. We also touch on a few others in Chapter 14 — positive thinking, prayer, and spirituality.

TIP

Check out the following overview of the alternative techniques most often used for easing arthritis pain:

>> **Acupuncture/acupressure:** Releasing energy blockages and pain by inserting fine needles or exerting pressure with the fingers, hands, or special tools on specific areas of the body.

>> **Aromatherapy:** Using fragrant aromas of substances called "essential oils" to calm the mind and the body.

>> **Bee venom therapy:** Alleviating arthritis pain with venom from bee stings.

>> **DHEA:** A hormone that may help ease fatigue, pain and inflammation in women with lupus.

>> **Herbs:** The roots, stems or leaves of plants that can act as anti-inflammatories, antirheumatics, sedatives, muscle relaxants, or pain relievers.

>> **Homeopathy:** The "like cures like" method of showing the body what's gone wrong so that it can correct itself.

>> **Hydrotherapy:** The use of hot or cold water, ice, and steam to stimulate or soothe the body and ease pain.

>> **Massage:** Rubbing, stroking, or kneading the muscles to ease muscular tension and pain.

>> **MSM:** An odorless crystalline powder, taken in capsule or tablet form or applied to the skin inas a lotion or cream to ease arthritis pain (see Chapter 19).

>> **Polarity therapy:** Balancing the body's energy systems through touching that ranges from light to firm.

>> **Reflexology:** Applying pressure to specific points on the soles of the feet to relieve pain in a corresponding part of the body.

>> **Reiki and touch therapy:** Two ways of channeling healing energy from the hands of the practitioner to the body of the patient, without actually touching.

Finding a Reputable CAM Practitioner

You should select a CAM practitioner with the same care that you give to finding the right medical doctor. You can find the names of practitioners of various alternative forms of health care in several ways:

>> Look for listings online.

>> Ask for recommendations from friends or alternative healers who you're already seeing.

>> Check the list of approved practitioners that your HMO or health insurance company may offer. (Some HMOs and health insurance companies pay for acupuncture services and perhaps other forms of alternative care.)

>> Get names from the various societies to which practitioners belong. (See Appendix B for the names of some of these organizations.)

>> Ask your doctor. A small number of medical doctors also practice alternative medicine, and those who don't may make recommendations.

Even if yours doesn't practice CAM or make recommenations, it's important that you let them know you're seeing a CAM specialist to ensure that what you're doing is safe.

After you put together a list of possibilities, treat them just as you would a list of physicians who you're considering. Ask the practitioners you're interested in the following questions:

>> Where did you study?

>> Do you have a license or certification?

>> What is your treatment philosophy?

>> What does treatment consist of?

>> What benefits can I expect from the treatment?

>> What are the side effects and how do you recommend handling them?

>> How will I know whether the treatment is working?

>> What is the cost of the treatment?

If you feel that your questions aren't answered forthrightly, or that you're being given the runaround, run out the door.

Checking credentials and certifications

Complementary and alternative medicine has a lot to offer, and it can fill in some of the gaps in conventional medical care. Unfortunately, CAM suffers from a lack of standardization. Herbs, for example, may vary greatly in purity and potency. Likewise, although some CAM healers are incredibly knowledgeable and skillful, while others are not.

Before selecting a complementary or alternative healer, make sure you do the following:

>> **See a physician (a medical doctor) to get an accurate diagnosis.** Some forms of arthritis are easy to recognize; others aren't. You need to know exactly what you're dealing with before undergoing any kind of treatment, conventional or CAM.

>> **Educate yourself.** Gather and study all the information you can about any given CAM therapy before subjecting yourself to it. Read books and articles, get information online, talk to people, and contact the professional organizations associated with the particular types of CAM that interest you.

Take all information with a grain of salt until you carefully consider its source. Is the person or group that offers this information knowledgeable? Do they have a solid educational background and/or practical experience? Are they an unbiased source or a salesperson?

>> **Ask for credentials.** Ask CAM therapists where they studied, whether they are licensed by the state, certified by a board, and so on. Don't be shy or afraid to ask questions. Any healer — conventional or CAM — who won't happily review their background with you isn't a good prospect. And don't be afraid to ask for the name and phone number of the school or society that issued the credentials so you can investigate that organization.

>> **Ask for references.** You might ask your CAM therapists if there are any clients they have worked with who you can contact for a reference. If so, contact these people; ask them what they were suffering from, what the CAM practitioner did for them, how well the therapy worked, what the side effects were (if any), and so on.

>> **Ask about the price.** Insurance doesn't cover most CAM therapies.

Identifying false claims

Everyone wants a miracle pill that can cure their ills. And everyone would like it even better if that pill were tiny and easy to swallow, worked instantly, didn't cost more than a pack of bubble gum, and had to be taken only once.

Unfortunately, such a cure doesn't yet exist for arthritis. However, this fact hasn't stopped some people from claiming that they have miracle cures for all your aches and pains.

Most alternative practitioners are honest and sincere, but hucksters will always happily tell you tales hoping to take your money. So safeguard your health and pocketbook by looking for the following warning signs:

>> **The "secret formula" trap:** Be wary if the cure offers no list of ingredients or is based on a secret formula. Claiming that something is secret can be an easy way for hucksters to avoid admitting that their "cure" doesn't contain anything remarkable. Reputable healers, on the other hand, are happy to tell you exactly what they're proposing that you take. And knowing what you're taking is important, for even if the stuff in the secret formula is helpful, it may

interact dangerously with a medicine or supplement you're already taking. Or perhaps you may be allergic to the secret stuff, or it's just not right for you.

>> **One–study wonders:** Proceed with caution if the health practitioner bases all claims for the treatment on only one study. It's true that only one study may be necessary to establish that a treatment works, but it's better if the therapy has been studied many times, with different patients and under different conditions. A therapy may work well in one study with, say, elderly and bedridden osteoarthritis patients, but not work so well when tested again with younger or more active subjects. The more studies, the better. Reputable healers know this, which is why they should want to cite as many studies as possible for their therapies.

>> **Catch-all cures:** Avoid cures that purport to work for all types of arthritis — and other diseases as well. Nothing is a cure-all. As you'll recall from the discussion of arthritis early in this book, the many different forms of the disease have widely different causes and symptoms. How could just one remedy work for all of them?

>> **The testimonial game:** Be wary of any therapy if its proof of effectiveness is made up entirely of testimonials (case histories). Although the case histories may be absolutely genuine, they aren't as valid as large-scale, long-term, carefully controlled scientific studies. After all, the patients in the case histories may not have had the same form of arthritis as you do, may have had complicating conditions, and may not have been given uniform doses of the therapy. The placebo effect may also account for the good results in the case histories. (That is, some of the patients may have gotten better primarily because they *believed* in the therapy.)

REMEMBER

A lack of studies doesn't necessarily mean a therapy is bad, and good study results by themselves don't guarantee that a treatment or therapy can work for you. Having a combination of both studies and case histories to review is best.

>> **Miracle cure myths:** Steer clear of practitioners who promise that their approach is the long-awaited *miracle cure,* the magic potion that erases all of your problems. Some standard and alternative cures are amazingly effective, but no one has yet developed a miracle cure that eases all our ills.

>> **Shady demands:** Avoid practitioners who tell you to throw away your crutches, stop taking your medicine, or ignore your physician's advice. Likewise, be wary of those who demand large amounts of money in advance or who don't want you to tell your physician what they're doing for you. In general, trust your instincts and don't do anything that you don't feel good about.

Working with Your Doctor

While around 30 to 40 percent of American arthritis patients use alternative therapies, perhaps three-quarters of them don't tell their physicians what they're doing. Many don't inform their physicians because they're afraid that their doctors may pooh-pooh their ideas, tell them that they're foolish, try to talk them out of it, or even refuse to continue working with them if they insist on using CAM.

WARNING

You, too, may be tempted to keep your CAM use a secret from your physician, but don't. Telling your physician everything you're doing, from taking herbs to using bee venom therapy, is important because you may inadvertently do something that clashes with one of your medical treatments. For example, combining St. John's wort with antidepressants can cause severe central nervous system depression and even be deadly.

Talking to physicians about CAM can be difficult. They have the weight of medical authority on their side. They've gone to medical school and can speak a language that you may not understand. But don't be intimidated. Doctors work for *you*; they're here to serve you. You have the right to ask questions and receive complete answers. To practice medicine effectively, a doctor must also practice good communication. Physician who close their ears toss away an important tool for understanding what you, the patient, needs. For more information about finding a doctor with great qualifications — and great ears — turn to Chapter 6.

TIP

Try these tips for discussing CAM with your physician:

>> **Begin with the assumption that your physician is supportive.** If you open your conversation with a challenge or disparaging remark, you probably won't get very far. Make it clear up front that you're not challenging or rejecting your doctor's ideas, but that you're simply looking for more information and help.

>> **Ask your physician what they know about the CAM that interests you.** Ask if the CAM is appropriate for your ailment, if you need to watch out for anything while participating in the therapy, and so on.

>> **If your physician doesn't know about the CAM that interests you, offer information.** Go online and get studies about the CAM, copy pages from articles and books, ask the CAM's professional organizations to supply you with information, and offer this information to help your doctor find out more about the CAM you're considering.

>> **If you don't have time to discuss CAM during this visit, ask for another appointment.** Offer to pay for the extra appointment, if necessary.

>> **If your physician gives you trouble, ask why.** Do they know for a fact that this CAM is dangerous? Have they had a bad experience with it or seen patients who experienced negative or dangerous results? Is the objection based on knowledge or simply a feeling that anything unconventional is bad?

>> **If your physician refuses to discuss CAM with you or work with you if you're already using a CAM, get a new doctor.** Closed-mindedness is a terrible trait in any healer and may limit your progress on the road to recovery.

REMEMBER

Be as open-minded as you want your physician to be. Take into consideration any bad reports about the CAM that interests you, as well as the good reports. No healing art, conventional or unconventional, is perfect. Each has its strengths and weaknesses, and it's best to know what your CAM can do for you — and what to watch out for.

Figuring Out Whether Alternative Medicine Is for You

Deciding whether or not to experiment with alternative therapies is a very individual matter and depends on many things: How dissatisfied you are with traditional Western therapies, how adventurous you are, how willing you are to try unproven or controversial methods, what your inner voice tells you, and how your body responds.

If you opt to try CAM, always remember that many of these therapies aren't supported by reams of scientific studies, so you'll be taking a chance. Always research any therapy you'd like to try, find the most qualified and highly recommended practitioner you can, consult with your physician before and during treatment, and make sure that your physician monitors your progress. But perhaps the most important thing is to listen to your body: Are you feeling better? Does this approach seem to be working? Sometimes even the most scientifically sound method won't help you, whereas something strange and virtually inexplicable will. Your body possesses its own brand of wisdom — when it speaks to you, make sure you listen.

Chapter **17**

Discovering Herbs and Homeopathy

Many people are frustrated by the inability of standard Western medicines to cure their arthritis or relieve their symptoms completely, so they look for relief from some of the older, more "natural" remedies. Two of the most popular remedies are herbal medicine and homeopathy.

Herbal medicine uses plants and plant parts to stimulate the body to return to a state of internal balance. Herbs used to treat arthritis generally fall into the classes of anti-inflammatories, antirheumatics (which are immunosuppressive and inflammation-fighting), sedatives/muscle relaxants, and pain relievers.

Homeopathy, on the other hand, is a system of medicine based on the idea that medications should be given to stimulate the body to cure itself, rather than counteract the symptoms of an illness. So a tiny bit of the "disease" is introduced to the body, which prompts the body to get to work on healing itself. Homeopathic remedies for arthritis usually target the swelling and tenderness caused by inflammation.

WARNING

A purely complementary and alternative medicine (CAM) approach to autoimmune/inflammatory arthritis (basically anything other than osteoarthritis) is dangerous and carries the risks of permanent joint damage and deformity. Thus, any CAM, including herbs and homeopathy, should be considered add-ons that you might try for relief. But they are not appropriate as sole treatments. Inform your doctor about any CAM that you are using or considering, to be sure that it's safe.

Digging into Medicinal Herbs

Ever since humankind began roaming the earth, healers have been using *herbs* — any plant whose leaves, seeds or flowers can be used for medicinal, flavoring, or aromatic purposes — to cure or at least alleviate what ails us. Some herbs are eaten in their natural form. Others are ground into powder, crushed, or squeezed to make oil or extract; brewed with boiling water to make an infusion; or mixed with beeswax, petroleum jelly, or cream to make ointments or balms.

TECHNICAL STUFF

What's the difference between a healing herb and a drug? Drugs are often stripped, highly refined versions of herbs. About one quarter of all our modern medicines come from herbs. To turn an herb into a drug, pharmacological researchers work with the herb, refining it and homing in on the main ingredient that produces the desired effect. This ingredient is separated from the rest of the plant, modified in some way, perhaps concentrated, and standardized so that each pill or capsule delivers an exact amount. Then it's sold as a drug.

The good part about this approach is that it allows us to extract the special part of the herb that cures a particular ill, like a great soloist in an orchestra. The bad part is the herb refinement lets us have only that soloist, casting aside the rest of the orchestra.

Doctors say drugs are better than herbs because the active ingredient is isolated, they're modified and pure, they're served up strong, and they work much faster than herbs.

Herbalists (those who practice the use of plants for medicinal and therapeutic purposes) say that herbs are better than drugs because the so-called active ingredient is only one of many substances that work in concert to relieve or cure ailments. Modifying and purifying the active ingredients makes them overly strong, dangerous, and more likely to cause side effects. Herbalists point out that some of the alleged impurities in herbs can actually make them gentler and safer. And although speed is sometimes necessary, many times it's not essential to effective treatment. Furthermore, drugs that work fast can also be overly harsh.

Although many pharmaceuticals are more potent and potentially more dangerous than most herbs, all herbs should also be considered "drugs" because they are a concentrated source of active ingredients. The fact that something is natural does not guarantee that it's safe. (Just think of arsenic.)

Getting the Lowdown on Herbs for Arthritis

Which herbs have medicinal value? How much should be used? Which are good for osteoarthritis and which for rheumatoid arthritis and gout? Should they be taken in powder form, rubbed on as ointment, or sipped in the form of an infusion? The answers to these and many other herbal questions may depend on whom you ask, and whether they are a doctor of Oriental medicine, an herbologist, a naturopath, or the clerk at the vitamin store. Unfortunately, no official board of herbology exists to set standards and doses, so the advice you receive about herbs to treat arthritis will undoubtedly vary from one healer to another. A variety of herbs may be prescribed, some specifically for your type of arthritis, others for joint problems in general, and still others for pain, depression, or strengthening the immune system.

For a short list of some common medicinal herbs and what they're used for, see the sidebar, "Inside the herbalist's toolbox," later in the chapter.

Keep in mind that some, but not all, of these herbs have been subjected to scientific studies of their effects on arthritis. The following herbs have shown the ability to ease certain symptoms of arthritis in some studies:

- Aloe
- Angelica
- Borage oil
- Boswellia
- Capsaicin
- Cat's claw
- Chinese Peony
- Chinese Thunder God Vine
- Curcumin
- Devil's claw
- Ginger
- Kava kava
- Stinging nettle

Many herbalists believe that the following herbs have benefits for arthritis sufferers but scientific evidence to support these claims is weak:

>> Alfalfa

>> Black cohosh

>> Bladderwrack

>> Burdock

>> Celery seed

>> Centaury

>> Fennel

>> Feverfew

>> Meadowsweet

>> Mustard

>> Sarsaparilla

>> Valerian

>> Wild yam

In addition to those herbs listed here, currently some 14 percent of Americans are using CBD (cannabidiol) products for pain relief. To find out about CBD's effects on arthritis pain, see the nearby sidebar "CBD and arthritis."

WARNING

Even though many people consider herbs to be safe, it's best not to self-medicate. You could do more harm than good to yourself, for these reasons:

>> You may have an allergic reaction.

>> The herb may interact with another medicine that you're taking, which could increase the intended effect of either one, create the opposite effect, produce a toxic effect, or otherwise affect the body in harmful ways.

>> You may have a medical condition that makes it dangerous for you to take a particular herb.

>> The herbal concentration may be too strong, too weak, or mixed with other ingredients that your body cannot handle. (The U.S. government does not regulate the content and quality of herbs, supplements, vitamins, and other non-drug alternatives, so you really *don't* know what you're getting.)

CBD AND ARTHRITIS

Cannabidiol (CBD) seems to be the latest and greatest way to relieve pain, at least according to some who have tried it. A chemical found in marijuana, along with THC (delta-9-tetrahydrocannabinol), and other chemicals, CBD is inhaled or taken in the form of an oil placed under the tongue. Most who have tried it report that CBD improves physical function, sleep, and a sense of well-being, and some have also reported improvement in pain and stiffness.

While a few animal studies have demonstrated CBD's anti-inflammatory and pain-relieving effects, and a review study found substantial evidence that cannabis (although not necessarily CBD) is an effective treatment for chronic pain, scientifically valid clinical trials of CBD have yet to be conducted. That said, CBD is generally considered safe when used as directed, with side effects including lightheadeness, drowsiness, dry mouth, and rarely, liver problems.

If you decide to try CBD, consult with your doctor first, find a brand with a "Good Manufacturing Practices" (GMP) certification, use the oral kind (not the inhaled kind), and start with a small dose taken at night. Also, be sure to continue taking your pre-scribed medication, and to have your progress monitored by your doctor.

Finally, don't turn to CBD as a first choice pain reliever. It should be used only if other treatments are not effective enough.

Avoid potential risk by checking with your health advisor before taking any herbs. Make sure your physician knows that you are taking herbs or planning to take them. Even if they are not an advocate of alternative healing methods, your physician should be aware of everything you're taking.

REMEMBER

In addition to the herbs listed in the following sections, your herbalist may suggest black willow, caraway seed, cinnamon, clove, couchgrass, dandelion, juniper berries, oats, nutmeg, poke root, prickly ash, skullcap, spearmint, star anise, wintergreen, wormwood, yarrow, and more! Suffice it to say, herbalists can draw from a lengthy list of herbs when recommending treatment for arthritis pain, inflammation, anxiety, depression, insomnia, skin rashes, muscle pains, and other symptoms.

Anti-inflammatories

Inflammation, which occurs when a part of the body becomes reddened, hot, swollen, and painful, is a major problem in several forms of arthritis and related conditions. Doctors can offer powerful anti-inflammatory drugs, like the corticosteroids, but many people prefer the gentle relief offered by herbs such as those listed below. Anti-inflammatory herbs don't actually suppress inflammation as much as they help the body reduce inflammation naturally.

INSIDE THE HERBALIST'S TOOLBOX

Herbal medicine is used to treat just about anything that can go wrong with the human body — from hemp for treating glaucoma, to fringe tree bark for fighting liver disease, to Essiac tea for combating cancer. A tremendous number of herbs may be found in the herbalist's little black bag, including:

- *Agrimony* for allergies
- *Cayenne pepper* to strengthen the immune system
- *Celery* for inflammation
- *Feverfew* for migraine headaches
- *Fringe tree bark* for liver disease
- *Garlic* for elevated cholesterol and blood pressure
- *Ginger* for nausea
- *Ginkgo biloba* for problems with memory and circulation
- *Goto kola* for varicose veins
- *Hemp* for glaucoma
- *Hyssop* for asthma
- *Kava kava* for anxiety and insomnia
- *Linden* for tension
- *Sambucol,* an elderberry extract, for cold and flu symptoms
- *Skullcap* for asthma
- *St. John's wort* for insomnia and depression
- *Turmeric* for inflammation
- *Valerian* for muscle and joint pain
- *Vervain* for headaches

Alfalfa

Rich in minerals, alfalfa is a folk remedy for arthritis favored in the Middle East for its ability to reduce swelling and inflammation. However, those who have lupus should know that there is some weak evidence that it might trigger flares. Alfalfa is scientifically known as *Medicago sativa.*

Angelica

Angelica, or *Angelica archangelica,* has been used to treat the inflammation associated with rheumatism. This herb is also believed to purify the blood and protect against contagious diseases.

Black cohosh

Scientifically known as *Cimicifuga racemosa,* black cohosh is a Native American remedy taken to reduce the inflammation and pain of rheumatoid arthritis.

Bladderwrack

Rising to prominence in the early 1800s, bladderwrack was originally used as a source of iodine. Today the herb, known by the scientific name *Fucus vesiculosus,* is used in compresses to help reduce arthritis inflammation.

Borage oil

Taken from the seeds of the starflower, borage oil has long been used to treat asthma, dermatitis, and rheumatoid arthritis. Rich in gamma linoleic acid (GLA), it has anti-inflammatory properties and is available as an oil, a softgel, or an herbal tea.

Boswellia

Known scientifically as *Boswellia serata,* boswellia comes from India, where its gummy resin has been used for thousands of years as an anti-inflammatory. Substances in boswellia, called *boswellic acids,* are believed to reduce inflammation and help relieve the pain of osteoarthritis and rheumatoid arthritis. It has also been used to treat psoriasis, ulcerative colitis, and allergies, and may also help lower high cholesterol and high triglyceride levels. Boswellia is used as an extract, cream, or ointment.

Cat's claw

An extract of the bark of a vine native to the Peruvian rainforest, cat's claw was used for generations by the Ashanica Indians of South America to treat colds, tumors, and cold sores. Known scientifically as *Uncaria tomentosa,* the herb is considered useful in combating arthritis symptoms in several ways; it may be recommended by herbalists to reduce inflammation, boost the immune system, and ward off free radical damage to the cells. Cat's claw is taken in the form of tea or capsules. The herb may also help counteract gastrointestinal damage caused by NSAIDs, discussed in Chapter 8.

Centaury

Also known by its scientific name, *Erythrina centaurium,* centaury was used by the ancient Egyptians to reduce high blood pressure, and later by German herbalists for anxiety and melancholy. Today, it's often recommended for cases of gout and rheumatism because of its ability to help relieve inflammation.

Chinese peony

In the 1990s, the anti-inflammatory effects of a substance found in the root of the Chinese peony plant (called *paeoniflorin*) were pitted against those of standard drug methotrexate in rheumatoid arthritis patients. Results showed that the peony extract had anti-inflammatory effects that were equal to those of the drug. However, unlike methotrexate, the peony extract also helped to normalize the patients' immune function, and produce noticeable improvements in their physical strength and quality of life. A third trial of the peony extract found that, in 80 percent of the RA patients, it eased morning stiffness, joint swelling and tenderness, while decreasing blood levels of RA factor.

Curcumin

A component of the spice turmeric, curcumin was shown in a 2019 study of patients with knee osteoarthritis to have anti-inflammatory and anti-pain effects equal to those of the standard drug diclofenac. The patients also reported fewer side effects with curcumin and an average weight loss of nearly 2 percent of their body weight. Although curcumin is found in turmeric, it accounts for only 3 to 5 percent of the weight of the spice. This means that getting large enough doses through ingestion of the spice is pretty difficult. Dietary supplements of curcumin can be an easy, more practical solution.

Devil's claw

Devil's claw, or *Harpagophytum procumbens,* is the root of an herb grown in Africa. An infusion made of devil's claw, which is believed to reduce joint inflammation and pain, is a folk remedy for arthritis, rheumatism, and gout. This herb is most commonly used in capsule, tea, and tincture form. Devil's claw contains harpagoside, which has pain-relieving and inflammation-reducing qualities that have been compared to cortisone and phenylbutazone.

Sarsaparilla

With the official name of *Smilax officinalis,* sarsaparilla originated in the New World and was brought to Europe in the 1600s. There, the herb was used to treat inflammation due to rheumatoid arthritis. Herbalists still use it today to relieve the pain and swelling of arthritis and to enhance overall well-being.

Wild yam

Known scientifically as *Dioscorea villosa,* wild yam is perhaps most famous as a traditional "female remedy," used for menstrual ailments and to prevent miscarriage. It also has anti-inflammatory properties, which is why herbalists may recommend it for rheumatoid arthritis and other forms of inflammatory arthritis.

Antirheumatics

Several herbs seem to be especially helpful in reducing the symptoms of rheumatoid arthritis (joint inflammation in a majority of joints, swelling in two matched joints, fever, fatigue, and so on) and related conditions.

Antirheumatics are not a substitute for rheumatoid arthritis medications.Any herbs should be taken in addition to your medications, under the supervision of your doctor. That said, here are a few of the better-known antirheumatic herbs.

Bogbean

Once used to prevent scurvy, this pretty wildflower is renowned for its ability to relieve the pain of rheumatism. Known to scientists as *Menyanthes trifoliate,* bogbean has mild sedative properties.

WARNING

Be careful, however, because large doses of bogbean may cause vomiting. It should not be used if you have inflammatory bowel disease.

Celery seed

Scientifically known as *Apium graveolens,* celery seed was used by Oriental healers to reduce elevated blood pressure. And the celery stalk was prized by Americans during the 1800s because it was so expensive. Today, celery seed and celery juice are used to rid the body of excess water and aid in digestion. The seed is also believed to ease both rheumatoid arthritis and gout.

Chinese Thunder God Vine

Used medicinally in China for over 400 years, an extract of the root of the Thunder God Vine *(Tripterygium wilfordii)* eases pain and inflammation safely and effectively in patients with treatment-resistant rheumatoid arthritis. The extract helps to "turn off" an overactive immune system and tone down the activity of certain inflammatory genes. Researchers believe that Chinese Thunder God Vine also has potential as a treatment for lupus, although more study is needed.

Meadowsweet

Meadowsweet (*Filipendula ulmaria*) contains a substance with aspirin-like properties. The herb has been used for hundreds of years to relieve arthritis pain and help combat rheumatic conditions.

Sedatives and muscle relaxants

Sleep can be a major issue for those with some forms of arthritis. How well can you sleep if you hurt, if movement is difficult, or if you're worried and stressed? The herbs in this category can help you relax and sleep better.

Kava kava

A popular treatment for insomnia and nervousness, kava kava (*Piper methysticum*) promotes relaxation of the muscles and nervous system without diminishing mental alertness. By helping you relax and perhaps sleep better, this herb can help you deal more effectively with the stress of arthritis.

Valerian

Known as *Valeriana officinalis,* valerian comes from the rootstock or roots of a perennial herb. It is typically used in the form of capsules and extracts. Valerian is recommended for arthritis patients because it helps ease pain and tension, and it also encourages sleep. In Germany, valerian is used as a mild sedative, and one study showed that it worked as well as a standard sedative drug with the added advantage of being non-addictive.

WARNING

Don't take more than the recommended dosage — very high doses can cause a weakened heartbeat and even paralysis. Check with your physician to see how much you should take.

Pain relievers

Pain is perhaps the most significant symptom of many forms of arthritis. Dull or sharp, constant or intermittent, achey or gripping, pain can make your life miserable. Here are some of the better-known herbs that can help relieve pain.

Aloe

Used internally or externally, aloe is a popular herbal cure for the pain of wounds, burns, and arthritis. Known to the scientific community as *Aloe vera* or *Aloe barbadenis,* it can also be used in the form of a fresh leaf, a gel, capsule, lotion, or liquid. In addition to relieving arthritis pain, aloe has been used to treat gastrointestinal problems and ulcers, as first aid for wounds and burns, and as a mild laxative.

WARNING

Taken internally, aloe may hamper or increase the action of certain medications, and cause uterine contractions or miscarriage in those who are pregnant.

Burdock

Burdock *(Arctium lappa)* is an ancient remedy that has been used to treat snakebites, dog bites, and a variety of other conditions thought to leave impurities in the blood. Today's herbalists have found that burdock has a diuretic effect and may ease arthritis pain as well as skin irritation due to psoriasis, eczema, and canker sores.

Capsaicin

Capsaicin, which comes from chili peppers, is the ingredient that makes the spice cayenne so darn hot. Capsaicin is believed to prompt the release of endorphins, the body's natural, built-in pain relievers, and to interfere with *substance P,* which is a compound produced by the body that helps transmit pain signals through the nervous system. Known scientifically as *Capsicum frutescens,* capsaicin is used to treat pain. It's typically applied as a cream or taken as a tea or capsule.

Fennel

Well-known among chefs, fennel has also been used to relieve stiff, painful joints. Herbalists and folk medicine healers often suggest that their patients apply fennel oil directly to their distressed joints and rub it in. This herb's scientific name is *Foeniculum vulgare.*

Ginger

The aromatic root of a tropical herb, ginger has been used by the Chinese to treat indigestion, stomach cramps, and stomach upset for over 2,000 years. Scientifically known as *Zingiber officinale,* ginger may be recommended by modern herbalists for arthritis patients. Studies have shown that taking ginger supplements or eating fresh ginger can help ease the pain, morning stiffness, and inflammation associated with some forms of arthritis, while increasing flexibility and range-of-motion.

Ginger is typically taken as a powder, capsule, extract, tea, or tincture. It can also be freshly grated and added to food or eaten as a side dish. Ginger compresses may be applied to painful joints.

Mustard (black)

A preparation of mustard, or *Brassica nigra*, has long been a favorite remedy for painful joints. Sometimes it's taken internally (often with honey), and sometimes it's applied directly to the joint. (Mustard oil plus rubbing alcohol can be applied to the skin to increase circulation to the affected area.) Black mustard is generally considered stronger and more effective than white mustard.

Stinging nettle

A prickly plant with stinging hairs that "inject" an irritant into the skin, stinging nettle has traditionally been used to treat allergies, insect bites, and wounds. Today it may be recommended to relieve joint pain and swelling; laboratory studies suggest that stinging nettle can counteract at least some part of the inflammatory response. A German study found stinging nettle plus a small amount of an NSAID to be as effective as the full dose of the NSAID in relieving symptoms of osteoarthritis. In addition, stinging nettle contains boron, a mineral important for bone health. Known scientifically as *Urtica dioica*, stinging nettle is typically taken as a capsule or extract. A poultice of cooked leaves may be applied to the painful area.

Stimulating the Body to Heal Itself with Homeopathy

Before drugs and surgery came to dominate Western medicine, healers called *homeopaths* flourished in the United States and Europe. Their guiding philosophy was *homeopathy*, which means "similar suffering."

The idea behind homeopathy, which was created by Dr. Samuel Hahnemann in the 18th century, is to stimulate the body's natural healing mechanisms by, in a sense, "showing" it a piece of what's wrong. This may sound odd; after all, we're accustomed to modern Western medicine killing disease with strong medicines. But Dr. Hahnemann believed that "like cures like." He theorized that if large amounts of a substance could cause the symptoms of a disease in a healthy person, then very small amounts of the same substance should be able to help the body recognize and eliminate the same ailment. These small doses would act something like vaccines to gently stimulate the body to heal itself.

For example, suppose that a large amount of Substance X caused constipation in healthy people. According to Dr. Hahnemann's homeopathic theory, a very tiny dose of the same Substance X would unlock the bowels in people who were already constipated. His idea was codified as homeopathy's *Law of Similars.*

Determining remedies according to your symptoms

While medical doctors try to suppress symptoms, doctors of homeopathy look upon them as helpful signs that the body is trying to heal itself. To the homeopath, symptoms are more than simply indicators that a certain disease is present. Instead, they are the body's way of describing what has gone wrong on a physical, mental, and emotional level. Probing beyond the symptoms (which is where most Western medicine stops), homeopaths look for the essence of their patients. Thus, they ask what the patients like to eat and drink, when and how well they sleep, whether they're day or night people, what they wish for and what they fear, what kind of weather they prefer, how they respond to stress, and so on.

If you complain of pain, a good homeopath looks beyond its location, intensity, and number of occurrences. They ask additional questions, such as:

>> When does it hurt?

>> What are you doing when it starts to hurt?

>> How are you feeling, emotionally, before the pain strikes?

>> What does the pain feel like? Is it sharp? Throbbing? An ache? Does it radiate? Is it constant? Does it come and go?

>> What makes the pain feel better? A warm bath? Eating certain foods? Going to work?

>> What makes it feel worse? Movement? Cold temperatures? Stress? Work? Family gatherings? Holidays?

These kinds of questions are designed to get to the essence of the problem: the physical and emotional state that allowed the disease to take hold and grow.

After the homeopath identifies the essential problem, it can be treated — but not with a medicine designed to destroy something. Instead, the homeopath looks for the single best remedy (homeopathic "medicine"). Which remedy is most effective depends mostly on the patient. If a patient has joint pain, for example, not just any remedy for pain will do. It has to be the remedy that best matches the patient's *constitutional makeup.* Every one of the 2,000 or so homeopathic remedies closely matches a particular temperament — including that person's fears and hopes, likes and dislikes, and sleep and behavior patterns.

In *classical homeopathy*, only the absolute minimum dose of a remedy is given, and only one remedy is prescribed at a time. If the right remedy is given, the patient's symptoms will begin to clear up in a few days. If not, a different remedy is selected. No new remedies are used after the body has begun to heal itself. Practitioners of *complex homeopathy*, however, prescribe more than one remedy at a time.

Discovering recipes for remedies

Homeopathic remedies are derived from a variety of sources: leaves, berries, fruits, bark, roots, minerals, and sometimes animals. But no matter where they come from, they're all processed in a very special way.

In keeping with the idea that small amounts are best, the remedies are diluted over and over again in solutions made of water and alcohol, lactose, or other diluents. And each time they're diluted, they are shaken and struck in a special way. The more diluted, shaken, and struck, so the theory goes, the stronger the remedy becomes. Indeed, a finished remedy may only contain one part per million of the active ingredient. Critics charge that very little or even none of the active ingredient remains after these successive dilutions, so the remedy couldn't possibly work. Supporters believe that either (1) what's left over is enough to do the trick; or (2) that the fluid retains a "molecular memory" of the medicinal substance and acts accordingly.

TECHNICAL STUFF

Remedies are rated according to their potency. When one drop of the medicinal substance is shaken and struck into 99 drops of diluent, the remedy has a potency rating of 1c. (This mixture is sometimes written as 1CH.) If one drop is taken out of this mixture and added to 99 drops of new diluent, the new remedy has a potency rating of 2c. If one drop of the 2c remedy is then diluted with 99 drops of a new diluent, the potency rating rises to 3c, and so on.

How potent the remedy should be depends on the state of the disease. Here are the general guidelines used in the United States and many other countries:

>> **Low potency:** Up to 6c, used when only physical symptoms or severe changes in the disease state exist.

>> **Medium potency:** From 12c to 30c, used when physical and mental/emotional symptoms exist.

>> **High potency:** Up to 200c or greater, used when the problem is long-standing or acute, or the symptoms are mental/emotional.

TECHNICAL
STUFF

Another, very similar rating system is based on 10 drops of diluent rather than 99. Instead of shaking and striking one drop of substance into 99 drops of diluent, you use only 9 drops of diluent. In this method, based on 10 drops, potencies are rated 1x (or D), 2x, 3x, and so on.

Homing in on homeopathic remedies for arthritis

Most homeopathic remedies come from minerals or plants, with only a few derived from animals. Homeopathic remedies are not highly concentrated; in fact, they're diluted again and again until only minuscule amounts of the original substance are left.

This method is counterintuitive to practitioners of Western medicine, who believe that medicines should have more of the active ingredient, not less. But remember, homeopaths argue that smaller portions are better, because larger portions can cause the arthritic problem. The tiny portions, they insist, help the body heal itself.

WARNING

Self-medicating is never a good idea and can lead to unintended consequences, interactions with other substances, and possible damage to your health. No matter how much you may have heard about the safety of homeopathic remedies, working with a medical doctor or doctor of homeopathy is essential when you're using them. If you are using any homeopathic remedies, be sure your physician knows exactly what and how much you're taking. Even if they don't believe in homeopathy, your physician should be aware of what you're taking.

The purpose of the homeopath is to find the best match between remedy and patient. The remedy that the homeopath selects depends as much on the patient's constitutional makeup as it does on the symptoms, which is why you can't just pull any old arthritis remedy off the shelf. The following are some of the homeopathic remedies used for arthritis:

>> *Actea spic:* May be indicated when the joints are swollen and pained, and the focus of the arthritis is in the hands and feet or the smaller joints.

>> *Aconitum napellus:* May be indicated for gout. The pain grows worse at night or when temperatures rise, and gets better when the patient rests or gets fresh air. The patient is anxious and imagines terrible things are happening.

>> *Ammonium carbonicum:* May be indicated when poor circulation to the hands exists, as in Raynaud's phenomenon (see Chapter 5).

>> **Apis mellifica:** May be indicated when the joints are stiff and swollen, when pressure makes the pain worse, and when the skin over the swollen joints feels stretched and tight.

>> **Arnica montana:** May be indicated when the patient has rheumatoid arthritis linked to cold and dampness, and soreness and bruising are problems. The patient is nervous and extremely sensitive, prefers to be alone, and denies that anything is wrong.

>> **Belladonna:** May be indicated for sudden, sharp pain, and red, swollen joints. Getting wet or chilled makes the pain worse, and the patient usually avoids any kind of stimulation.

>> **Benzoic acid:** May be indicated when rheumatoid arthritis settles in the smaller joints, and nodular swellings exist.

>> **Bryonia alba:** May be indicated for gout with greatly swollen joints. Heat, movement, or touch makes the pain worse; cold, rest, and pressure help.

>> **Calcarea carbonica-ostrearum:** May be indicated for rheumatoid arthritis in the shoulders and upper back. Wetness and dampness worsen the pain and fear and perhaps confusion engulfs the patient.

>> **Causticum:** May be indicated when arthritic joints are stiff and tight. Lying on the afflicted joints increases the soreness, and the patient is restless at night.

>> **Chamomilla:** May be indicated for severe pain when anger and restlessness are present.

>> **Cimicifuga racemosa:** May be indicated when pain is centered more in the muscles than the bones. Restlessness, talkativeness, and an unstable mood often accompany the pain.

>> **Ledum palustre:** May be indicated when pain is primarily in the smaller joints and travels up the body, with little or no swelling. Pain is worse when patient is in a warm bed.

>> **Ruta graveolens:** May be indicated when the patient suffers from bursitis (see Chapter 5).

>> **Sabina:** May be indicated when the patient is suffering from gout, and the gouty joints have nodules. The pain worsens with heat and movement, feels better with cool air, and is usually accompanied by depression.

>> **Sambucus:** May be indicated when the patient is suffering from poor circulation to the hands, as in Raynaud's phenomenon. The hands are blue and cold, and the patient sweats excessively while awake, but not while sleeping.

Finding homeopathic help

No one has proven why or how homeopathy may work, and while some studies suggest that it's significantly more effective than a placebo, others have found it unimpressive. Although all the evidence is not yet in, many people are convinced that homeopathy is right for them. Homeopathy is practiced by a variety of healers in the United States: naturopaths, herbalists, dentists, acupuncturists, and even certain medical doctors and doctors of osteopathy (DOs). The level of training and skill, however, varies from healer to healer, so be forewarned!

The National Center for Homeopathy offers a directory of homeopaths in the United States; see Appendix B for contact information. You can also find homeopaths by asking for referrals from certain physicians and other health professionals, searching online, or contacting homeopathic pharmacies.

» Understanding the theory behind each therapy

» Knowing what to expect during a therapy session

» Getting to know the possible benefits of each therapy

» Finding a competent practitioner

Chapter **18**

Hands-On Healing Methods

For thousands of years, healers have known that the "laying on of hands" can have a powerful therapeutic effect on the body. And why wouldn't it? Human beings are made to be touched. Babies fail to thrive if they're not touched enough. Huddling together against the cold was undoubtedly a survival technique for scores of our ancestors, and lovemaking is perhaps one of life's most fulfilling, restorative activities. Therefore, looking to hands-on methods for healing your body when it's ill or in pain makes sense. This type of therapy doesn't necessarily cure the disease, but it can help relieve pain, increase vital circulation, ease mental stress, relax tensed muscles, increase overall relaxation, and aid the body in its struggle to rebuild itself.

Various methods of hands-on therapy, from the ancient art of acupressure to the relatively new trigger point therapy, are explored in this chapter. Keep in mind, however, that if you decide to engage in any of these therapies, you should use them in addition to — not in place of — standard medical treatment, and discuss your preferred therapy method with your physician in advance.

Unblocking the Energy Flow: Eastern Hands-On Healing Methods

These therapies, which are rooted in either Chinese or Japanese medicine, are designed to remove blockages and restore balance to the body's energy flow. Once balance is restored, so the theory goes, the body can begin to heal itself.

Pinpointing the pain with acupuncture

An important part of traditional Chinese medicine, *acupuncture* has been used for thousands of years to prevent and treat disease by balancing the body's energy flow.

In traditional Chinese medicine, disease is thought to be the result of an imbalance or blockage of energy or *chi* (pronounced "chee") in one or more parts of the body. (While air and food will supply us with energy, the stresses and strains of living will diminish it.) Acupuncturists believe that manipulating specific points on the body can unblock the energy flow and restore the body's balance.

According to traditional Chinese medicine theory, energy flows through the body along invisible channels called *meridians.* Twelve major meridians run through your body to deliver energy and sustenance to your tissues, but these channels can become obstructed. When they do, the obstructions act like tiny dams, blocking or slowing the flow of energy and serving as major causes of pain and disease. Luckily, the meridians near the surface of your skin at some 300 different locations called *acupuncture points,* and by manipulating and stimulating these points, an acupuncturist can remove the obstructions and reestablish the healthy flow of chi throughout your body.

When you first visit an acupuncturist, they will probably interview you extensively about your symptoms, level of pain, medical history, diet, bowel habits, quality of sleep, and so on. The acupuncturist may also examine your eyes, tongue, skin, or fingernails; take your pulse; and listen to your voice, breathing, and bowel sounds.

During your visit, you will either lie or sit on a padded table for the treatment, but you won't have to remove all your clothing, just loosen it and uncover the areas to be treated. Your acupuncturist will then stimulate and manipulate certain acupressure points, but just a few — not all 300 of them! The following list explains the various methods your acupuncturist may use to do this:

>> **Inserting fine needles:** Your acupuncturist may insert anywhere from 2 to 15 ultra-thin needles into certain points and leave them in place for a period

of time (usually 10 to 20 minutes). They won't necessarily insert the needles directly into the area that's bothering you, but rather along the meridian that affects that area. So don't be surprised if your feet are manipulated to ease your back or neck pain! The needles are so fine, you may not feel them, but if you do, you will usually feel just a moderate sting that disappears quickly. Your acupuncturist may insert needles shallowly (just under your skin) or as deep as an inch or more.

>> **Adding a low-level current (electroacupuncture):** Many acupuncturists have found that the addition of a low-level electrical current can make the treatment more powerful. A small electrode is attached to the acupuncture needles after the needles are inserted, allowing a low amount of electricity to run through the electrode to the acupuncture points. Your acupuncturist will adjust this current by turning a dial. You should feel a light buzzing at your acupuncture points. If the buzz is annoying or uncomfortable, tell your acupuncturist, and they will turn down the "juice" until it no longer bothers you.

>> **Using heat and herbs (moxibustion):** To stimulate the flow of chi and strengthen the blood, your acupuncturist may burn a small amount of an herb called *mugwort* (or *moxa* in Chinese) over your acupuncture points, being careful not to burn your skin.

>> **Cupping:** Small glass cups are heated and placed over your acupuncture points where they create a vacuum-like effect. As the cups cool, they promote an increase in blood circulation, with the goal of relieving muscle tension, promoting cell repair and aiding in overall regeneration.

Discovering what acupuncture can do for you

According to the National Center for Complementary and Integrative Health, an estimated 35 million Americans undergo acupuncture treatments regularly. The therapy is used to treat ailments ranging from asthma to ulcers, but its primary use is pain relief. Many people with osteoarthritis, rheumatoid arthritis, gout, fibromyalgia, and Raynaud's phenomenon swear by acupuncture, and some studies have shown that it can relieve pain caused by osteoarthritis and/or fibromyalgia. Although no scientific explanation for its effectiveness exists, acupuncture does produce real responses in the body, including stimulation of the immune and circulatory systems and the release of endorphins, the body's natural painkillers.

You may require several acupuncture sessions (perhaps as many as six) before you begin to notice a difference, but once the beneficial effects set in, they often last for weeks, months, or even longer. Unfortunately, acupuncture doesn't work for everyone.

Finding a good acupuncturist

To find a good acupuncturist, begin looking for one who is licensed by your state, if your state happens to be one that does this. (Some states don't.) It's also a good idea to look for a practitioner certified by the National Certification Commission for Acupuncture and Oriental Medicine (NCCAOM), acupuncture's equivalent to the American Medical Association. Some 17,000 practitioners have been certified by the NCCAOM, so you can probably find at least one in your area.

Or, if you like the idea of receiving acupuncture from someone with a medical degree, contact the American Academy of Medical Acupuncture (AAMA). It can provide you with a list of MDs or DOs (doctors of osteopathy) who have completed 200 hours of medical acupuncture training, had two years of medical acupuncture clinical experience, and performed at least 500 medical acupuncture treatments. (See Appendix B for more contact information on NCCAOM and AAMA.)

Finally, ask the members of your health care team for referrals, as more members of the traditional Western medical community are now aware of the benefits of acupuncture. (Who knows? Maybe some of them see acupuncturists themselves!) It doesn't hurt to ask, and your medical team members may be able to give you some good leads.

Pressing your buttons with acupressure (shiatsu)

Acupressure (which the Japanese call *shiatsu*) is a lot like acupuncture, but instead of needles, the therapist presses on your acupuncture points using the fingers, hands, or special tools to unblock your energy flow and restore balance. Because acupressure involves hands-on manipulation, it's often considered another form of massage instead of a version of acupuncture. And because it's actually a combination of these two methods, both acupuncturists and massage therapists often use acupressure.

Instead of lying on a padded table as you do during an acupuncture session, during acupressure you will lie on a mat on the floor for better resistance against the pressure exerted during treatment. Using the thumbs, fingers, whole hand, elbows, or feet, the practitioner will apply pressure and manipulate your body along meridians to improve your flow of *chi*. They may also use tools, such as wooden rollers, balls, or pointers. As the practitioner works to unblock your *chi*, they will also work to transmit some of their own energy into your body. Your acupressure session may include stretching or other kinds of massage, and some practitioners also give diet and lifestyle tips.

Discovering what acupressure can do for you

Acupressure is designed to produce the same pain relieving and energizing results as acupuncture — without the needles, of course! Like massage, acupressure has a calming and soothing effect, and that alone may help ease some of your symptoms almost immediately. Although good studies demonstrating its effectiveness as an arthritis treatment don't currently exist, acupressure does work for some people, without side effects (when it's properly done). At the very least, your acupressure session should be a pleasant experience.

Finding a good acupressurist

Contact the National Certification Commission for Acupuncture and Oriental Medicine (NCCAOM) to find a certified acupressurist. (See Appendix B for more contact information.)

TIP

You may also find referrals through your health care team, rehab center, or pain management center.

Restoring healing energy with Reiki

The word *Reiki* (pronounced "ray-kee") is a combination of two Japanese words — *rei*, meaning a higher intelligence or spiritual consciousness, and *ki* (or *chi* in Chinese), meaning the life force or energy that animates all plants and animals. Therefore, *Reiki* is a healing energy guided by a higher intelligence or a spiritual power.

The basic principle of Reiki is that universal life energy, which creates and maintains all forms of life, can be channeled into a patient by a practitioner as a force for healing. The Reiki practitioner will administer the treatment by laying hands on specific parts of your body and applying little or no pressure. (You remain fully clothed.) Some practitioners won't actually touch you, but rather place their hands directly above your body. The practitioner will then channel healing energy into you to help relieve energy blockages and balance the life force within your body. This technique is sometimes used along with some form of massage.

Discovering what Reiki can do for you

Enthusiasts say that Reiki can help ease the pain and other symptoms of virtually every kind of illness and injury while increasing the effectiveness of many kinds of therapy. Although the practitioner may not actually touch the patient, those who have experienced Reiki say they feel a glowing radiance flowing throughout their bodies after a 60- to 90-minute session. Stress reduction, relaxation, and an increased sense of well-being are typical benefits of a session.

Finding a good Reiki practitioner

Check out The International Association of Reiki Professionals web site: www. iarp.org. (See Appendix B for more contact information.) Here you will find a list of Reiki practitioners in your area.

Realigning and Releasing Tension: Western Hands-On Healing Methods

While Eastern therapies are based on releasing energy blockages and restoring the chi, Western therapies contain a potpourri of approaches, ranging from manipulating the alignment of the spine to applying pressure to specific points on the sole of the foot. Each is based on a different theory, and each takes a completely unique approach to pain relief.

Rubbing away muscle tension with massage

Massage is the manipulation of body tissues by rubbing, stroking, kneading, or tapping using the hands or other instruments such as rollers, balls, or pointers. For most kinds of massage, you will lie on a padded table, wearing little or no clothing, covered by a soft flannel sheet. Your body will remain covered by the sheet throughout the massage, except for the area that's actually receiving the treatment.

If you're uncomfortable with the idea of disrobing in front of the therapist, remember that you only need to take off enough clothing to reveal the areas that you want massaged. Keeping your underwear on is definitely okay! It's also possible to be massaged while sitting in a chair, completely clothed. (Sometimes this is done in the workplace.)

The therapist should ask you what kind of massage you'd like (invigorating, relaxing, and so on), if and where you're experiencing any pain, and how firm or soft a touch you'd prefer. If you like, the therapist may darken the room and play soft music during the massage. Oil or lotion (usually pre-warmed) will be used so the therapist's hands will glide over your skin without causing friction.

REMEMBER

Speak up! It's not necessary to get a whole body massage unless that's what you want. If you just want work done on your neck, feet, and hands, for example, say so. And don't be afraid to give your therapist feedback during the massage: Tell him or her what's painful, what's soothing, what you'd like more or less of, what kind of pressure feels best, and so on. The therapist should adjust the technique and pressure accordingly. The whole point of massage is for you to relax and feel comfortable, so be clear about what you need.

Here are some of the most popular kinds of massage:

>> **Swedish massage:** Also known as *effleurage,* Swedish massage involves the gentle kneading and stroking of muscles, connective tissue, and skin, using oils or lotions. Sometimes clapping or tapping movements are also used. Therapists can make this method of massage as gentle or as vigorous as you like. If you have fibromyalgia, rheumatoid arthritis, or another particularly painful form of arthritis, a gentle Swedish massage may be just what you need to help you relax.

>> **Shiatsu:** Also known as acupressure. (See the section titled "Pressing your buttons with acupressure (shiatsu)," earlier in this chapter.)

>> **Deep tissue massage:** This method involves the exertion of intense pressure to relieve chronic tension deep within the muscles. Using fingers, thumbs, and, sometimes, elbows, your aching, knotted, or chronically tense muscles will be slowly stroked across the grain to release tension and induce relaxation. Deep tissue massage can be painful and may cause soreness during and after the session. But if you develop chronic tension in other parts of your body because you're favoring certain painful joints, deep tissue massage may be a way to release the tension.

>> **Rolfing:** Rolfing was developed in the 1950s by Ida P. Rolf, a biochemist who discovered therapeutic bodywork when an osteopath successfully treated her for a respiratory problem. Dr. Rolf's treatment is based on the idea that both physical and psychological health are affected by the alignment of the body. If the body is out of line, poor physical, mental, and emotional health results.

To correct body misalignment, the Rolfing practitioner stretches and manipulates the thin membrane called the *fascia* that covers each bone, muscle, organ, nerve, and blood vessel. The fascia can become tight in response to stress, injury, or chronic misuse. To release this tightness, the practitioner will use their fingers, knuckles, or elbows to apply intense pressure. Administered in one-hour sessions once a week for ten weeks, Rolfing is uncomfortable at best; at worst, it's quite painful. But proponents of this method claim that it can produce marked improvement in muscle function and reduced strain on the joints. Combined with special breathing techniques, Rolfing may also help release the buried emotions that create chronic physical tension.

>> **Myofascial release:** Myofascial release is a milder form of Rolfing, in which the practitioner applies gentle but steady pressure to the fascia to stretch it and release tension.

>> **Sports massage:** This form of massage is intended to ease soreness; assist in healing sports injuries such as sprains, strains, tendinitis, or muscle soreness; and prevent future injury. Like Swedish massage, sports massage involves kneading and stroking the muscles and connective tissue, with an emphasis on the areas of your body most affected by the sport (for example, the shoulder and arm of a baseball pitcher or the knees and legs of a football player). If you have an injury or an inflamed joint, make sure that your massage therapist is a qualified expert in this type of massage.

>> **Trigger point therapy:** Using the fingers to apply prolonged, deep tissue pressure to specific points on knotted, painful muscles, trigger point therapy relieves tension and helps muscles relax. This therapy causes the pain sensors in the pinpointed area to "overload," so they either send fewer pain messages or stop sending them altogether. In some cases, trigger point therapy can be a helpful treatment for fibromyalgia.

Trigger point therapy is one of those treatments that feels so good — when it stops! Let's say, for example, that you have chronic tension in your neck that you just can't seem to release. To perform trigger point therapy, your massage therapist will ask you to lie face down on a padded table, and then proceed to apply intense thumb pressure to a specific point where your neck and shoulders meet. (Yes, it hurts!) Your therapist will maintain this pressure for a good 30 to 45 seconds (or as long as you can stand it), but after the pressure is released, your chronic neck tension should be gone (or at least, greatly reduced).

WARNING

Most kinds of massage, including shiatsu, deep tissue release, Rolfing, myofascial release, sportgs massage, and trigger point therapy are not recommended for those with autoimmune or inflammatory forms of arthritis as they can promote inflammation and make these conditions worse. Check with your doctor before engaging in any kind of massage.

REMEMBER

Injured and/or inflamed joints should not be massaged directly, as injured tissue may be further damaged, and the increased circulation brought about by massage may make any swelling worse. Don't engage in any kind of massage that doesn't feel really good.

Discovering what massage can do for you

Like most kinds of hands-on therapy, massage can significantly affect your well-being — at least temporarily. A slower heart rate, increased endorphin levels, decreased pain levels, and improved relaxation are just a few of the positive results. Like a nice warm bath, a good massage can increase your circulation, then go two steps further. It helps your body clear away by-products of metabolism that can irritate nerve endings, and ease pain by increasing your level of endorphins — the body's natural morphine.

Some types of massage may not be appropriate for your type of arthritis. Consult your doctor for guidelines before getting massage therapy, especially if you have rheumatoid arthritis, osteoarthritis, or ankylosing spondylitis. Also, avoid massage if you've got a fever or infection, if you're having an arthritis flare, or if you're coming down with an acute illness.

TIP

Be sure to drink plenty of water prior to and following a massage. Massage can help release built-up toxins in the muscles, and you can help your body flush them out by keeping well-hydrated during this period.

Finding a good massage therapist

Locating a skilled massage therapist who is experienced in treating clients with arthritis should be one of your top priorities. Fortunately, your physical therapist or doctor may be able to steer you to someone suitable.

But just as important as technical qualifications is the chemistry between you and your therapist. The sex of the therapist, in fact, is an issue for many people. If you feel a little strange about being massaged by a man, for example, you should automatically narrow your search to include women only. Remember, if you don't feel completely comfortable with the therapist you choose, you won't be able to enjoy all the benefits of massage. So shop around; you may want to try several therapists before deciding on one person. Keep in mind that many massage therapists will come to your home with their massage tables and all the accoutrements in tow. All you have to do is pick up the phone!

Promoting energy balance with polarity therapy

Like traditional Eastern systems of healing, *polarity therapy* is based on the belief that the body contains energy systems that must remain balanced because unbalanced or blocked energy leads to pain and disease. The aim of polarity therapy is to find these blockages and release them by using the hands to touch specific points on the body to help restore balance. After balance is achieved, the body should return to a healthy state.

During your first visit, the practitioner will interview you, observe your body and the way you move, and manually feel certain areas of your body to determine the location and degree of your energy blockages. The therapy itself will involve touches that can vary from light to firm, but you won't have to disrobe, and the touching will be guided by your verbal feedback. A typical session will last from an hour to an hour and a half.

Discovering what polarity therapy can do for you

Your polarity therapy practitioner will work to help you increase your awareness of *subtle energetic sensations*. For example, you may feel mild waves of energy coursing through your body, tingling, warmth, or general relaxation. Your practitioner may also offer advice on diet and lifestyle. The aim of polarity therapy is to relieve your pain and help your body heal itself, although no scientific studies confirm that polarity therapy can achieve these goals.

Finding a good polarity therapy practitioner

To find a practitioner of polarity therapy, see the American Polarity Therapy Association web site: https://polaritytherapy.org to get a list of referrals.

Relieving pain and encouraging healing with reflexology

Reflexology involves applying pressure to specific points on the soles of the feet, the palms of the hands, or the ears that are believed to correspond with various organs and other parts of the body. Reflexology theory maintains that the body is divided into ten zones, each running lengthwise from head to foot and down one arm through one of the ten fingers. Applying pressure on one part of the zone is believed to help relieve pain and encourage healing in another part of that zone.

The reflexologist manipulates a specific area — most commonly on the bottom of the foot, but sometimes on the palm of the hand or the ear — that corresponds to the diseased or painful area. They use a map of the foot, hand, or ear that indicates the points that can stimulate healing in the heart, stomach, lung, pancreas, kidney, colon, eyes, ears, throat, and even the tonsils. For example, your reflexologist may press an area just outside the middle of the ball of your foot to stimulate your lungs. Reflexologists will use special thumb, finger, and hand techniques, without the addition of oils or lotions, to stimulate your body parts. For most people, reflexology is a relaxing and pleasant experience.

Discovering what reflexology can do for you

No scientific studies prove that reflexology is an effective treatment for arthritis. But, like most kinds of massage, reflexology may be helpful in reducing the stiffness seen in osteoarthritis and rheumatoid arthritis. It may also help increase circulation, which is helpful if you have Raynaud's phenomenon.

Finding a good reflexologist

You can search a directory of reflectologist on the homepage of the Reflexology Association of America web site: `https://reflexology-usa.org`. You may also get referrals from your massage therapist or another healing arts professional.

Transmitting healing energy through touch therapy

In *touch therapy*, also known as therapeutic touch, energy is transmitted from the practitioner's hands to the patient's body in order to speed the healing process and ease pain. Like certain Eastern philosophies, therapeutic touch is based on the belief that the body possesses an energy field and the energy within this field must be ordered and balanced to maintain health. When the energy becomes unbalanced, disease results.

Although the practitioner won't actually touch your body, they can discern where problems exist in your energy field by meditating while holding their hands over your body to feel the vibrations. The practitioner will then channel energy into your body to help ease your pain and speed healing. One session usually takes about 30 minutes.

Discovering what touch therapy can do for you

Some studies have found that therapeutic touch is effective, including one performed on 25 patients with osteoarthritis. The participants in this study were divided into three groups: One received standard Western medical care, another received therapeutic touch, and a third received a simulated version of touch therapy. The participants who received bona fide touch therapy experienced a significant decrease in pain along with an increase in mobility, while the other study participants did not. Several studies have shown that touch therapy helps ease pain, including the pain associated with arthritis, while others have found it has little or no effect. Still, therapeutic touch is taught at more than 100 colleges and universities in 75 countries, is used by many nurses, and is the subject of a great deal of scientific research. If you're in pain, you may want to give it a try.

Finding a good touch therapy practitioner

To find a good touch therapy practitioner, go to the Therapeutic Touch International Association web site at `https://therapeutictouch.org`.

Chapter **19**

Other Alternative Approaches

Y ou're probably already familiar with herbs and homeopathy. (If you aren't, check out Chapter 17.) But did you know that many people utilize other alternative methods (besides herbs and homeopathy) to ease the symptoms of arthritis? In this chapter, we introduce you to some of these therapies, how they're performed, what some say these methods can do for you, and where you can begin your search for a competent, qualified therapist.

REMEMBER

Even if you're lucky enough to find both a therapy that works and an excellent practitioner, you will still need to continue to work with your physician and the other members of your health care team. Studies have shown that people with arthritis who completely ignore traditional medicine in favor of alternative methods find that their health deteriorates at an alarming rate. If an alternative therapy is used, it should be a *complement* to traditional medicine, not a substitute for it.

Breathing In the Healing: Aromatherapy

Aromatherapy utilizes a wide variety of fragrant substances called *essential oils* to treat physical and emotional ills. These oils are taken from the fruit, flowers, bark, or roots of plants producing deliciously enticing smells, such as basil, bergamot, black pepper, camphor, cedar wood, chamomile, fennel, frankincense, hyssop, jasmine, juniper, lavender, patchouli, and rose. The unique aroma of each essential oil is believed to trigger beneficial physiologic and emotional responses in those who inhale it. Lavender, for example, is believed to be soothing and relaxing, which is why it's recommended for people who are stressed or anxious. Ginger, on the other hand, is thought to be energizing and warming and is sometimes used as a mild aphrodisiac.

Understanding how it works

Massage is perhaps the most effective delivery system for aromatherapy when it is performed with *carrier oils* that contain a small amount of one or more essential oils. Carrier oils are plain, unscented oils that do not irritate the skin (such as soy oil or corn oil) which account for the majority of the solution applied to the skin, with only a drop or two of essential oil added for aromatic purposes. (With the exception of lavender oil, essential oils are never applied directly to the skin in their undiluted state because they are too strong and irritating.)

As pleasurable as an aromatherapy massage may be, it's certainly not the only way to enjoy the benefits of essential oils. They can also be dropped into a pot of boiling water, with their aromas allowed to escape into the air in the form of steam, or the steam itself can be inhaled after the solution has cooled somewhat.

WARNING

When inhaling steam, be sure to remove the pot from the stove and allow it to cool until the steam can be inhaled comfortably. Inhaling the steam from a boiling pot can cause burns!

Discovering what aromatherapy can do for you

Aromatherapy is an ancient healing art dating back over 4,000 years to the ancient Egyptians who used fragrant oils to cure the ills of both mind and body. Plant oils were also used throughout the Middle Ages to treat wounds and help heal disease. And modern proponents of aromatherapy insist that it can help treat acne, arthritis, bronchitis, poor circulation, skin problems, and many other conditions. Because it acts on the central nervous system, aromatherapy may also help to ease anxiety and depression, reduce stress, induce relaxation or sedation, lessen pain, give you a lift, or even act as a mild stimulant.

The essential oils most often prescribed for arthritis pain include basil, bergamot, citrus, eucalyptus, frankincense, ginger, jasmine, lavender, peppermint, and turmeric. One study found that arthritis patients who used aromatherapy were able to reduce their intake of painkillers while maintaining their current level of comfort.

Finding out where to get aromatherapy

Many people perform aromatherapy on their own, but it's a good idea to see a professional first to find out how to do it safely and effectively. You can find a certified aromatherapist through the National Association for Holistic Aromatherapy, web site https://naha.org.

Fighting Pain with Bee Venom Therapy

Believe it or not, this therapy actually uses the venom from bee stings to help alleviate pain! Although the preferred method of administering bee venom therapy (BVT) is through the sting of a live bee, the venom can also be administered via an injection, although this method is thought to be less effective than a bee sting.

WARNING

Be warned that bee venom therapy may cause *anaphylaxis*, a severe potentially life-threatening allergic reaction. It may also cause *thrombocytopenia*, or a low blood platelet count. Since platelets help your blood clot, mild to serious bleeding can occur when they're in short supply. Also, since the FDA hasn't approved BVT as an antidote to pain, you may have trouble finding a health care practitioner who will give you the bee venom injections, should you want to avoid being stung by a live bee. However, bee venom acupuncture therapy (using venom applied to the tips of acupuncture needles, which are inserted into acupoints) is now practiced by some acupuncturists.

Understanding how it works

The bee venom is administered either directly on or near the site of your pain, or on specific acupuncture points or trigger points. While the injections are pretty straightforward, applying the live sting of a bee is an interesting procedure. The bee, held in long tweezers, is placed on the designated spot and allowed to do its thing. (The area to be stung may be iced beforehand to dull your pain.) Unfortunately, the process may need to be repeated several times before you experience any arthritis pain-relieving results. And, as you can imagine, it hurts.

Discovering what bee venom therapy can do for you

Surprisingly, bee venom has powerful pain-relieving and anti-inflammatory effects. Because bee venom therapy is quite popular in Asia and Eastern Europe, and many people swear by its ability to ease the symptoms of their arthritis. In 2018, researchers in China pitted bee venom acupuncture against the standard drug, methotrexate, to measure its ability to allieviate the signs and symptoms of rheumatoid arthritis in 120 RA patients. Bee venom acupuncture was just as effective in improving RA symptoms as methotrexate. It's an interesting finding, although more human studies need to be done. And, of course, you should never substitute bee venom acupuncture for your RA medications.

WARNING

This treatment can be fatal if you develop an allergic reaction to the bee venom. Before beginning bee venom therapy, ask your doctor to test you for an allergy to bee stings. If you are allergic, do not use this treatment! And even if you aren't, it's imperative that you make sure someone is with you when you are stung, and you have an anaphylaxis emergency treatment kit (available by prescription only) in case you suddenly develop an allergic reaction.

Finding out where to get bee venom therapy

It's best to start with a physician or an acupuncturist who will give you bee venom injections or acupunture, which are less painful than the bee stings. And in case anything goes wrong, you'll already be in the presence of a healthcare practitioner. Since bee venom isn't FDA-approved for this kind of therapy, you may need to rely on word-of-mouth referrals or recommendations from a pain clinic to find a willing physician or acupuncturist.

For live bee sting therapy, contact a beekeeper or other proponent of bee venom therapy. The American Apitherapy Society web site www.apitherapy.org can provide you with more information on this unusual therapy. (See the appropriately named Appendix B for additional contact information.)

Replacing the Hormone DHEA

This therapy is based on the belief that some kinds of arthritis may be related to the lack of a hormone called DHEA (dehydroepiandrosterone). Although DHEA is a male hormone (an androgen), it's manufactured in both male and female bodies.

The body then uses DHEA to make several other hormones, including estrogen and testosterone. Levels of DHEA have been found to be low in some people with lupus, juvenile arthritis, and rheumatoid arthritis.

So far, results have been positive when DHEA was given to women with mild to moderate forms of lupus. In one study of 191 women with lupus, 200 milligrams of DHEA per day helped ease fatigue, pain, and inflammation, allowing the women to cut back on their medication. Unfortunately, no scientific studies have yet shown the same positive results for rheumatoid or juvenile arthritis.

Understanding how it works

Researchers don't know exactly how DHEA works against lupus. What they do know is the immune system "goes wild" in lupus and mistakenly attacks the body's own tissue, and that androgens tend to suppress immune function. And, in both test tube and animal studies, DHEA reduces the production of cytokines, which promote inflammation, thus reducing lupus flares. Thus, DHEA may help combat some symptoms of lupus by keeping the immune system's "bad behavior" in check. But while it might reduce disease activity in those with severe or active lupus, it is not a cure for the disease.

Discovering what DHEA can do for you

Besides helping to relieve symptoms of lupus, high levels of DHEA in the blood have been linked to a lower risk of heart disease, stroke, cancer, diabetes, Alzheimer's disease, and Parkinson's disease. Blood levels of DHEA decline rapidly after the age of 30, so keeping them high may help ward off degenerative diseases and age-related problems.

WARNING

DHEA is a drug and may cause side effects, like headache, fatigue, insomnia, and acne, so a physician should always monitor its use. In some people, DHEA may actually *increase* the risk of certain types of cancer (breast, ovaries, and prostate) and heart disease. Don't take DHEA if you're pregnant or breastfeeding, or currently taking azathioprine (Imuran) or methotrexate, as the combination can cause liver damage.

Finding out where to get DHEA

Begin by asking your health practitioner about DHEA. If they agree that it may be worth a try, get a prescription. DHEA (generic name, prasterone) is a drug and a physician should always monitor its use. Some people need a dose of about 200 milligrams per day to see positive results, but try starting on a lower dose and see what happens.

WARNING

DHEA is widely available online, in health food stores, and at other commercial enterprises, although some of these brands contain significantly less DHEA than they claim.

TIP

You may come across wild yam products that claim to be natural, unprocessed sources of DHEA. But although these products may be natural, your body can't absorb DHEA until it has been chemically altered, so don't waste your money.

Another form of androgen supplementation is a transdermal patch. The patch is placed on your skin, and your body absorbs the hormone at a steady rate. You replace the patch every three days. Testosterone is the main hormone delivered in this manner, but others may soon be available.

Although doctors have much more to learn about the benefits and risks of this supplementation, there seems to be a possible benefit for certain people with the rheumatic diseases, specifically those in which androgen levels are decreased. Benefits can include fewer flares, increased bone mineral density, less depression, and improved joint function. The main areas of concern are increased risks of cardiovascular disease and cancer. The first step is to have the levels of the androgen hormones measured in your blood

Fighting the Pain and Disability of RA with MSM

MSM (methylsulfonylmethane) is an organic, sulfur-containing compound that is often used to fight inflammation and ease the joint and muscle pain seen in osteoarthritis and rheumatoid arthritis. It is also a potent antioxidant and free-radical scavenger that can play a critical role in supporting the immune response. Animal studies have shown that osteoarthritic joints have a lower sulfur content than normal joints and that mice with arthritis given MSM had less joint deterioration. A 2017 review study showed that MSM is effective in reducing arthritis-related inflammation and protecting cartilage from being degraded by suppressing two inflammatory cytokines, TNF-a and IL-1b. MSM was also found to reduce exercise related muscle damage, due to its antioxidant effects.

TECHNICAL STUFF

Antioxidants are substances that may protect your cells against unstable molecules called *free radicals*, which play a role cellular damage, aging, heart disease, cancer and other diseases. Free radicals are produced during normal cell metabolism and when you're exposed to environmental stressors like tobacco smoke and radiation. *Free radical scavengers* interact with free radicals and neutralize them, preventing them from causing damage to the cells.

Understanding how MSM is used to treat arthritis

Oral forms of MSM are available in capsule or powder form, and it can also be applied to the skin in the form of a gel. The Arthritis Foundation recommends a dosage of 1,000 to 3,000 milligrams per day in two or three divided doses, although optimal doses have not been set for either OA or RA. To be safe, you might start by taking 500 milligrams a day divided into two or three doses, and watch for side effects such as headaches, low energy, aches and pains, and depression. If you experience any of these symptoms, lower your dose and wait until the symptoms subside. Once they do, you can gradually increase the amount until you reach the standard dose.

WARNING

Always consult with your healthcare pracitioner before taking MSM, and don't stop taking your other arthritis medication(s) unless they advise you to do so.

Discovering what MSM can do for you

MSM has been used as an additional treatment for reducing the pain and inflammation seen in osteoarthritis, rheumatoid arthritis, tendinitis, tenosynovitis (inflammation of the lining of the sheath that surrounds a tendon), fibromyalgia, bursitis, and carpal tunnel syndrome, although evidence of its effectiveness is still scant.

What clinical research has shown is that MSM taken orally (1.5 to 6 grams per day in divided doses), either alone or combined with glucosamine, modestly reduced OA pain and swelling and improved joint function or physical function. It is believed to work by supplying the body with extra sulfur to form collagen and create the amino acid methionine, which helps the body synthesize connective tissue and absorb nutriients.

Finding out how to get MSM

MSM is widely available in online, at health food stores, and at other commercial enterprises.

WARNING

Don't take MSM if you are pregnant or breastfeeding, as not enough is known about the safety of MSM in these circumstances. Since it is a sulfa drug, do not take MSM if you have allergies to sulfa.

Whirling the Pain Away with Hydrotherapy

Hydrotherapy is an ancient treatment using water (both hot and cold), steam, and ice to stimulate and soothe the body, rearrange its energies, and encourage healing.

Understanding how hydrotherapy is used to treat arthritis

Water is either applied to the entire body or to specific areas in the form of liquid, steam, or ice. It may be delivered via showers, baths, *sitz baths* (baths in which you're immersed only up to waist level), warm and cool compresses, wet sheet wraps, hot wet blankets, steam baths, and other techniques. Hydrotherapy can also be performed internally by drinking water and/or taking colonics (enemas that flush out the colon).

Discovering what it can do for you

Hydrotherapy is an age-old therapy for arthritis. The Romans were famous for their public baths, where people "took the waters" to ease the pain of their arthritic joints. A modern hydrotherapist may recommend a variety of treatments including drinking plenty of water to flush toxins away, taking short cold baths or showers to increase circulation, using warm baths or steam rooms to increase circulation and sweat out toxins, and applying cold compresses to ease joint pain.

TIP

Although bathing in mineral waters (and sometimes drinking them) has long been touted as a health aid, evidence suggests that bathing in plain old warm water works just as well!

Finding a good hydrotherapist

To find a specialist in hydrotherapy, ask your physical therapist or other health-care practitioner for referrals or search online for "hydrotherapist near me." Be sure to look for someone experienced in treating arthritis, as some forms of hydrotherapy may be detrimental to your condition (for example, cold water therapy for Raynaud's may further constrict blood vessels that are already overly-constricted).

Peering into the Possibilities of Prolotherapy

Prolotherapy, which involves injecting an inflamed joint or the area surrounding a joint with dextrose (sugar) water, is a nonsurgical way to treat several musculo-skeletal conditions. "Prolo" is short for "proliferation," and this therapy is believed to promote the proliferation (growth) of new ligament tissue surrounding joints where weakened and damaged tissue is causing joint instability and chronic pain.

Understanding how it works

Prolotherapy fights inflammation by creating even more inflammation — much like fighting fire with fire. Ligaments, the structures that connect the bones within a joint and hold those bones in place, can become injured and have a hard time healing. Since the blood supply to the ligaments is limited, the healing process can be slow and incomplete, leaving them loose, damaged, and weak. Unfortunately, the ligaments have plenty of nerve endings, ensuring that you'll feel plenty of pain. Injecting sugar water into the area surrounding the ligament where it attaches to the bone increases inflammation, bringing extra blood, nutrients, and oxygen to the weakened tissue, which may help the healing process.

Discovering what prolotherapy can do for you

Although there are only a few small studies on prolotherapy, it appears to improve joint function and ease pain in a lot of different conditions, including osteoarthritis; ligamentous laxity (loose or improperly healed ligaments), and chronic back and neck pain.

A 2017 systematic review of ten studies of the effects of prolotherapy on knee osteoarthritis found that all of the studies produced positive outcomes and high patient satisfaction. A 2020 review of current injectable therapies found that pro-lotherapy likely provides at least some benefit, although as the review stated, the quality of available data makes this statement hard to prove.

Finding out where to get prolotherapy

If you're interested in prolotherapy, ask your doctor or healthcare practitioner if this treatment is appropriate for your condition and, if so, if they can provide it. If you need to find a doctor who specializes in prolotherapy, go to www.getprolo. com/ to find a listing of prolotherapy physicians.

5
The Part of Tens

This part of the book is a kind of "distilled" way of presenting some key information about managing your arthritis.

We include new treatments that you might not have heard about yet, tips for traveling with arthritis, ways to save prescription dollars, and health professionals who can help you fight arthritis.

Chapter **20**

Ten Crackerjack New Treatments

In the not-too-distant future, physicians may be able to diagnose arthritis by looking at a map of the patient's genes and treating the ailment through subtle genetic manipulation. In fact, doctors may be able to prevent arthritis by studying an infant's genetic code and tweaking it to ensure that the young one's joints never begin the process of deterioration.

We're certainly not there yet, but medical researchers have developed a host of new treatments. Some are modern twists on older therapies; others are entirely new ideas.

Janus Kinase Inhibitors for Rheumatoid Arthritis

Janus kinase (JAK) inhibitors are part of a family of drugs known as the disease-modifying antirheumatic drugs (DMARDs) used to treat chronic inflammatory conditions like rheumatoid arthritis.

People with RA have overactive immune systems that are flooded with cytokines. Some of these cytokines attach to receptors on immune cells and, with the help of enzymes known as *Janus kinases*, they force the cell to make even more cytokines. JAK inhibitors work by blocking the activity of these enzymes so the messages can't get through, causing cytokine production to fall. This calms the immune system and decreases RA pain, swelling, and joint damage.

In recent years, three JAK inhibitors have been FDA-approved to treat RA (and sometimes other conditions such as ankylosing spondylitis) in those who have not responded to or cannot tolerate one or more tumor necrosis factor (TNF) inhibitors:

>> Xeljanz (tofacitinib)

>> Olumiant (baricitinib)

>> Rinvoq (upadacitinib)

See the next section, "New Drug Treatments for Psoriatic Arthritis" for more on Xeljanz.

REMEMBER

The JAK inhibitors have several benefits. They are oral medications, while most of the traditional DMARDs and biologics are available only as injectables or infusions.They may start working quickly, in as little as a few days for some people, while it can take several weeks for the DMARDs and biologics to kick in. They are just as effective as DMARDs and biologics, and they can be used in combination with other nonbiologic DMARDS to get better results.

For more on the JAK inhibitors, see Chapter 8.

WARNING

The FDA has concluded there is an increased risk of heart attack or stroke, cancer, blood clots, and death with the use of Xeljanz, so they are adding this information to the Boxed Warning on Xeljanz, as well as on Olumiant and Rinvoq because they work in the same way as Xeljanz does. The FDA is also limiting all approved uses of these drugs to patients who have not responded or cannot tolerate one or more TNF inhibitors. If you're taking or considering taking one of the JAK inhibitors and you are a current or past smoker, and/or have a current or recent history of cancer, a heart attack or other heart problems, a stroke, or blood clots in the past, tell your health care professional, as these medications may put you at higher risk of developing serious problems.

New Drug Treatments for Psoriatic Arthritis

Almost a third of those who have psoriasis go on to develop psoriatic arthritis (PsA), with symptoms of joint pain, stiffness and swelling that can range from mild to severe. Foot pain, lower back pain, and swollen fingers and toes are just a few of PsA symptoms.

The disease has no cure and treatment is currently geared toward controlling symptoms and preventing joint damage, which can cause disability without treatment.

Fortunately, some new drugs have been FDA-approved in recent years for the treatment of PsA symptoms, including Orencia, Simponi and Simponi aria, Xeljanz, Rinvoq, and Tremfya.

Here's a brief overview of each:

>> **Orencia** (abatacept) was approved by the FDA in 2017 to treat symptoms of psoriatic arthriti in adults. It works by inhibiting the activation of T cells, which play an important role in promoting inflammation. Although various studies have shown that Orencia is effective in treating adult PsA, it may be less effective in those with moderate to severe psoriatic skin symptoms. Orencia is also FDA-approved to treat adult RA, polyarticular JIA, and the prevention of acute graft host disease.

>> **Simponi and Simponi aria** (golimumab) are TNF inhibitors, both of which are FDA approved for the treatment of adult forms of PsA, rheumatoid arthritis, and ankylosing spondylitis. Simponi aria is also approved to treat PsA and polyarticular JIA in children age 2 years or older. One major difference between the two is Simponi aria is given as an intravenous infusion while Simponi is given as an injection. Both work by targeting a protein called TNF which causes inflammation. A 2017 double-blind study (see the nearby sidebar for more on what this means) of 480 patients with PsA published in *Arthritis & Rheumatology* found that 75 percent of the patients given Simponi aria experienced at least a 20 percent improvement in signs and symptoms of PsA by week 14. Another study found that Simponi plus methotrexate is superior to methotrexate alone in inducing remission in those with PsA.

DOUBLE-BLIND STUDIES AND PLACEBOS

A double-blind study is a medical study involving human participants randomly assigned to one of two groups:

- The treatment group (those who received the treatment that is being tested)

- The control group (those receiving a placebo, which is a harmless medicine or procedure)

Since none of the participants know which group is getting the treatment, there is less risk of bias.

WARNING

The TNF inhibitor medications can bring about dramatic results, but they are also costly and can produce some serious side effects. A very small percentage of patients who were apparently prone to infections have developed deadly diseases, such as tuberculosis, while taking these medications. Because of the possibility of developing tuberculosis, you must be screened for active/latent tuberculosis, hepatitis B and C viruses, and HIV infection before taking TNF inhibitors. Your vaccinations should be up to date before treatment begins, and once you begin taking TNF inhibitors you should not receive any live immunizations.

» **Xeljanz** (tofacitinib) is a Janus kinase (JAK) inhibitor FDA-approved for treating psoriatic arthritis in 2017. The first JAK inhibitor to be approved for treating this disease, Xeljanz works by blocking the activity of JAK enzymes, which stimulate a kind of inflammatory protein know as the cytokines. Since all JAK inhibitors are taken in pill form, Xeljanz offers an oral alternative to the injectable or infused medications usually prescribed to treat this condition, like Humira and Remicade. Xeljanz is also FDA-approved as a treatment for ankylosing spondylitis, rheumatoid arthritis, ulcerative colitis, and polyarticular JIA.

» **Tremfya** (guselkumab), a new interleukin blocker, was FDA-approved in 2020 for the treatment of psoriatic arthritis and plaque psoriasis in adults. It is the first treatment for psoriatic arthritis that targets a cytokine called interleukin-23 (IL-23), which plays a critical role in producing PsA-related inflammation. A 2021 meta-analysis comparing the generic form of Tremfya (guselkumab) to other interleukin blockers as well as several TNF inhibitors found that guselkumab is just as effective as the other treatments for PsA and is often better at improving skin symptoms. Another study found that guselkumab may be particularly helpful in easing inflammation of the sacroiliac joints, which link the pelvis to the lower spine.

>> **Rinvoq** (upadacitinib), a Janus kinase (JAK) inhibitor, was FDA-approved in 2021 to treat psoriatic arthritis in adults who had unsuccessfully used TNF inhibitors, such as Humira. Many people with psoriatic arthritis have found relief when using TNF inhibitors, although not everyone can tolerate them. To find out if Rinvoq worked as well as Humira and might be used as a substitute, researchers performed a 12-week study involving 1,704 psoriatic arthritis patients comparing the effects of these drugs. The results showed that up to 71 percent of those given 30 milligram Rinvoq daily improved by at least 20 percent, while just 65 percent of those given Humira met this benchmark. The Rinvoq group also showed greater improvements in physical function and skin symptoms. And, since Rinvoq is an oral medication, it is much easier to take than Humira, which must be injected.

Matrix-Induced Cartilage Implantation for Knee Osteoarthritis

Matrix-Induced Cartilage Implantation (MACI) is a newer method of a cartilage implantation procedure known as *autologous chondrocyte implantation* that was FDA approved in 2016 for the repair of cartilage defects in the knee. Otherwise, it sounds as tho the defects occurred in 2016. For this procedure, cells taken from a patient's cartilage are grown in the lab until there are enough of them to form an implant. These new cartilage cells are then surgically placed over the patient's damaged cartilage and secured. In the past, the securing process involved using a membrane that was sutured into place. It was a time consuming, difficult process that caused scar tissue to form in surrounding areas.

With MACI, however, the new cartilage cells are applied to a *scaffold* (actually, it's a piece of collagen membrane taken from a pig) that is carefully cut to fit the area where the damaged tissue has been removed. The scaffold, with cartilage cells in place, is secured to the area using fibrin glue, instead of sutures.

The MACI procedure is simpler, less time intensive, and less likely to cause trauma to surrounding tissues than earlier forms of cartilage transplantation. And because the implant can be shaped to fit the damaged area exactly, MACI can be used to treat multiple areas of the knee and reach hard-to-access areas of damaged cartilage. The good news is that MACI's success rates in easing knee OA pain and restoring function are 90 percent or better. The cost of MACI is steep (around $40,000), but the majority of national insurance companies now include it in their plans.

Bone Marrow Aspirate Concentrate (BMAC) Therapy for Damaged Cartilage

Bone marrow, the soft, spongy substance that resides in the inner cavities of bones where blood cells are produced, also contains stem cells. The stem cells have the ability to generate many different kinds of cells under the right conditions, and these cells are used to create new tissue, including cartilage.

Aspirate is matter that was drawn from the body by suction. In BMAC, the matter happens to be bone marrow fluid collected from the fatty tissue inside a large bone such as the pelvic bone, using a needle. This fluid, known as *bone marrow aspirate concentrate* (BMAC), is processed in a lab to produce a concentration of stem cells that can then be injected into the affected area to help form new tissue.

REMEMBER

Besides forming new tissue, BMAC may ease inflammation, improve cartilage function, treat osteoarthritis, and delay arthritis progression. BMAC can be used in almost any joint, and only one treatment is usually needed.

While BMAC therapy has been studied in just a few clinical trials, a 2021 study of 505 patients with OA of the knee published in the journal *Applied Sciences* found that BMAC was superior to injections of either hyaluronic acid or autologous conditioned serum in improving knee OA pain and symptoms of the disease. After dividing the patients into three groups, each group received one type of injection repeatedly over the course of a year. At the end of the year, all three groups showed improved pain and knee OA symptoms. But BMAC was found to be the most effective, especially in patients who had more severe cases of the disease.

Platelet-Rich Plasma Injections for Knee Osteoarthritis

Platelet-rich plasma (PRP) is a combination of plasma (the liquid part of the blood) and platelets, a type of blood cell that contains clotting factors and growth factors. When injected into a damaged area, the platelets are believed to stimulate the regeneration of the tissue through cell reproduction. The plasma part of PRP is the delivery vehicle made from a substance your body won't reject. You can think of platelet-rich plasma as blood with a higher concentration of platelets than normal.

PRP is created by taking some of your own blood and spinning it inside a centrifuge to separate the platelets from the other blood cells, leaving only plasma and a high concentration of platelets.

This solution is then injected into the area being treated (most often the knee), to ease pain and accelerate the healing process. Some studies have shown that PRP can ease joint pain and stiffness by decreasing inflammation, promote healing, and shorten injury recovery time.

Although more studies are needed, two things are certain:

>> It takes several weeks for treatment results to reach their peak.

>> The results are not permanent. Symptom improvement typically lasts for six to nine months.

Hyaluronic Acid for Osteoarthritis

Hyaluronic acid (HA) is a major component of connective tissue. A clear, gooey substance, HA primarily keeps the body's tissues moist and well-lubricated. Within the joints, it forms a slippery, gel-like solution that helps the cartilage-tipped bone ends to slide easily across each other. And it draws water into the cartilage, preventing it from drying out and cracking, which are early signs of cartilage breakdown.

Some studies have shown that hyaluronic acid can be helpful in easing OA pain when taken either as an oral supplement or an injection into the affected joint(s). It's believed to work by tamping down inflammation, increasing the number of cartilage-producing cells, and inhibiting the release of enzymes causing cartilage breakdown. Several double-blind, placebo-controlled studies have found that taking oral doses of 80 to 200 milligrams of HA daily for at least two months significantly reduced knee pain in people with OA, especially those between the ages of 40 and 70 years old. (For an explanation of double-blind studies and placebos, see the sidebar of the same name earlier in this chapter.)

WARNING

Injections of HA are used primarily to ease inflammation and help lubricate and cushion painful joints. Treatment consists of either a single injection or three to five injections, each spaced one week apart. While HA injections are FDA-approved for knee osteoarthritis, study results are mixed. A 2018 review involving over 12,000 adults found only a modest reduction in pain, with relief felt after five weeks of treatment. However, other studies have shown that HA injections may work even better than painkillers for some people with OA. What's fairly certain is that HA injections work better in some people than in others, with lesser results experienced by older people and those with severe OA.

Cooled Radiofrequency Ablation for Knee Osteoarthritis

When your body suffers trauma, disease, or injury, the nerves in the affected area transmit pain signals to your brain. Usually, the pain signals stop once the disease runs its course or the injury heals. But sometimes the pain just keeps on going. Cooled radiofrequency ablation (CRFA) uses a small, insulated needle to deliver a heated, high-frequency electrical current to the affected nerves, deactivating them so the pain signals are no longer sent. Cool water is circulated along with the heated electrical current to eliminate the burning sensation, which makes the procedure more comfortable.

CRFA and hyaluronic acid (HA) injections are commonly used techniques for controlling knee OA pain and stiffness and improving knee function. But which one works best? To find out, in 2019 researchers conducted a 12-month trial comparing HA to a brand of CRFA called COOLIEF, the first and only radiofrequency treatment to be cleared by the FDA for moderate to severe OA knee pain. Of 175 patients with knee OA who had responded well to a nerve block, approximately half were treated with COOLIEF in four nerves in the knee, while the rest were given a single HA injection to the knee. Six months later, 71 percent of those in the COOLIEF group had experienced at least a 50 percent reduction in pain compared to 38 percent in the HA group. Function had improved by 48 percent and quality of life went up 72 percent in the COOLIEF group, compared to 23 percent and 40 percent in the HA group.

Because CRFA is minimally invasive and involves no incisions, most patients feel pain relief within one or two weeks and experience an increased quality of life much sooner than they would with surgery. While CRFA has a reported 70–80 percent effectiveness rate in those who respond well to nerve blocks, evidence supporting this technique as a long-lasting, reliable way to relieve knee OA pain is still quite limited.

Vagus Neurostimulation for Rheumatoid Arthritis

The *vagus nerve*, which runs from the brainstem to the abdomen, is an important communication highway that links the brain, immune system, cardiovascular system, and gut. And apparently it can also do much to reduce the pain, swelling, and lack of mobility seen in RA.

Containing 80,000 nerve fibers, the vagus nerve signals the brain when its time to produce hormones and neurotransmitters, and it also regulates stress reactions.

In 2002, Dr. Kevin Tracey discovered that the vagus nerve also has the ability to reduce inflammation. It does this by tamping down the release of key cytokines like TNF, which cause inflammation. Apparently the vagus nerve contains a kind of "off switch" that can keep TNF from being overproduced. And all you have to do to flick that switch into the "off" position is to stimulate it.

Vagus nerve stimulation, which has been used since the 1990s on more than 100,000 epilepsy patients to lessen and/or control their seizures, is now FDA-approved to treat both epilepsy and depression. And recently it was shown to be effective in treating rheumatoid arthritis.Dysfunctional autonomic nervous systems (of which the vagus nerve is a major component) affect an estimated 60 percent of RA patients. But several studies have shown that stimulating the vagus nerve with a small implanted device can reduce symptoms of RA, and bring TNF levels down to almost normal. All of this without using any drugs!

REMEMBER

More studies need to be done, but don't be surprised if vagus nerve stimulation turns out to be the latest and greatest non-drug treatment for RA.

Robotic-Assisted Surgery for Hip Replacements

As surgical techniques have become more refined in recent years, hip replacement surgeries have greatly improved. Today, instead of slicing straight through muscles to get to defective hip bones, surgeons carefully separate the muscle fibers and wend their way through, reaching the bones that they need to replace while cutting very little tissue. Thanks to these muscle-sparing techniques, patients now experience less pain, a faster return to function, and a more rapid discharge from the hospital than ever before.

Now, the use of robot-assisted surgery is taking the hip replacement to a whole different level.

Software attached to the robotic equipment creates a personalized surgical plan for each patient, using information generated by specialized 3-D images. The plan tells the surgeon exactly where to make the incisions and how to position the artificial hip joint for maximal hip function. The software can also exactly match the length of the leg receiving the hip replacement to the other leg, a critical part of a successful hip replacement. Robot-assisted surgery is reportedly five times more accurate at matching leg length than any of the methods used in conventional surgery. It also does a better job of inserting the new hip joint at the correct angle.

During the surgery, the robotic arm acts as a co-pilot and navigator for the surgeon, showing where the cutting instruments and the "safe zones" are at all times. Should the instruments drift away from the safe zone, the robot will sound an alert and shut off. This markedly decreases the risk of accidentally damaging bone and surrounding tissues, while vastly improving surgical accuracy. The robot also allows the surgeon to confirm, once and for all, that both the leg length and the alignment of the joint are correct before closing the surgical wound.

While robot-assisted surgical devices are already FDA-approved for use in certain types of surgical procedures, including hysterectomy, prostatectomy, and colectomy, they have not yet been approved for use in hip replacements. Most likely, it's just a matter of time.

New Drug Combination for Treatment for Uncontrolled Gout

Gout, a form of inflammatory arthritis resulting from excess uric acid in the blood, can cause painful attacks in the joints, especially the joint of the big toe. Left untreated, it can cause severe damage and disability. Treatment of gout involves lowering the body's uric acid levels, but there aren't a lot of therapies that do this. Allopurinol and febuxostat help lower the amount of uric acid the body makes. And probenecid aids the kidneys in removing uric acid from they body. If none of these work, and the gout remains uncontrolled, infusions of pegloticase can be used to convert uric acid into a harmless chemical eliminated through the urine. Unfortunately, pegloticase can trigger a potent immune response in people with uncontrolled gout.

In 2020, researchers hoping to lower the dangerous immune response seen with pegloticase decided to add the drug mycophenolate mofetil (MMF) the treatment. MMF is normally used for immunosuppression in transplant patients. Thirty-two subjects were randomly given either MMF or a placebo before receiving their pegloticase infusions, which were administered every two weeks for six months. After three months of treatment, the dangerous immune response to the pegloticase decreased, as expected. But the uric acid levels had also decreased — a lot! The combination of MMF and pegloticase *doubled* the decrease in uric acid levels seen with pegloticase alone, a stunning 86 percent as opposed to 42 percent in those who didn't get MMF.

This new drug combination could be the safe and effective treatment for uncontrolled gout that, up until now, has been out of reach.

Chapter **21**

Ten Tips for Traveling with Arthritis

ew things are more exciting and invigorating than packing your bags and hitting the road, bound for some exotic destination, or just getting out of Dodge for a while to clear your head! Yet traveling with arthritis can be a whole different animal, what with the additional strain on your joints, skyrocketing stress levels, change in routine, long hours sitting in cramped seats, jet lag, and having to haul loads of luggage and other travel paraphernalia. But don't worry — you *can* still travel when you've got arthritis, and you can even have a good time! You just need to plan a little more carefully than you may have in the past. Consider this chapter the Ten Commandments of Traveling with Arthritis.

Talking to Your Doctor

Tell your doctor about your travel plans: where you're going, for how long, what you plan to do, the kind of climate you'll be experiencing, and the kinds of foods you plan to eat. Then ask if they have any cautions for you. Should you limit yourself to certain kinds of activities? How much time should you spend resting every day? Should you be responsible for carrying your own luggage or ask others to carry it? Should you arrange for a wheelchair at the airport? Is pain the best indication of when to stop an activity? Or should you stop before the pain sets in?

It could also be helpful to find out whether a good doctor or health facility is near your destination. Ask your doctor about the possibility of bringing a prescription for any medicines you may need in case you run out, and get a letter from them describing your condition.

TIP

If you need to bring injection medications in a cooler, ask your doctor to include this in the letter. Then there should be no problems getting your meds through the airport, and the cooler should not count as a carry-on.

You may also want to check with your medical insurance company to find out if you're covered during travel and once you've arrived at your destination. If so, how does your insurance work? If, for example, you have an arthritis flare in Belgium, how do you pay for a visit to the doctor, and how do you get reimbursed? If your insurance doesn't cover you, find out about purchasing additional coverage for the short-term.

Reviewing Your Medications and Supplements

Make a list of every medication, vitamin, mineral, herb, supplement, potion, cream, rub, or liniment that you use. Then bring all of them! Try to follow your normal routine as closely as possible; don't start tossing out what seems to be superfluous right before you go on a trip. That "superfluous" item may be just the thing that can help you avoid or clear up a flare. Bring along familiar over-the-counter aids for pain so you don't have to start experimenting with strange brands when you're in unfamiliar territory. If you're flying, pack your medications in a carry-on bag so you have them with you even if your luggage gets lost.

After you have everything assembled, count the days you're going to be gone and make sure you take enough of everything to last the entire trip. Then pack a little extra. They may not have what you need where you're going!

WARNING

Before you travel to another country, try to find out which drugs it considers illegal. For example, Japan frowns on stimulants, while Greece and Turkey are strict about opiates such as codeine. Be sure to carry all of your medications (prescription, over-the-counter, and even vitamins) in their original containers. If you're taking along syringes or narcotic drugs, get a letter from your doctor explaining why you need them. The last thing you want is endless delays or interrogations because you're carrying the "wrong" medication!

Preplanning to Reduce Stress

Think through your trip and try to anticipate and solve any problems before you leave, so you can travel without worry. For example, if you have trouble walking, request a wheelchair or motorized cart in advance. Keep your carry-on bag light and easy to manage, and make sure all of your luggage has wheels and is well-balanced. (Imagine the aggravation caused by a rolling suitcase that keeps toppling over!)

Make a daily plan that includes alternating periods of activity and rest, and plenty of time to sleep. Schedule some time to exercise and to soak in a hot bath, if you find these activities helpful. Build in an extra day to give yourself time to recover from jet lag. In other words, don't just rush headlong into the unknown (meaning your trip) without a plan. If you do, your body may not be getting all that it needs. And that can translate to arthritis flares and pain.

Finally, plan an "emergency exit" procedure in case you need to cut your trip short. For example, you might want to purchase trip insurance, if it's available. Or get open-ended plane tickets. One thing is certain: You won't enjoy being far away and unable to go home when you're not feeling well.

Eating Wisely and Well

Eating a healthful, balanced diet is always important, but especially when your body is stressed by an ongoing condition such as arthritis compounded by the strain of traveling. Some foods may increase inflammation (especially if eaten in large amounts) and actually make your condition worse. Luckily, other foods may help relieve certain symptoms.

In general, no matter what your destination, you should try to do the following:

>> Eat a wide variety of foods, focusing on whole grains, fresh fruits, and fresh vegetables, with smaller amounts of meat, fish, poultry, (4 to 6 ounces per day maximum) and dairy products.

>> Limit your intake of cholesterol, fat, sugar, and salt (sodium).

>> Take it easy on the alcohol.

>> Use olive oil, canola oil, flaxseed oil, and other oils high in the "good" fatty acid (linoleic acid), which can help lessen inflammation.

>> Watch your intake of foods that contain the "bad" fatty acid (arachidonic acid) such as meat, poultry, egg yolks, and full-fat dairy products.

>> Eat fish that contain omega-3 fatty acids (mackerel, herring, salmon, and so on) a couple of times weekly.

Exercising, Even Though You're on Vacation!

We just can't stress this enough! Regular physical activity strengthens joint supporting structures, helping them take some of the pressure off the joint itself, while nourishing and moisturizing the cartilage. Aerobic activity can tone you all over, strengthen your heart, increase bone density, and help keep your weight under control (very important, especially for those with arthritis of the knee). Flexibility (stretching) exercises increase and maintain your range of motion, loosen up your muscles, and make your tendons and ligaments more resilient. At the same time, these exercises help release tension and promote relaxation — translating into less pain and stiffness, greater ease of movement, and an improved mental attitude. In addition, exercise can increase your physical abilities, help prevent joint deformities, boost your immune system, improve your balance, and help you maintain your independence.

Get plenty of exercise before you leave, to help carry you through the trip. If traveling by car, get out and stretch every 90 minutes or so. If traveling by plane, try to get out of your seat and walk up and down the aisle every so often to ease joint stiffness and prevent *deep vein thrombosis* (a potentially life-threatening condition in which a blood clot forms in one of the deep veins of the body, usually in the leg). If you can find room, try doing a few stretches and some range-of-motion exercises.

While on the trip, set aside some time each day to stretch and do relaxation exercises. And if your trip doesn't include plenty of walking, start each day with a brisk 20- to 30-minute walk. It's a great way to greet the day, and the scenery will be brand new to you!

Using Joint-Protection Techniques

When traveling, the way you use (or abuse) your joints becomes crucial. Remember (and apply) these joint–protection techniques recommended by the Arthritis Foundation:

>> Respect pain.

>> Avoid joint stressing postures or positions.

>> Avoid staying in one position for a long time.

>> Use the strongest and largest joints and muscles for the job.

>> Avoid sustained joint activities.

>> Maintain muscle strength and joint range of motion.

>> Use assistive devices or splints, if necessary. (See the next section.)

Using Assistive Devices

Splints, supports, canes, pillows, carts, and anything else that takes a load off your joints can be invaluable when you're traveling. Be sure to take advantage of the many "little helpers" designed to make your life easier and more comfortable. For example:

>> Use a horseshoe-shaped pillow to support your head and relieve neck pain while riding in a car or flying.

>> Support your back by wedging a lumbar pillow between the back of your waist and the seat.

>> A small pillow atop the armrest in a plane or a car can make it easier and more comfortable for you to prop up your upper body.

>> Wear your knee supports, or wrap your affected joints in elastic tape for greater stability.

>> If you're planning on visiting museums or galleries but your knees hurt when you stand for long periods of time, bring along a small campstool so you can pull up a chair whenever you need to.

>> Use canes, walkers, motorized carts, and wheelchairs as needed.

Renting an Arthritis-Friendly Car

The right car can minimize physical exertion, ease joint stress and strain, and make a driving trip a whole lot more comfortable. Call your rental car company at least six weeks before your trip to request a car that has these arthritis-friendly features:

» Automatic seat belts

» Cruise control

» Six-way seats that adjust for maximum comfort

» Four doors

» Hand controls

» Lightweight doors

» Plenty of legroom

» Button ignition instead of a key

» Big mirrors for a better view

» Seat belt extenders, making them easier to grab

» Tilt steering wheel

Flying with Finesse

Flying is often uncomfortable even for those who don't have arthritis, but it can be torture for those with chronically stiff, achy joints. To make your flight as tolerable as possible, try the following:

» If your budget allows it, fly first-class or business-class. It's a lot more comfortable — from the seats and the amount of space you have, to the service. But it can be mighty costly.

» If you're flying coach (like most of us), make your reservations early and request a seat in the first row or an exit row, to ensure more legroom.

» Spend the extra five bucks and get a skycap to handle your luggage or use curbside check-in.

» Request a wheelchair or motorized cart in advance if walking is a problem for you.

>> Ask for preboard status so you can take your time to get settled. The airlines will be happy to accommodate you.

>> Arrange for a nonstop flight when possible, to avoid the hassle of getting on and off two planes, and to cut down on the duration of the trip.

>> Get up and move as much as possible during the flight to ease joint stiffness.

>> Drink plenty of water during the flight, as the atmosphere inside the plane is extremely dehydrating.

>> Travel during the less busy times (midweek or midday, evening, and late at night) to avoid the crush of a crowd.

Taking a Test Run

If you're concerned about taking a long trip, try a smaller one first. Think of it as a test run. You'll find out what works for you and what you need to work on to make a bigger trip more successful. Make a detailed list of what you brought and what you were lacking. Once you get home, revise your list so you know exactly what to take next time.

Each time you travel, make a note of what was missing and revise your list when you get home. Then refer to the list the next time you pack. You'll become a seasoned traveler in no time. Happy wandering!

» Finding out about prescription drug assistance programs

» Cutting drug costs by buying generic, buying in bulk, or splitting pills

» Finding reputable online pharmacies

Chapter **22**

Ten Ways to Save on Prescriptions

The high cost of prescription drugs can be a real problem if you've got a chronic condition that requires a steady supply of medication, such as arthritis. Luckily, you can do several things to lower the cost of your meds, including sorting through what you're currently taking to see what you really need, buying generic forms of the drugs you really do need, buying in bulk, and splitting pills. Then, take a look at the many drug discount programs that are available, some of which offer certain drugs for free. Other good ideas include shopping around for the best price, getting assistance with paying your Medicare drug coverage from Medicare's Extra Help program, and buying from certain reputable online pharmacies. You may be surprised how much you can do to slash the cost of your prescription drugs.

Review Your Medications

Over time, that assortment of medications you're taking can start to resemble an overstuffed closet. You may have some you no longer need, some that no longer fit your condition, some that are duplicates, and some that clash with others.

TIP

For the sake of both your health and your pocketbook, compile a list of every drug you're currently taking, plus dosage and frequency, and ask your doctor to review it. Better yet, just bring all of your pill bottles to show to your doctor. Find out which, if any, can be eliminated, and which can be replaced with over-the-counter varieties (which can sometimes cost less than your prescription drug copay).

If you pay for your medications out of pocket, or your copayment is a hefty one, be sure to tell your doctor. They may be able to prescribe a less expensive version of the same drug, or fill out prior authorization paperwork to ensure that it's covered by your insurance. And because many insurance companies have a preapproved list of covered medications, show a copy of the list of medications your company covers to your doctor. If your doctor knows which drugs are on the "green-light" list, chances are they will be able to prescribe one appropriate for your needs that won't break the bank.

Ask Your Doctor for Free Samples

Almost all doctors have closets full of drug samples that were given to them by pharmaceutical companies. So, instead of investing a lot of money in a medication that may not work for you or has side effects you just can't tolerate, ask your doctor for some free samples. They will not only save you money, they'll also save you a trip to the pharmacy.

Check Out Medicare's Extra Help Program

Extra Help is a program that helps pay for your Medicare drug coverage, including plan premiums, deductibles, and the cost of filling prescriptions (copays or coinsurance). If you qualify for Extra Help, you may be able to pay less for your plan premium and yearly deductible, or nothing at all.

REMEMBER

How do you qualify? As of 2021, Extra Help is available to individuals with a yearly income of $19,320 or less, and married couples with a combined income of $26,130 or less, as long as their resources (money in checking or savings accounts, stocks, or bonds) are no greater than $14,790 for an individual and $29,520 for a married couple. Others who qualify for Extra Help include those on Medicare who are receiving: full Medicaid coverage; help from their state Medicaid program in paying Part B premiums; or Supplemental Security Income (SSI) benefits.

To apply for Medicare's Extra Help Program, visit the U.S. Social Security Administration web site at https://secure.ssa.gov/i1020/start. If you need help in completing the application, call Social Security at 1-800-772-1213 (TTY 1-800-325-0778). If you need information about Medicare Savings Programs, Medicare Prescription Drug plans, or how to enroll in a plan, call 1-800-MEDICARE (TTY 1-877-486-2048) or visit www.medicare.gov.

Look Into Patient Assistance Programs (PAPs)

If you can't afford to buy the medications you need, there are a great many patient assistance programs (PAPs) that may be able to help. PAPs are run by pharmaceutical companies, pharmacies, nonprofit organizations, or states, and may be able to provide you with free or low-cost medication. They typically require that applicants show proof of residence in the United States, have no prescription insurance coverage, and meet the program's income guidelines.

TIP

To find a list of PAPs and their contact information, visit https://www.rxhope.com/PAP/info/ProgramList.aspx and click on the name of the pharmaceutical company that manufactures the drug(s) followed by "patient assistance program." You'll find contact information, eligibility requirements, the drugs the PAP supports, and a link to the application.

Consider a Pharmacy Discount Card

Pharmacy discount cards can save you a lot of money, especially if you take several medications. Fortunately, these discount cards are easy to access. For example:

>> AARP offers a free prescription discount card to both members and non-members (although members get more benefits), available for use at 64,000 pharmacies. AARP claims their discount card can save you up to 61 percent on FDA-approved medications, as well as prescribed over-the-counter drugs. You can also view the cost of what you'd pay at other pharmacies on their web site. For more information, see https://aarppharmacy.com.

>> Amazon Prime offers a free discount card to Prime members that saves consumers an average of 78 percent of the full price of generics and 37 percent of the full price of select brand medications. The discount card

can't be combined with insurance or any other secondary payer (such as a PAP), but you still may end up paying less than you would with your insurance copay. The Amazon Prime discount card can be used at over 60,000 participating retail pharmacies in the U.S. and Puerto Rico, including Amazon Pharmacy. For more information see https://amzn.to/3fzJGDu.

>> Costco offers members and their eligible dependents discounts on prescription drugs, so long as they do not have drug coverage insurance, or their insurance doesn't cover the prescription drug in question. The Costco program cannot be used by anyone who receives Medicare or Medicaid. Estimated savings range from 2 percent to 40 percent. For a list of participating Costco Pharmacies and member inquiries, call 1-800-806-0129.

Some stores also have discount pharmacy services that are worth looking into. For example, for an annual fee of $36, members of the Kroger Rx Savings Club have access to over 100 common medications that will cost you $3, $6, or nothing at all. Walgreen's offers discounts of up to 80 percent of the retail cost of thousands of prescriptions, available to insured and uninsured alike.

Other well-known prescription discount cards that you might want to check out include ScriptSave WellRx (www.wellrx.com), SingleCare (www.singlecare.com) and GoodRx (www.goodrx.com).

Buy the Generic Version

A generic drug contains the exact same active ingredient(s) as its corresponding brand name drugs. It has the same potency, chemical makeup, dosage, quality, intended use, and performance. But it can cost between 25 and 75 percent less! So instead of buying brand name medications, ask your doctor to prescribe the generic equivalent. Pharmacists are legally allowed to substitute generic drugs for many brand name products, but they must first ask if this is all right with you.

TIP

Buying generic is also a great way to save money on over-the-counter medications. For example, Advil or Motrin (generic name ibuprofen) are much more expensive than the generic equivalent (which is often the store name brand), even though both contain exactly the same active ingredients.

Buy in Bulk

If you will be taking a medication for more than a month (usually the case if you have a chronic disease like rheumatoid arthritis or lupus), you might consider ordering your drugs in bulk to save money. Most pharmacies charge less per individual pill if you buy a 90-day supply as opposed to a 30-day supply, and online pharmacies are famous for selling medications in bulk.

Of course, there's a small catch: For most insurance companies, there is a copayment charge for every 30-day supply. In these cases, getting a 90-day supply without using your insurance (especially if you have a prescription drug discount) may actually be cheaper than paying three copayments. Check the figures before you buy. And make sure your doctor is not planning to adjust the type of medication you take or its dosage before you order three months' worth.

Double the Strength and Split the Pills

Getting medication at a higher dose and splitting the pills is a good way to save money. In fact, in some cases it can result in a 50 percent savings! You'll need to get your doctor on board, of course, to get that higher-dose prescription. And pill-splitting doesn't work with time-release medications or pills in capsule form. Although you can buy a pill splitter and cut each pill in half yourself, it will be safer if you get your pills split by a pharmacist.

Compare Prices at Different Pharmacies

If you're paying more than a set copayment for your medications, it may be worth your while to shop around for the pharmacy that offers the best price. That's right — pharmacies don't necessarily charge the same thing for the same drug! Some routinely offer discounted prices because they don't provide extra services like home delivery. Others may be running special deals on certain drugs.

To find out what a given pharmacy charges, simply call and ask. Be sure to provide the exact name, amount, and dosage of your medication. Or visit https://aarppharmacy.com and click on "Find a drug price." If you find the drug in question at a cheaper price than you'd pay at your regular pharmacy, your pharmacy may try to match it. If not, go elsewhere.

Consider Using Online Pharmacies

Unbeatable convenience and hefty discounts have made ordering medications online an attractive prospect for many people. Even if the cost of the medication is the same, you may be able to save money by ordering a 90-day supply for the same amount you'd pay in copays for three 30-day supplies from a retail pharmacy. You'll also save the cost of having to travel and from to the pharmacy and the annoyance of standing in line. Most prescription insurance companies have an online (mail-order) option for medications.

WARNING

For better or worse, many people look to Canada and other countries as sources of less expensive drugs. But this can be risky. According to Canada's National Association of Pharmacy Regulatory Authorities, only 1,400 of the 35,000+ online pharmacies around the world are safe and legal. This means just 4 percent can be trusted! You could wind up with the wrong product, an incorrect dose, a contaminated drug, a pill with zero medicinal ingredients, or one that does nothing to treat your condition. And even though Canada may seem like a very modern, health-conscious country, the Canadian government admits that some 74 percent of Canadian online pharmacies source their medications from outside the country.

If you do want to order from an online Canadian pharmacy, find out if it's legitimate before you buy. On its web site, locate the Canadian pharmacy's business address (usually under "Home" or "Contact Us"). Then go to the the web site of Canada's National Association of Pharmacy Regulatory Authorities (NAPRA) (https://napra.ca/pharmacy-regulatory-authorities), click on the appropriate province or territory, and click on "Find a Pharmacy." If the pharmacy is listed, it's licensed. If you can't find a business address for the pharmacy, look for one that does show an address and repeat the process.

You can also find valuable information about buying drugs over the internet from Health Canada at https://bit.ly/3IiAU92.

REMEMBER

In the United States, you can confirm the legitimacy of an online pharmacy by contacting the Pharmacy Verified Websites Program at https://nabp.pharmacy/programs/accreditations-inspections/dotpharmacy/and clicking on "View our list of Pharmacy verified websites," or visiting https://safe.pharmacy to check to see if a web site is safe

Chapter **23**

Ten Professionals Who Can Help You Fight Arthritis

You probably know that taking charge of your arthritis isn't just a matter of seeing your doctor once in a while and popping a few pills. Because arthritis is a multi-faceted disease, your fight takes place on many fronts, including the physical, the mental, the emotional, and the practical day-to-day business of living. To be effective, you will probably need to assemble a team of health care professionals (think of them as "generals") to help you attack arthritis in several ways.

The most important member of the team (after you) is the *rheumatologist,* a doctor who specializes in arthritis and other diseases of the joints, muscles, and soft tissues. But other members of the team, including the pharmacist, physical therapist, occupational therapist, social worker, massage therapist, and others will also play vital roles. Assembling a team is up to you and you alone. So research all you can about what these experts do and find the best ones you can to help you win the war against arthritis pain and joint destruction.

Rheumatologist

A *rheumatologist* is a doctor who specializes in diseases of the internal system (an *internist*) and has additional training and experience in the diagnosis and treatment of arthritis and other diseases of the joints, muscles, and soft tissues. The rheumatologist treats arthritis and related diseases such as fibromyalgia, lupus, scleroderma, and Sjögren's syndrome (usually referred to simply as Sjögren's). The goal is to alleviate pain, ease inflammation and other symptoms and, as much as possible, ward off further damage to your joints.

Treatment by a rheumatologist can be particularly crucial for those with rheumatoid arthritis. Taking DMARDs (disease modifying antirheumatic drugs; see Chapter 8 for details) is considered a first-line treatment for newly diagnosed RA patients. Studies have shown RA patients treated with DMARDs and other biologics have less joint damage, better joint function and a significantly reduced mortality rate compared to those who aren't treated with these medications. RA patients seen by a family practitioner or an internist are much less likely to be prescribed this important medication than those seen by a rheumatologist.

For referrals to rheumatologists in your area, ask your primary care physician, contact your health insurance company, or search the Medicare web site at www.medicare.gov/care-compare/#search, click on "Doctors and Clinicians" and type "Rheumatology" in the search box.

Primary Care Physician

Even though you may be seeing a rheumatologist, you will still need to maintain a relationship with your primary care physician, who is most likely the first health care professional you see when troubled by joint pain. Your primary care doctor (a family practitioner, internist, or geriatric specialist) will continue to be responsible for your overall health and well-being, even though they may refer you to a rheumatologist or other specialists.

The primary care physician's role is crucial. Many rheumatologists and other specialists don't provide regular health maintenance, which is essential for arthritis patients. Important examples include cancer screenings like pap smears, breast exams, and mammograms, which are especially important because many of the drugs used to treat arthritis and related conditions increase the risk of cancer. Paying attention to the prevention and treatment of heart disease is also vital, as more and more research suggests that patients with inflammatory arthritis of any kind are at increased risk of heart problems. Your primary care physician can also treat any coexisting diseases (keeping tight control of blood pressure in a lupus patient with kidney disease helps the person's kidneys survive longer), and primary care physicians also can provide vaccines. (Most patients who are taking immunosuppressants should get a yearly flu shot.) Patients receiving the best care often have close communication between their rheumatologist and their primary care physician.

For referrals to primary care physicians in your area, contact your health insurance company or visit the Medicare web site at `www.medicare.gov/care-compare/#search`, click on "Doctors and Clinicians" and type "Primary Care" in the search box.

Orthopedic Surgeon

Orthopedic surgeons are specially trained to surgically treat bone and joint problems that affect movement such as arthritis. They may specialize in treating disease of the hip, knee, spine, hands, feet, or other joints in the body.

REMEMBER

Naturally, not everyone who has arthritis will need the services of an orthopedic surgeon. Surgery is reserved for those with particularly severe forms of arthritis who haven't been sufficiently helped by more conservative treatments. The goal of surgery is to relieve pain and improve function while correcting whatever deformities may be creating the pain.

The most common orthopedic procedures for arthritis, including joint replacement, arthroscopic surgery, and *osteotomy* (the surgical cutting or removal of a bone or a piece of bone).

For referrals to orthopedic surgeons in your area, contact your health insurance company or visit the Medicare web site at `www.medicare.gov/care-compare/#search`, click on "Doctors and Clinicians" and type "Orthopedic Surgery" in the search box.

Pharmacist

Your pharmacist can do a lot more than just fill your prescriptions. These highly educated professionals are like walking encyclopedias when it comes to information on interactions between two or more drugs, drugs and foods, or drugs and herbs or supplements. They can give suggestions for maximizing drug effectiveness and minimizing or avoiding side effects. They will automatically keep track of all medications you're taking (assuming you get all of your medications from the same pharmacy), and they can look for potential problems or overdoses. Some pharmacists can even check your blood pressure, screen you for osteoporosis or high cholesterol, and administer flu shots or COVID vaccinations.

TIP

Bring your medication-related questions to your pharmacist, who can be a gold mine of free, accurate, and trustworthy information.

WARNING

If your pharmacist gives you information about a medication that scares you, or recommends that you avoid taking a medication your doctor has prescribed, talk to your doctor before you decide what to do. It's possible that the pharmacist has given you the wrong information, has overreacted, or hasn't factored in the risk/benefit ratio of taking the medication.

Physical Therapist or Exercise Physiologist

A physical therapist or exercise physiologist can help you put together a program of the best possible exercises to strengthen the muscles supporting your painful joints. They will show you how to do these exercises correctly, without inflicting more joint damage. Either one can also help you increase joint and muscle flexibility, restore range of motion, and pump up your endurance without putting undue strain on your joints. The services of both a physical therapist and an exercise physiologist may be covered by your insurance plan if you get a referral.

Although you won't need the services of either of these professionals forever, it does take several weeks to get you on track with a good exercise program and to supervise your exercising and stretching to make sure that you're not doing more harm than good to your body. You may also find techniques using heat, cold, or water therapy that can help you manage pain and improve your mobility.

For referrals to physical therapists or exercise physiologists in your area, contact your primary care physician or your health insurance company.

Occupational Therapist

An occupational therapist (OT) can show you how to overcome arthritis-related movement limitations through the use of special techniques or assistive devices that can ease the performance of daily activities. The OT will interview you and watch you in action, and then come up with recommendations that can make it easier for you to get dressed, groom yourself, get around, shop, do housework, drive, or work. They may also design special splints or supports for you and show you techniques to reduce joint stress and help prevent further joint damage.

To find occupational therapists in your area, contact your primary care physician or health insurance company.

Registered Dietitian

If you have osteoarthritis and are overweight, nutrition therapy can be an important component in your recovery. OA of the knee is often a direct result of carrying too much weight, and losing as little as 5 pounds can do much to prevent arthritis of the weight-bearing joints or, at least, dramatically reduce the symptoms. But losing weight, as we all know, is a lot easier said than done, and getting the help of a professional may be well worth the cost. A good dietitian can help you figure out how to eat regular, well-balanced meals consisting of standard size portions; distinguish between eating/food-related behaviors and feelings/psychological problems; and help you gradually lose weight and keep it off.

For referrals to dietitians in your area, contact your primary care physician, your health insurance company, or visit the Academy of Nutrition and Dietetics web site at www.eatright.org.

Social Worker

A social worker can help you deal with serious illness or disability, solve personal and family problems, locate community resources, and recommend support groups or other special services. They can also help you apply for public assistance, find a home health care worker, access after-hospital services such as meals-on-wheels or hospital equipment, and locate valuable community resources.

TIP

Several different kinds of social workers are available, but the ones who may be of most use to you are those specializing in clinical, health care, or gerontology social work. Clinical social workers offer psychotherapy and counseling. Medical social workers can help you and your family cope with chronic illness and work through the paperwork and red tape involved in applying for health care benefits. Gerontological social workers can advise those who are over 65 about senior citizen housing, transportation, and long-term care options.

For referrals to social workers in your area ask your primary care physician, contact your health insurance company or visit the Medicare web site at v www. medicare.gov/care-compare/#search. (Medical and gerontological social workers aren't included in this search.)

Mental Health Professional

A mental health professional can help you cope with the depression, anger, anxiety, relationship problems, or other emotional fallout that you may experience due to chronic illness. They can help you understand the origins of your emotional troubles, find new ways of handling these problems, and address coexisting conditions, such as alcoholism, drug abuse, or prescription drug dependence.

REMEMBER

Although anyone can call themself a "therapist" and set up a practice, a licensed mental health professional (psychologist, social worker, or psychiatrist) is your best bet. Social workers have a master's or doctoral degree in social work, and psychologists hold a master's degree or a doctoral degree in psychology. Both must perform thousands of hours of supervised counseling before they can be licensed. Psychiatrists are physicians and are therefore the only mental health professionals who can prescribe medication. But most mental health professionals can refer you to a psychiatrist if medication is needed.

For referrals to mental health professionals in your area, contact your primary care physician or health insurance company, or the National Register of Health Service Psychologists at www.findapsychologist.org.

Massage Therapist

If you have osteoarthritis, your other muscles may be working overtime to favor the joints that hurt. A good massage therapist can help ease the pain that can settle in the muscles doing double duty. Massage may also relieve some of your s pain by easing tension in the muscles surrounding your painful joints and improving joint range of motion. In general, by increasing circulation, helping your body release the metabolic byproducts that can irritate nerve endings, pumping up endorphin levels, and relieving tension, massage can be an effective way of helping you let go of some of the pain, stress, and the extra tension in locked-up muscles.

Massage is not recommended for autoimmune/inflammatory types of arthritis, is it can worsen these conditions by increasing inflammation and pain.

If you decide to enlist the services of a massage therapist, find one who is skilled in treating arthritis patients. Some kinds of massage may be too rough or painful to be beneficial to those with arthritis. And if you've got an infection or a fever, or you're coming down with an illness, avoid a massage because it increases circulation and therefore can increase inflammation. To find referrals for a massage therapist in your area, contact your primary care physician or the American Massage Therapy Association at at www.amtamassage.org.

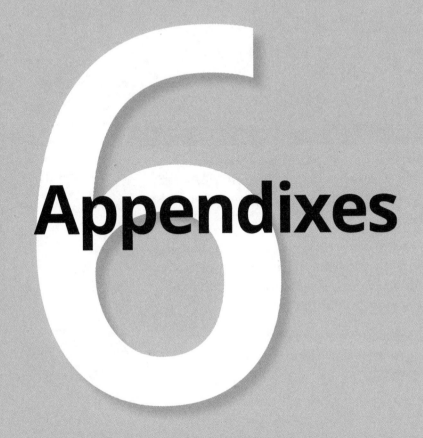

6 Appendixes

In Appendix A, we give you a glossary that defines the most frequently used terms related to arthritis, terms you'll probably encounter as you read and talk to others about arthritis.

Appendix B is a list of resources — associations where you can find a practitioner, get more information, find support groups, and more. A lot of good, free information can be found online as well.

And in Appendix C, we tell you how to take stress off your joints by reaching and maintaining a healthy weight.

Appendix A

Glossary

Acupressure (Shiatsu): A Japanese form of massage that aims to restore health by normalizing the flow of energy and blood in the body.

Acupuncture: A part of traditional Chinese medicine that uses the insertion of very fine needles to help balance the flow of energy in the body.

Acute pain: Pain that typically strikes severely and suddenly, builds, and then fades away. It occurs in response to injury, inflammation, surgery, and so on, and usually doesn't last long.

Alternative medicine: Healing techniques that fall outside of the realm of conventional, Western medicine.

Analgesics: Pain relievers that reduce or relieve headaches, arthritis pain, muscle soreness or other types of pain. Although Sold over-the-counter or as prescription drugs, they include acetaminophen (Tylenol), opiods such as oxycodone, combinations of Tylenol plus an opiod, and the non-steroidal anti-inflammatory drugs (NSAIDs), such as aspirin. The NSAIDS, however, are often considered a separate class of pain reliever because they interfered with the inflammation process, while Tylenol and the opiods change the body's reaction to pain signals.

Ankylosing spondylitis: A disease that causes inflammation and stiffness of the spine and its joints and that can result in the fusing or "locking" of those joints.

Antioxidants: Substances manufactured by the body and found in foods and supplements that help control the oxidation and free radical activity that can damage body tissue and cause or worsen certain disease states.

Anti-TNF drugs: Also known as TNF inhibitors (or blockers), or biologic therapies, these drugs block the action of tumor necrosis factor, a substance overproduced by the body in those who have rheumatoid arthritis, psoriatic arthritis, ankylosing spondylitis and other inflammatory forms of arthritis. Anti-TNF drugs (including adalimumab, etanercept, and infliximab) are made from human or animal tissue in a lab (and therefore are considered "biologics"). Taken via injection, infusion or (in some cases) orally, they cause a reaction in the immune system that blocks inflammation.

Aromatherapy: An alternative healing system based on the belief that inhaling certain aromas or scents can help the body heal itself.

Arthritis: A group of diseases (formerly called rheumatism) that strikes the joints and/or nearby tissues. The word arthritis means *joint inflammation,* although not all forms of arthritis cause inflammation.

Arthrodesis: Surgically immobilizing a joint so that the bones grow together and "lock" into position. This procedure is sometimes performed in cases of rheumatoid arthritis.

Arthroplasty: Surgical reconstruction of a joint using a combination of natural tissues and artificial parts; most commonly performed on the hip and knee.

Arthroscopy: Visual examination of the inside of a joint performed by using a special "scope" that is passed through a small incision. Arthroscopy can be used to diagnose certain types of joint disease and in some cases, make repairs surgically.

Autologous chondrocyte implantation: The transplantation of healthy cartilage cells from a normal joint to a damaged one, so that they can grow and supplement or replace ailing cartilage.

Ayurvedic healing: An ancient Indian healing art that uses diet, exercise, internal cleansing, herbs, massage, crystals, aromatherapy, color therapy, gems, and other modalities to eliminate illness and restore balance to the body.

Bee venom therapy: The use of bee venom to relieve pain and inflammation. The venom may be delivered via the sting of a live bee or through an injection.

Biofeedback: A method for helping one learn to exert some control over certain physiological functions, such as muscle tension or blood pressure. During a biofeedback session, you're hooked up to a machine that provides audio and visual feedback, as for example, muscle tension increases or decreases. Feedback from the machines shows you how certain body functions change as you relax.

Biologics: Also known as biological agents, these are substances made from living organisms use to treat auto-immune disease, cancer, and other diseases. They include antibodies, interleukins, and vaccines.

Biomechanics: In a non-technical sense, it is the study of the way the body deals with its own weight — for example, the impact of walking or running on the weight-bearing joints. Using proper biomechanical techniques, one can greatly minimize the stress placed on the joints while moving, lifting, or even sitting.

Borrelia burgdorferi: The bacteria that causes Lyme disease, transmitted to humans by infected ticks.

Bursitis: A painful condition resulting from inflammation of the bursae, the fluid-filled pouches that keep certain joints moving smoothly. Shoulder joints are likely targets of bursitis.

Calcium pyrophosphate dihydrate crystals: Crystals that can accumulate in a joint and cause the symptoms of pseudogout.

Capsaicin: The hot part of chili peppers. Capsaicin fights pain by stimulating nerve cells to release large amounts of substance P, which sensitizes the receptors that originate the pain signals. When the cells run out of substance P, pain signals subside.

Carpal tunnel syndrome: A condition caused by pressure on the median nerve as it runs through the *carpal tunnel,* a narrow opening between the ligaments and bones in the wrist. Symptoms include pain, weakness, tingling, burning, and muscle atrophy.

Cartilage: Connective tissue found in the joints and elsewhere in the body. Joint cartilage helps protect bone ends that would otherwise rub against each other and produce pain and other problems.

Chondroitin sulfate: A supplement that, studies suggest, can relieve symptoms of osteoarthritis. Often used in conjunction with glucosamine, chondroitin sulfate helps pull water into the cartilage and fight cartilage-eating enzymes that can damage this precious tissue.

Chronic pain: Pain that lasts weeks or months, that accompanies long-term disease, or that keeps recurring. It may continue long after the apparent cause has disappeared, and can significantly reduce the quality of life.

Complementary medicine: Nonstandard healing approaches designed to work with conventional Western medicine.

COX-2 Inhibitors: A relatively new form of NSAID with the same pain-relieving and anti-inflammatory benefits as other NSAIDs, but with fewer side effects.

Dermatomyositis: A disease that produces muscle pain plus skin rashes and other problems.

DHEA (dehydroepiandrosterone): A hormone that the body uses to make testosterone, estrogen, and other hormones, DHEA is sometimes used by alternative healers to treat lupus and other ailments. Sometimes called the mother of all hormones, it is produced primarily in the adrenal glands.

Discoid lupus erythematosus: A "limited" form of lupus that may produce a rash and other skin problems, weakening of the immune system, and other symptoms, but isn't as severe as systemic lupus erythematosus.

DMARDs: Disease-modifying, antirheumatic drugs used for rheumatoid arthritis, psoriatic arthritis, and other forms of the disease. DMARDs appear to work by altering the behavior of the immune system.

Fibromyalgia: A disease characterized by inflammation of the connective tissue, including the ligaments, tendons, and muscles. Symptoms include chronic achy pain, stiffness, disturbed sleep, depression, and fatigue.

Glucosamine: A supplement that studies suggest can relieve symptoms of osteoarthritis. Often used in conjunction with chondroitin sulfate, glucosamine is used by the body to manufacture proteoglycans, which draw water into the cartilage and keep it moist.

Gonococcal arthritis: The most common form of infectious arthritis, caused by the *gonococci* bacterium.

Gout: A type of arthritis caused by an accumulation of uric acid crystals in the joint, often the bunion joint of the large toe. Symptoms of gout include terrible pain, joint stiffness and swelling, and possibly fever, chills, and an elevated heart rate.

Herbalism (phytotherapy): The use of the roots, bark, stems, flowers, or other parts of selected plants to relieve the symptoms of illness and/or strengthen the body.

Holistic medicine: An approach to healing and health based on treating a patient's mind, body and spirit, rather than simply trying to counteract the disease or relieve symptoms.

Homeopathy: An alternative healing system developed in the eighteenth century, based on the belief that "like cures like." Thus, for example, patients suffering from nausea would be treated with very small doses of a substance that can cause nausea when given in large amounts to healthy people.

Hydrotherapy: The use of water, both hot and cold or in the form of steam, ice, compresses, and so on to relieve symptoms and help the body heal itself.

Immunosuppressants: Drugs that dampen the immune system. These may be used to treat rheumatoid arthritis, lupus, and other diseases in which the immune system is malfunctioning.

Infectious arthritis: Arthritis that is caused by the invasion of bacteria, viruses, or fungi.

Interleukin (IL) inhibitors: Immunosuppressive agents that inhibit the action of a type of cytokine in the blood called interleukins. The interleukins play a key role in regulating the immune system and when they aren't working correctly there can cause an overblown inflammatory response, the kind seen in autoimmune diseases like rheumatoid arthritis, psoriatic arthritis. IL inhibitors interrupt the inflammation. Examples of IL-inhibitor drugs include guselkumab (Tremfya) and secukinumab (Cosentyx).

Janus kinase (JAK) inhibitors: Janus kinase (JAK) inhibitors are used to treat chronic inflammatory conditions like rheumatoid arthritis. People with RA have overactive immune systems that are flooded with cytokines, a kind of protein that can stimulate the immune system When these cytokines attach to receptors on immune cells and, they can force the cell to make even more cytokines, with the help of enzymes known as Janus kinases. JAK inhibitors work by blocking the activity of these enzymes so the messages can't get through. This calms the immune system and decreases RA pain, swelling, and joint damage.

Joint: The place where two bones meet. Joints can be moveable or fixed. There are gliding joints such as the spinal vertebrae, hinge joints such as the elbows, saddle joints such as the wrist, and ball-and-socket joints such as the hip.

Juvenile idiopathic arthritis (JIA): The most common form of arthritis to strike children, producing pain or swelling in the joints, fever, anemia, and other symptoms.

Lyme disease: A disease caused by the *borrelia burgdorferi* bacteria, which is transmitted to humans through the bite of an infected tick. Lyme disease can produce a large bull's-eye shaped rash at the bite site, swelling and pain in the joints, fever, fatigue, muscle aches, nausea, swollen lymph nodes, and other symptoms.

Mediterranean diet: The standard diet consumed by people living in the Mediterranean areas of Greece, Italy, southern France, and parts of Spain, made up of plenty of fresh vegetables, fruits, whole-grain breads, pasta and cereal, nuts and legumes, plus good amounts of olive oil. This diet may help ease RA-related pain and swelling.

MSM (methylsulfonylmethane): MSM is a popular dietary supplement used most often as an anti-inflammatory agent.

Naturopathy: A healing art based on the belief that all diseases have natural causes and that the body has very strong, natural healing powers. Naturopathic physicians use diet, herbs, exercise, stress reduction, acupressure, and other modalities to help increase the body's healing prowess.

NSAIDs: Nonsteroidal anti-inflammatory medications designed to reduce pain and inflammation, often prescribed for various forms of arthritis.

Occupational therapist: A licensed professional who can help you cope with the day-to-day problems of living with arthritis (and other ailments) by finding easier ways for you to accomplish tasks, designing splints, recommending assistive devices, teaching you ways to protect your joints, and so on.

Omega-3 fatty acids: Sometimes called fish oil because their major source is certain types of fish, these substances can help reduce inflammation and other symptoms of rheumatoid arthritis, and possibly other forms of arthritis.

Omega-6 fatty acids: Found primarily in salad or cooking oils, these fatty acids can increase the inflammatory response. The exception is an omega-6 called gamma-linolenic acid (GLA), which helps calm inflammation. GLA is found in evening primrose oil, as well as black currant seed oil and borage seed oil.

Orthopedic surgeon: A medical doctor specially trained in the surgical treatment of bone and joint problems that affect movement, such as arthritis.

Orthopedist: A medical doctor specializing in diagnosing and treating problems of the bones, joints, muscles, and related tissues.

Osteoarthritis: A type of arthritis caused by the breakdown of cartilage, most often in the hips, knees, and other weight-bearing joints. Osteoarthritis may be due to injury, obesity, metabolic errors, heredity, or other factors.

Osteotomy: A surgical procedure during which a piece of bone is removed to improve joint alignment. It is sometimes used to treat osteoarthritis or ankylosing spondylitis.

Paget's disease: A disease in which the body inappropriately breaks down and rebuilds bone, resulting in weaker bones, bone deformity, and other problems. Many patients with Paget's disease are middle aged or older.

Physical therapy: The use of massage, exercise, hydrotherapy, electrical stimulation, and other modalities to help relieve pain, increase range of motion, strengthen muscles, and stimulate healing.

Polarity therapy: An alternative healing art based on the idea that the body contains energy systems that must be kept in balance. Polarity therapists attempt to find and release energy blockages by touching specific points on the body, and sometimes use gentle massage.

Polymyalgia rheumatica: A rheumatic condition characterized by severe, sudden stiffness in major joints, plus headaches, difficulty swallowing, coughing, and other symptoms.

Polymyositis: A disease that produces inflammation of the muscles and loss of strength. There may also be joint pain, weight loss, Raynaud's phenomenon, and other symptoms. Polymyositis is like dermatomyositis, without the skin problems.

Pseudogout: A from of arthritis similar to gout, but caused by the accumulation of calcium pyrophosphate dihydrate crystals (rather than uric acid crystals) in the affected joint.

Psoriatic arthritis: Striking about 5 percent of those who have the skin condition known as psoriasis, psoriatic arthritis can cause inflammation, swelling, and sometimes joint deformity.

Raynaud's phenomenon: A disease in which arterial spasms cause pain, burning, tingling, numbness, and/or discoloration, primarily in the fingers and toes. Raynaud's disease is more the common and often milder form; Raynaud's phenomenon is triggered by another ailment, such as lupus or scleroderma.

Reactive arthritis: A disease that may develop after an infection, reactive arthritis can produce mild to severe pain in the joints, inflammation of the eyelid, eyeball, and urethra, and other problems.

Reflexology: An alternative healing system based on the idea that specific areas of the feet are linked to parts of the body. Manipulating the point on foot corresponding to the lungs, for example, is believed to help relieve some of the symptoms of asthma.

Reiki: A Japanese healing art in which the practitioner channels energy into the patient by laying his hands lightly on or directly above the patient's body to help restore the body's flow and balance of energy.

Rheumatoid arthritis: The second most common form of arthritis, rheumatoid arthritis is brought about when the immune system attacks the body. The result can be joint pain and inflammation, generalized soreness and stiffness, fever, difficulty sleeping, and joint deterioration. The disease can also attack the lungs, blood vessels, and other parts of the body.

Rheumatoid factor (RF): An antibody found in some 80 percent of those with rheumatoid arthritis. Its presence strongly suggests that one has rheumatoid arthritis, although it's possible to have RF and not develop the disease.

SAMe (S-adenosyl-L-methione): A product of body metabolism, SAMe (pronounced *sammy*) is used in supplement form to combat depression and the symptoms of osteoarthritis.

Scleroderma: An autoimmune disease in which the body produces and stores excess collagen, resulting in damage to the skin, joint pain and swelling, difficulty swallowing, digestive difficulties, injury to the blood vessels, and damaged organs.

Sjögren's syndrome: Usually referred to simply as Sjögren's, this is a disease that produces dryness of the eyes and mouth and certain other parts of the body. Depending on the extent of the dryness and which parts of the body are affected, problems can range from the manageable to the very serious. A fair number of those with Sjögren's also develop arthritis, but this arthritis is most often a separate entity.

Soft tissue rheumatism: An old term indicating inflammation or pain in the bursae, tendons, ligaments, and other tissues surrounding supporting the joints. Carpal tunnel syndrome is an example of soft tissue rheumatism.

Steroids: A group of hormones naturally produced by the body that have wide ranging effects on metabolism, water balance, and organ function. The man-made versions have powerful anti-inflammatory properties but also have some serious side effects.

Swedish massage: The gentle kneading and stroking of muscles, connective tissue, and skin to relieve stress and soothe pained muscles.

Synovectomy: A surgery in which an overgrown, inflamed joint lining is removed; it may be performed for rheumatoid arthritis.

Synovial membrane: Part of the capsule surrounding certain joints, this membrane releases a lubricating fluid into the joint.

Systemic lupus erythematosus: An autoimmune disease that tends to attack women of childbearing age. Systemic lupus erythematosus can cause a variety of symptoms, including joint pain and inflammation, fever, rash, hair loss, anemia, weakness of the immune system, depression, and nervous system disorders. It can be fatal.

Tendonitis: Inflammation of a tendon, characterized by pain to the touch or upon movement. The upper arms, hands, fingers, and backs of the ankles are common targets of tendonitis.

TENS: Transcutaneous electrical nerve stimulation — the use of mild electrical currents to deliver small jolts to painful areas of the body. The electricity overrides pain signals.

Trigger finger: The locking of a finger in a bent position caused by swelling and inflammation of a tendon.

Trigger point therapy: Prolonged, deep tissue pressure applied to specific, tender and hard points on muscles to relieve tension and pain. The therapy may include injections of local anesthetic into trigger points.

Tumor Necrosis Factor: Also known as TNF, tumor necrosis factor is a substance in the body that causes inflammation. Drugs that block the action of TNF (anti-TNF drugs or TNF inhibitors) have been shown to be beneficial in reducing the inflammation in auto-immune diseases such as rheumatoid arthritis, psoriatic arthritis, and ankylosing spondylitis. These drugs include infliximab (Remicade), etanercept (Enbrel), and adalimumab (Humira), to name just a few.

Urethritis: An inflammation of the *urethra,* the tube urine passes through to get from the bladder to the outside of the body.

Uric acid crystals: The offending agents in gout that accumulate in the joint, causing pain and other symptoms.

Vasodilators: Medications that relax blood vessels and help blood flow more freely.

Appendix B

Resources

Organizations

Acupuncture/Acupressure

American Academy of Medical Acupuncture (AAMA), 2512 Artesia Blvd, Ste 200, Redondo Beach, CA 90278; phone (310) 379-8261; email info@medicalacupuncture.org; web site https://medicalacupuncture.org

National Certification Commission for Acupuncture and Oriental Medicine (NCCAOM), 2001 K Street, NW, 3rd Floor North, Washington, D.C. 20006; phone (888) 381-1140 or (202) 381-1140; email info@thenccaom.org; web site www.nccaom.org

Alexander Technique

Alexander Technique International (ATI), PO Box 30558 Indianapolis, IN 46230; phone (317) 932-3570; email office@alexandertechniqueinternational.org; web site www.alexandertechniqueinternational.com

American Society for the Alexander Technique (AmSAT), 11 West Monument Avenue, Suite 510, Dayton, OH 45402-1233; phone (800-473-0620) or (937) 586-3732; email info@AmSATonline.org; web site www.amsatonline.org

Alternative Medicine

National Center for Complementary & Integrative Health (NCCIH) Clearinghouse, 9000 Rockville Pike, Bethesda, Maryland 20892; phone (888) 644-6226; email info@nccih.nih.gov; web site www.nccih.nih.gov/health/nccih-clearinghouse

Aromatherapy

National Association for Holistic Aromatherapy (NAHA), 6000 S. 5th Ave., Pocatello, ID 83204; phone (877) 232-5255; email info@naha.org; web site https://naha.org

Arthritis Information and Management

American College of Rheumatology, 1800 Century Place, Suite 250, Atlanta, GA 30345-4300; phone (404) 633-3777; email pr@rheumatology.org; web site www.rheumatology.org

American Juvenile Arthritis Organization, 1330 West Peachtree St., Atlanta, GA 30309; phone (800) 568-4045 or (404) 965-7624; email help@arthritis.org; web site www.arthritis.org

Arthritis Foundation, 1355 Peachtree St. NE, 6th Suite, Atlanta, GA 30309; phone (800) 283-7800; online help https://www.arthritis.org/i-need-help; web site www.arthritis.org

Fibromyalgia Network, change to: **National Fibromyalgia Association**, 3857 Birch St., Suite 212, Newport Beach, CA 92660; phone (714) 921-0150; email nfa@FMaware.org; web site https://FMaware.net

Lupus Foundation of America, Inc., 2121 K Street NW, Suite 200, Washington, DC 20037; phone 202-349-1155; email info@lupus.org; web site www.lupus.org

The Myositis Association, 6950 Columbia Gateway Drive, Suite 370, Columbia, MD 21046; phone (800) 821-7356; email TMA@myositis.org; web site www.myositis.org

National Institute of Arthritis and Musculoskeletal and Skin Diseases (NIAMS) Information Clearinghouse, National Institutes of Health, 1 AMS Circle, Bethesda, MD 20892-3675; phone 877-226-4267 (toll free) or 301-495-4484; email NIAMSinfo@mail.nih.gov; web site www.niams.nih.gov

The National Psoriasis Foundation, 6600 SW 92nd Ave., Suite 300, Portland, OR 97223-7195; phone 800-723-9166; web site www.psoriasis.org

The Paget Foundation, P.O. Box 24432, Brooklyn, NY 11202; phone (800) 237-2438; email PagetFdn@aol.com; web site hwww.paget.org

Scleroderma Foundation, 300 Rosewood Dr., Suite 105, Danvers, MA 01923; phone (800) 722-4673 or (978) 463-5843, email sfinfo@scleroderma.org; web site www.scleroderma.org

Sjögren's Foundation,10701 Parkridge Blvd., Suite 170, Reston, VA 20191; phone (301) 530-4420; email info@sjogrens.org; web site www.sjogrens.org

Spondylitis Association of America, 16430 Ventura Blvd., Suite 300, Encino, CA 91436; phone (800) 777-8189 or (818) 892-1616; email info@spondylitis.org; web site https://spondylitis.org

Bee Venom Therapy

American Apitherapy Society, 15 Heights Rd., Northport, NY 11768; phone (631) 470-9446; email aasoffice@apitherapy.org; web site www.apitherapy.org

Biofeedback

Association for Applied Psychophysiology and Biofeedback (AAPB), 4400 College Blvd, Suite 220, Overland Park, KS 66211; phone (800) 477-8892 or (303) 422-8436; email info@aapb.org; web site www.aapb.org

Biomechanics Experts

American Academy of Osteopathy, 3500 DePauw Blvd., Suite 1100, Indianapolis, IN 46268 -1136; phone (317) 879-1881; email info@academyofosteopathy.org; web site www.academyofosteopathy.org

Help for Caregivers

Family Caregiver Alliance, 101 Montgomery St., Suite 2150, San Francisco, CA 94104; phone (800) 445-8106 or (415) 434-3388; email info@caregiver.org; web site www.caregiver.org

Caregiver Action Network, 1150 Connecticut Ave. NW, Suite 501, Washington, DC, 20036-3904; phone (202) 454-3970; email info@caregiveraction.org; web site https://caregiveraction.org

Homeopathic Medicine

National Center for Homeopathy, P.O. Box 1856, Clarksburg, MD 20871-1856; phone (703) 548-7790; email info@homeopathycenter.org; web site www.homeopathycenter.org

Hypnotherapists

American Council of Hypnotist Examiners (ACHE), 7183 Navajo Rd., Ste. E, San Diego, CA 92119; phone (619) 280-7200; email: hypnotistexaminers@gmail.com; web site https://hypnotistexaminers.org

National Guild of Hypnotists, Inc. P.O. Box 308, Merrimack, NH 03054-0308; phone 603-429-9438; email ngh@ngh.net; web site www.ngh.net

Massage Therapists

The American Massage Therapy Association (AMTA), 500 Davis Street, Suite 900, Evanston, IL 60201; phone (877) 905-2700; email info@amtamassage.org; web site www.amtamassage.org

Associated Bodywork & Massage Professionals (ABMP), 25188 Genesee Trail Rd., Suite 200, Golden, CO 80401; phone (800) 458-2267; email expectmore@abmp.com; web site www.abmp.com

National Certification Board for Therapeutic Massage & Bodywork, NCBTMB, 1333 Burr Ridge Parkway, Suite 200, Burr Ridge, IL 60527; phone (800) 296-0664; email info@ncbtmb.org; web site www.ncbtmb.org

Medical Societies

American Academy of Orthopaedic Surgeons (AAOS), 9400 West Higgins Rd., Rosemont, Illinois 60018; phone (847) 823-7186; email – use contact form on web site; web site www.aaos.org

American Academy of Physical Medicine and Rehabilitation, 9700 W. Bryn Mawr Ave., Suite 200, Rosemont, IL 60018; phone (847) 737-6000; email info@aapmr.org; web site www.aapmr.org

American Board of Medical Specialties (ABMS), 353 North Clark Street, Suite 1400, Chicago, IL 60654; phone (312) 436-2600; email info@abms.org; web site www.abms.org

American Board of Surgery, 1617 John F. Kennedy Blvd., Suite 860, Philadelphia, PA 19103-1847; phone 215-568-4000; email abscomms@absurgery.org; web site www.absurgery.org

American Medical Association, AMA Plaza, 330 N. Wabash Ave., Suite 39300, Chicago, IL 60611-5885; phone (312) 464-4782; email – use contact form on web site; web site www.ama-assn.org

American Occupational Therapy Association, 6116 Executive Boulevard, Suite 200 North Bethesda, MD 20852-4929; phone (301) 652-6611; email – use contact form on web site; web site www.aota.org

American Physical Therapy Association, 3030 Potomac Ave., Suite 100, Alexandria, VA 22305-3085; phone (800) 999-2782 or (703) 684-2782; email – use contact form on web site; web site www.apta.org

The Mind/Body Connection

American Meditation Institute, 60 Garner Road Averill Park, NY 12018, phone (518) 674-8714; email info@americanmeditation.org, web site https://americanmeditation.org

The Center for Mind-Body Medicine, 5225 Connecticut Ave., Suite 414, Washington, DC 20015; phone (202) 966-7338; email – use contact form on web site; web site https://cmbm.org

Naturopathic Medicine

The American Association of Naturopathic Physicians, 300 New Jersey Ave. NW, Suite 900, Washington, DC 20001; phone (202) 237-8150; email – use contact form on web site; web site https://naturopathic.org

The Homeopathic Academy of Naturopathic Physicians (HANP), 600 West Emma St., Lafayette, CO 80026; phone (303) 665-2423; email info@hanp.net; web site https://hanp.net

Nutritional Counseling

Academy of Nutrition and Dietetics (formerly the American Dietetic Association), 120 South Riverside Plaza, Suite 2190, Chicago, IL, 60606-6995; phone 800-877-1600 or (312) 899-0040; email nis@eatright.org, web site www.eatright.org/find-a-nutrition-expert

OnPoint Nutrition (online nutritional counseling), 774 South Street #132, Philadelphia, PA 19147; (215) 867-9424; email https://www.aanc.net; web site www.onpoint-nutrition.com/online-nutritionist

Pain Management

American Chronic Pain Association, P.O. Box 850, Rocklin, CA 95677; phone 800-533-3231; email ACPA@theacpa.org; web site www.theacpa.org

American Academy of Pain Medicine, 1705 Edgewater Dr., #7778, Orlando, FL 32804; phone (800) 917-1619 ext. 102; email info@painmed.org; web site: https://painmed.org

U.S. Pain Foundation, Inc., 15 North Main St., Unit 100, West Hartford, CT 06107; phone (800) 910-2462; email contact@uspainfoundation.org; web site https://uspainfoundation.org

Polarity Therapy

American Polarity Therapy Association, 318 Avenue I, #17, Redondo Beach, CA 90277; phone (336)574-1121; email aptaoffices@polaritytherapy.org; web site https://polaritytherapy.org

Psychotherapy

American Psychological Association, 750 First St., NE, Washington, DC 20002-4242; phone (202) 336-5500; Web site www.apa.org

Association for Applied and Therapeutic Humor (AATH), 220 East State Str. FL G, Rockford, IL 61104; phone (815) 708-6587; email info@aath.org; web site www.aath.org

National Register of Health Service Psychologists, 1200 New York Ave. NW, Suite 800, Washington, D.C. 20005; phone (202) 783-7663; email support@nationalregister.org; web site www.nationalregister.org

Reiki

The International Association of Reiki Professionals (IARP), 20 Trafalgar Square S405, Nashua, NH 03063; phone (603) 318-1888; email – use contact form on web site, web site www.iarp.org

Reflexology

Reflexology Association of America, 1809 Rutledge, Madison, WI 53704; phone (608) 571-5053; email infoRAA@reflexology-usa.org; web site https://reflexology-usa.org

Social Workers

National Association of Social Workers (NASW), 750 First St. NE, Suite 800, Washington, DC 20002; phone (800) 742-4089; email naswdc@socialworkers.org; web site www.socialworkers.org

Support Groups Online

National Mental Health Consumers' Self-Help Clearinghouse, 1211 Chestnut Street, Suite 1100, Philadelphia, PA 19107; phone (800) 553-4539 or (215) 751-1810; email info@mhselfhelp.org; web site: www.mhselfhelp.org

Arthritis Online Community (WebMD), web site www.webmd.com/arthritis/arthritis-online-community

Mental Health America (MHA), 500 Montgomery St., Suite 820, Alexandria, VA 22314; phone (800) 969-6642 or (703) 684-7722; email — use contact form on website; web site www.mhanational.org

My RA Team, Social network for those living with rheumatoid arthritis. web site www.myrateam.com

Therapeutic Touch

Therapeutic Touch International Association, Box 130, Delmar, NY 12054; phone (518) 325-1185; email ttia@therapeutictouch.org; web site https://therapeutictouch.org/

The Trager Approach

United States Trager Association, 3755 Attucks Dr., Powell, OH 43065; phone (440) 834-0308; email exec@tragerus.org; web site www.tragerapproach.us

Assistive Devices — Online Retailers

AccessTR.com (Adaptive recreation equipment for the physically challenged), 8 Sandra Court, Newbury Park, CA 91320-4302; phone (800) 634-4351 or (805) 498-7535; email CustomerService@AccessTR.com; web site https://accesstr.com

Aids for Arthritis, Inc. (products useful for those with arthritis, fibromyalgia, multiple sclerosis and/or aging in general), 1019A Industrial Dr., West Berlin, NJ 08091; phone (800) 654-0707; email orders@aidsforarthritis.com; web site www.aidsforarthritis.com

American Discount Home Medical Equipment (lift chairs, mobility scooters, walkers and more), P.O. Box 24827, San Jose, CA 95154; phone (800) 956-6616; email (none listed); web site www.home-med-equip.com

ArthritisSupplies.com (arthritis aids for daily living), The Wright Stuff, Inc., 111 Harris St., Crystal Springs, MS 39059, phone (601) 892-3115; email for customer inquiries customercare@thewrightstuff.com or for other inquiries info@thewrightstuff.com; web site www.arthritissupplies.com

Assistive Technology Services (products and solutions to help customers live independently), 8023 Franklin Road, Murfreesboro, TN 37128; phone (615) 562-0043; email questions@atscares.com; web site www.assistivetechnologyservices.com

Brownmed (gloves, splints, cushions and egonomic products for arthritis relief), 4435 Main St., Suite 820, Kansas City, MO 64111, phone (877) 853-5518, email — use contact form on web site, web site www.brownmed.com

Dr. Leonard's Healthcare Corp., P.O. Box 7821, Edison, NJ 08818-7821, phone (800) 455-1918, email — use contact form on web site; web site www.drleonards.com

Performance Health, (gloves, splints, supports, utensils, assistive devices), 28100 Torch Parkway, Suite 700, Warrenville, IL 60555; phone (800) 323-5547, email customersupport@performancehealth.com; web site: www.performancehealth.com

Rehabmart.com, (rehabilitation products and solutions), Rehabmart, LLC, 3651 Mars Hill Rd. Bldg. 2400, Watkinsville, GA 30677-6042; phone (800) 827-8283; email assistance@rehabmart.com; web site www.rehabmart.com

SoftFLEX Computer Gloves, (for carpal tunnel syndrome), Four Points Products, Inc., 4230 Winding Willow Dr., Tampa, FL 33618; phone 800-216-8415; email info@softflex.com; web site: www.softflex.com

Books

21-Day Arthritis Diet Plan: Nutrition Guide and Recipes to Fight Osteoarthritis Pain and Inflammation. Reisdorf, A., Rockridge Press, 2020.

Mayo Clinic Guide to Arthritis: Managing Joint Pain for an Active Life. Peterson, L.S., Mayo Clinic Press, 2020.

Meals That Heal: 100+ Everyday Anti-Inflammatory Recipes in 30 Minutes or Less. Williams, C., Tiller Press, 2019.

The Rheumatoid Arthritis Healing Plan: A Holistic Guide and Cookbook for Inflammation Relief. Samson, C., Rockridge Press, 2019.

The Holistic Fibromyalgia Treatment Plan. Mendez, A., Rockridge Press, 2020.

Books/DVDs from the Arthritis Foundation

To find the following titles, see the Arthritis Foundation web site at www.arthritis.org, click on **Store** and then **Arthritis Foundation Books** or **Arthritis Foundation DVDs.**

Raising a Child with Arthritis

Tips for Good Living with Arthritis

Walk with Ease

Arthritis Friendly Yoga DVD

Tai Chi for Arthritis DVD

Appendix C

Weight Loss and Management Guide

Even if you're eating a balanced diet, getting plenty of omega-3s, and avoiding danger foods, you need to take one more step — the one that puts you on a scale. And if what you see when you look at the numbers doesn't look good, you need to lose weight.

TIP

If you're overweight or obese, one of the best things you can do for your aching joints is to lose weight. Trimming away extra pounds will take a tremendous burden off the joints that have to bear your weight, such as your hip and knee joints. According to the Arthritis Foundation, for every pound an overweight or obese person loses, four pounds of pressure are removed from their knees. This means that losing just ten pounds can relieve a stunning 40 pounds of pressure on the knee joints! And not only does weight loss take the pressure off, strong evidence suggests that dropping down to your ideal weight can help ease or prevent osteoarthritis (especially OA of the knee and hip), as well as reduce the risk of developing rheumatoid arthritis.

The Framingham Study, which tracked knee osteoarthritis in independently living elderly people for over 35 years using X-rays, found that obesity precedes knee OA and increases the risk of developing it. But in overweight women of normal height, every 11 pounds of weight loss reduced the risk of knee OA by 50 percent. Not surprisingly, both the Arthritis Foundation and the American College of Rheumatology strongly recommend weight loss for patients with knee and/or hip OA who are overweight or obese.

Figuring Out Whether You're Too Heavy

On average, adult Americans have packed on an additional 15 pounds in the past 20 years, and we're continuing to grow, with an average yearly weight gain of 1.1 to 2.2 pounds. That can really add up over time!

Medical experts agree that being slim is better, especially where arthritis is concerned. But what's slim?

TIP

For years, people have looked at height-weight charts to see if they should drop a few pounds, but these charts were only rough guidelines. Then a division of the National Institutes of Health issued a set of guidelines based on the *body mass index* (BMI), a comparison of height and weight. Now you just need to look for one number, your BMI, to see whether or not you need to lose weight. Here are the standards:

>> If your BMI is between 18.5 and 24.9, you're fine.

>> If it's between 25 and 29.9, you're overweight. Those extra pounds are beginning to challenge your health and put extra pressure on your joints.

>> If it's 30 or above you're obese. Your weight is causing or likely will cause health problems.

So you want your BMI to be no more than 24.9, and certainly less than 30. The formula for determining BMI is simple: Multiply your weight in pounds by 703 and divide the answer by your height in inches squared. Well, maybe it's not so simple when put like that! Table C-1 helps you skip the figuring and get a fairly good idea of where you stand.

REMEMBER

The BMI isn't an absolutely perfect guide to weight. It only compares height to weight; not taking into account that fact that some people appear "fatter" and have higher BMIs because they have lots of muscles. For others, the reverse can be true, because they don't have much muscle. Still, the BMI is a good starting point.

TABLE C-1

Body Mass Index Chart

Height	Weight That Gives a Healthy BMI of 24.9 or Less	Weight That Puts You in the Overweight BMI Range	Weight That Gives an Obese BMI of 30
5'0"	127	128-148	153
5'1"	131	132-153	158
5'2"	135	136-158	164
5'3"	140	141-168	169
5'4"	144	145-173	174
5'5"	149	150-179	180
5'6"	154	155-185	186
5'7"	158	159-190	191
5'8"	163	164-198	197
5'9"	168	169-202	203
5'10"	173	174-208	209
5'11"	178	179-214	215
6'0"	183	184-220	221
6'1"	188	189-226	227
6'2"	193	193-232	233

Losing Weight the Safe and Healthy Way

The bad news is that we can't provide you with a quick, simple, guaranteed way to lose weight. The gimmicks don't work, and the fad diets don't live up to their promises. Oh yes, you'll lose weight on almost any fad diet, primarily because they all get you to restrict your intake in one way or another. And with many of them you'll quickly lose lots of water weight. But most people quickly regain all the water weight — and all the other weight as well. The overwhelming majority of people who drop pounds on fad diets gain them back — plus a few more. And to make matters worse, a fair number of fad diets are nutritionally unbalanced: Eating what these diets recommend for long periods of time can lead to trouble.

The good news is that you *can* lose weight without sacrificing nutrition or your health. While we can't go into great detail on losing weight, because this isn't a diet book, there are many books available that present safe, sensible, and effective diets.

Most people already know how to lose weight. Notwithstanding the hype in the fad diet books, the basic principles for healthy people are quite simple: Eat a well-rounded diet emphasizing fresh vegetables, whole grains, and fruits; keep your fat content down to reasonable levels; enjoy sweets as occasional treats only; and burn lots of calories through physical activity and exercise. In short, burn more calories than you take in.

Aiming for long-term benefits

Don't diet. "Dieting" is a bad word, because it means giving up your favorite foods and eating a lot of stuff you don't like, or, even worse, starving yourself. Both are short-term fixes designed to be discarded as soon as possible.

Instead, eat for lifelong good health. Focus on the slow, steady, and permanent weight loss that comes when your diet and activity/exercise habits are in alignment.

Eating fruits and vegetables

Eat a variety of vegetables, fruits, and whole grains to ensure that you get all the numerous nutrients in foods. No single food or food group gives you all you need, as there's no such thing as a magic food. Eat moderate amounts of meat, poultry, and dairy products, and when you do, eat many different kinds.

Limiting your intake of certain foods

Take it easy on cholesterol, saturated fat, sugar, and salt.

Eat sweets sparingly. Many people have found that the more they cut back, the less they crave these foods. Don't look upon it as depriving yourself: Just cut back a little bit at a time. You may be surprised to find that your desire for sweets falls off as your consumption decreases.

Read the labels on your food cans and packages carefully. You may be surprised at how many calories food makers squeeze into some foods you thought were fairly "lite."

Using psychological strategies to get through

Put smaller portions on your plate. That way, you can clean your plate without stuffing yourself.

Avoid places and settings that normally cue to you overeat. For example, if you're always eating plates loaded with fried tortilla chips and gooey, fatty cheese dip when you meet your friends at a Mexican restaurant after work, try going to a restaurant that doesn't have such temptations.

Don't shop when you're hungry, because your growling stomach will make you much more likely to buy sweets and fattening foods.

TIP

Set a reasonable goal. Don't try to lose 30 pounds a month or squeeze into that teensy bathing suit by next week. People who lose weight that fast usually put it on again almost as rapidly. If you stick to a good eating and exercise plan and only lose a quarter or a half pound a week, you'll be doing well.

Don't be too hard on yourself if you don't meet all of your goals exactly on schedule. You're only human; give yourself some leeway. And remember: you're eating for life; you're in it for the long haul. You don't have to sprint; just stay on the right track.

Oh, and when you do something great, be sure to reward yourself with something other than food.

Understanding that it's not just what you eat . . .

Remember that what you do or do not eat is only half the equation. You must also burn up calories with physical activity and exercise.

Eat slowly. It takes a while for your brain to register a feeling of fullness in your stomach, so it's easy to eat more than you want or need to when you're shoveling it in. Take your time, and let your brain become aware of the feeling of satiety. You'll eat less that way.

"Pre-eat" a little bit before going to parties, movies, and other places where you can't get healthy food. If you eat a small portion of health-enhancing food before you go out, you won't be tempted to overdo it on the fatty hors d'oeuvres and tempting sweets after you're there. Instead, you can enjoy a little taste, as a special treat.

Eyeballing those portions

Many diets suggest specific portion sizes, such as 3 ounces of fish, 1/2 cup of vegetables, or 8 ounces of milk. But because few of us carry little food scales or measuring cups, we're often forced to estimate. Eyeballing the correct amount can be difficult, because most people tend to underestimate the portion size of foods they enjoy eating and overestimate those they don't like. (Ever notice how 1/2 cup of ice cream looks like nothing, but 1/2 cup of beets looks like way too much?)

Table C-2 offers some tips for eyeballing food portion sizes. The tips are easy to remember, or if you like, you could take a photo of the table on your phone and always have it close at hand.

TABLE C-2 ## Visual Food Portion Guidelines

Quantity	Visual Aid
How big is a 3-ounce serving?	About the size of a deck of cards.
What's one serving of pancake or waffle?	A pancake or waffle the size of a 4-inch DVD.
How much is 1 teaspoonful?	About the size of the tip of your thumb.
What's 1/2 cup serving of veggies, rice, pasta, or cereal?	Cooked, a mound about the same size as a small fist (or baseball).
How big is a small baked potato?	Roughly the size of a computer mouse.
What's a medium apple or orange?	One about the size of a baseball.
What's an ounce of cheese?	About the size of four dice.

Index

A

AARP, 333

Abdul, Paula (singer), 27

Academy of Nutrition and Dietetics, 341, 359

AccessTR.com, 362

acetaminophen, for treating osteoarthritis, 37

aconitum nappellus, 285

actea spic, 285

Actemra (tocilizumab), 52, 119–120

Actonel (risedronate), 120

acupressure (shiatsu), 263, 292–293, 295, 347, 355

acupuncture, 263, 290–292, 347, 355

acute gouty arthritis, 58

acute pain, 158–161, 347

adalimumab (Humira), 52, 68, 128

age
  as a cause of arthritis, 20
  as a risk factor of osteoarthritis, 35

aggression control, as a treatment option, 26

Aids for Arthritis, Inc., 362

air travel, 328–329

Alexander, F. Matthias (actor), 222

Alexander Technique International (ATI), 355

The Alexander Technique, 222, 355

alfalfa, 277

allergies, food, 182

aloe, 280

aloe vera, for inflammation, 189

alpha-linoleic acid, 179

alternative medicine
  about, 261, 263, 301
  aromatherapy, 263, 302–303, 347, 356
  bee venom therapy (BVT), 263, 303–304, 348, 357
  choosing, 269

defined, 347

dehydroepiandrosterone (DHEA), 264, 304–306, 349

finding CAM practitioners, 264–267

hydrotherapy, 264, 308, 350

methylsulfonylmethane (MSM), 306–307, 350

organizations for, 355

prolotherapy, 309

types of, 262–264

working with doctors, 268–269

Amazon Prime, 333–334

American Academy of Medical Acupuncture (AAMA), 292, 355

American Academy of Orthopedic Surgeons (AAOS), 358

American Academy of Osteopathy, 357

American Academy of Pain Medicine, 360

American Academy of Physical Medicine and Rehabilitation, 358

American Apitherapy Society, 304, 357

American Board of Medical Specialties (ABMS), 358

American Board of Surgery, 359

American Chronic Pain Association, 360

American College of Rheumatology, 101, 356

American Council of Hypnotist Examiners (ACHE), 358

American Discount Home Medical Equipment, 362

American Juvenile Arthritis Organization, 356

American Medical Association (AMA), 94–95, 359

American Meditation Institute, 359

American Occupational Therapy Association, 359

American Physical Therapy Association, 359

American Polarity Therapy Association, 298, 360

American Psychological Association, 360

American Society for the Alexander Technique (AmSAT), 355

The American Association of Naturopathic Physicians, 359

The American Massage Therapy Association (AMTA), 343, 358

ammonium carbonicum, 285

Amoxil (amoxicillin), 121

amphiarthrodial joints, 10

analgesics, 24, 116–117, 347

Anaprox-DS (naproxen sodium), 121

anchovies, 174

anemia, as s symptom of Sjögren's syndrome, 83

angelica, 277

ankle rotations, 206–207

ankylosing spondylitis (AS)
  about, 14, 67
  defined, 347
  diagnosing, 68
  symptoms of, 67–68
  treating, 68

Ansaid (flurbiprofen), 121

antibiotics
  for gonococcal arthritis, 65–66
  for infectious arthritis, 65
  for Lyme disease, 78
  for reactive arthritis, 76

antibody abnormalities, as s symptom of Sjögren's syndrome, 83

anti-DNA test, 108

anti-inflammatories, 275–279

anti-malarial drugs, for discoid lupus erythematosus (DLE), 72

antinuclear antibody (ANA), 48, 108

antioxidants, 306, 347

antirheumatics, 279–280

anti-Sm test, 108

anti-TNF drugs, 347

apis mellifica, 286

apples, 174

arachidonic acid, 182

Arava (leflunomide), 121–122

arm, extending, 201–202

arnica montana, 286

aromatherapy, 263, 302–303, 347, 356

artgrodesis, 347

arthralgia, 8

arthritis

  about, 7–8, 57

  ankylosing spondylitis, 67–68

  causes of, 20–21

  compared with arthritis-related conditions, 14–19

  conditions linked to, 69–90

  defined, 347

  effect on joints of, 8–13

  famous sufferers of, 27–28

  gonococcal arthritis, 65–66

  gout, 58–60

  infectious arthritis, 64–65

  juvenile idiopathic arthritis, 62–64

  organizations for information and management of, 356–357

  pseudogout, 61–62

  psoriatic arthritis, 66

  signs and symptoms of, 19–20

  statistics on, 21–23

  treatment options for, 23–26

Arthritis Foundation, 94, 101, 184, 219, 257, 356, 363

Arthritis Online Community (WebMD), 361

arthritis-related conditions, 14–19

ArthritisSupplies.com, 362

arthrodesis, 147–148

arthroplasty, 148–151, 348

arthroscope, 147

arthroscopy, 110, 143, 348

Arthrotec (diclofenac sodium/misoprostol), 122

Aspirin, 122

assistive devices, 254–255, 327, 362–363

Assistive Technology Services, 362

Associated Bodywork & Massage Professionals (ABMP), 358

Association for Applied and Therapeutic Humor (AATH), 243, 360

Association for Applied Psychophysiology and Biofeedback (AAPB), 357

autologous chondrocyte implantation (ACI), 154, 317, 348

Ayurvedic healing, 348

azathioprine (Imuran), for treating polymyositis, 89

Azulfidine (sulfasalazine), 123

B

back leg, extending, 206

Ball, Lucille (actress), 27, 46

ball-and-socket joints, 13

B-cell inhibitors, for rheumatoid arthritis (RA), 52

bee venom therapy (BVT), 263, 303–304, 348, 357

belladonna, 286

benzoic acid, 286

biofeedback, 241, 348, 357

biologics, 24, 52–53, 118, 348

biomechanics, 222–223, 348, 357

biopsy of rheumatoid nodules, for rheumatoid arthritis (RA), 49

black cohosh, 277

bladderwrack, 277

The blamer, 245

blood chemistries, 108

blood tests, 78, 107–109

board certified, 95

body alignment, 225–229

body mass index (BMI), 366–367

body weight, secondary osteoarthritis and, 34

bogbean, 279

bone cement implantation syndrome (BCIS), 152–153

bone disease, secondary osteoarthritis and, 34

bone end damage, secondary osteoarthritis and, 34

Bone Marrow Aspirate Concentrate (BMAC) therapy, for cartilage, 318

bones, 9

bony growths, as symptom of osteoarthritis (OA), 32

books, as resources, 363

borage oil, 277

boron, 186

borrelia burgdorferi, 77, 78, 107, 348

boswellia, 277

Bouchard's nodes, 32

Bradshaw, Terry (athlete), 27

breath control, 242

broccoli, 174

bromelain, 190

Brownmed, 362

bryonia alba, 286

burdock, 280

bursae, 9

bursitis, 17, 79–80, 348

C

calcarea carbonica-ostreorum, 286

calcitonin, for treating Paget's disease, 85

calcium pyrophosphate deposition disease (CPPD), 61–62, 348

cannabidiol (CBD), 274–275

cantaloupe, 175

capsaicin, 165, 190–191, 280, 348

car rentals, 328

cardiovascular endurance, exercise for, 196–198, 217

Caregiver Action Network, 357

caregivers, organizations for, 357

The caretaker, 245

carpal tunnel syndrome, 18, 86, 348

cartilage

  about, 10, 30–31

  autologous chondrocyte implantation (ACI), 154

  Bone Marrow Aspirate Concentrate (BMAC) therapy for, 318

  causes of breakdown, 33–35

defined, 349

hydrolyzed collagen for, 187–188

cat posture, 208–209

cat's claw, 277–278

ceftriaxone, for gonococcal arthritis, 65–66

celecoxib (Celebrex), 51, 123

celery seed, 279

centaury, 278

The Center for Mind-Body Medicine, 359

certifications, checking, 265–266

cevimeline (Evoxac), for treating Sjögren's syndrome, 83

chair dancing, 212–213

chair exercises, 212–214

chair fencing, 213–214

chair marching, 212

chair running, 212

chamomilla, 286

Cheat Sheet (website), 3

check-ups, 103–106

child's pose, 211

Chinese peony, 278

Chinese Thunder God Vine, 279–280

chlamydia trachomatis, 76

chondrocytes, 30, 33

chondroitin sulfate, 192–193, 349

chores, minimizing, 252–256

chronic pain, 158–161, 349

cimicifuga racemosa, 286

Cimzia (certolizumab pegol), 52, 123

citrus fruits, 175

classes, exercise, 219

Clinoril (sulindac), 124

cognitive behavioral therapy (CBT), 243

ColBenemid (probenecid/ colchicine), 124

colchicine, 61, 124

cold, applying, 164

cold compresses, for rheumatoid arthritis (RA), 50

collagen, 30, 33

complement, 108

complementary and alternative medicine (CAM) practitioners, 262–267

complementary medicine, 262, 349

complete blood count (CBC), 48, 108–109

conditions, linked to arthritis, 69–90

conjunctivitis, as a symptom of reactive arthritis, 76

Conn, Doyt
"Red Flags," 101–102

conserving energy, 248–249

control group, 316

cool, for treating osteoarthritis, 39

cool-down, 218

cooled radiofrequency ablation (CRFA), for knee osteoarthritis, 320

corticosteroids, for rheumatoid arthritis (RA), 53

cortison injections, 102

Cosentyx (secukinumab), 125

Costco, 334

cousticum, 286

COX-2 inhibitors, 349

"cracking" joints, as symptom of osteoarthritis (OA), 32

C-reactive protein (CRP), 48, 108

credentials, checking, 265–266

CT scans, 74, 106–107

cupping, 291

curcumin, 278

curry, 175

cutaneous lupus erythematosus (CLE), 71–72

cyclic citrullinated peptide (CCP), 48, 109

cycling, as exercise, 197

Cymbalta (duloxetine), 125

Cytoxan (cyclophosphamide), 125

D

Daypro (oxaprozin), 126

day-to-day living
about, 247
joining support groups, 256–257
minimizing chores, 252–256
taking care of yourself, 248–251
workplace, 257–258

Decadron (dexamethasone), 126

deep tissue massage, 295

dehydroepiandrosterone (DHEA), 264, 304–306, 349

Deltasone (prednisone), 126

depression
controlling, as a treatment option, 26
effect on pain of, 237–240

dermatomyositis, 89–90, 349

designing workout programs, 216–219

devils claw, 278

diagnosing
ankylosing spondylitis (AS), 68
bursitis, 79–80
dermatomyositis, 90
discoid lupus erythematosus (DLE), 72
gonococcal arthritis, 65–66
gout, 60
infectious arthritis, 64–65
juvenile idiopathic arthritis (JIA), 63–64
Lyme disease, 78
osteoarthritis (OA), 36–37
Paget's disease, 85
polymyalgia rheumatica (PMR), 84–85
polymyositis, 89
pseudogout, 61–62
psoriatic arthritis, 66
Raynaud's phenomenon, 82
reactive arthritis, 76–77
rheumatoid arthritis (RA), 47–49
Sjögren's syndrome, 83–84
systemic lupus erythematosus, 71
systemic scleroderma, 74–75
tendonitis, 81
tenosynovitis, 81

diet
for rheumatoid arthritis (RA), 50
during travel, 325–326
as a treatment option, 25

digestive difficulties, as a symptom of systemic scleroderma, 74

disability benefits, 258

Disalcid (salsalate), 126–127

National Register of Health Service Psychologists (website), 243, 342, 360

The National Psoriasis Foundation, 356

natural irritants, 161

natural pain management, 161

naturopathic medicine, 359

naturopathy, 351

neck, stretching, 201

nerve conduction tests, for diagnosing polymyositis, 89

niacin, for Raynaud's phenomenon, 188

nightshades, 181–182

noninvasive therapies

about, 162

cold, 164

heat, 162–164

hot paraffin wax treatments, 163

joint manipulation, 166

splints, 166–167

supports, 166–167

topical pain relievers, 165–166

transcutaneous electrical nerve stimulation (TENS), 168, 353

water therapy, 164–165

nonsteroidal anti-inflammatory drugs (NSAIDs)

about, 24, 102, 117, 166

for ankylosing spondylitis (AS), 68

for bursitis, 79

defined, 351

for Lyme disease, 78

for osteoarthritis, 37

for pseudogout, 61

for reactive arthritis, 76

for rheumatoid arthritis (RA), 51

for systemic scleroderma, 74

for tendonitis, 81

for tenosynovitis, 81

nonsurgical treatments, 143

noradrenaline, 161

norepinephrine, 161

nutritional counseling, 359–360

nuts, 175

O

occupational therapist (OT), 160, 248, 340–341, 351

oligoarthritis, as a symptom of juvenile idiopathic arthritis (JIA), 63

olive oil, 177

Olumiant (baricitinib), 133, 314

omega-3 fatty acids, 178–180, 351

omega-6 fatty acids, 178, 180–181, 351

O'Neal, Tatum (actress), 27

online pharmacies, 336

OnPoint Nutrition, 360

opiate-containing analgesics, 117

Orencia (abatacept), 52, 134, 315

organ meats, 182

organizations, as resources, 355–361

orthopedic surgeon, 143, 339, 351

orthopedist, 351

osteoarthritis (OA)

about, 15, 29

boron for, 186

cartilage, 30–31

causes of cartilage breakdown, 33–35

chondroitin sulfate for, 192–193

compared with rheumatoid arthritis (RA), 55–56

defined, 351

diagnosing, 36–37

glucosamine sulfate for, 192–193

hyaluronic acid (HA) for, 319

risk factors of, 35–36

signs and symptoms of, 31–32

treating, 37–40

vitamin D for, 187

osteotomy, 147, 351

outside help, 255–256

overuse, as a cause of arthritis, 20

oxidants, 184–186

oysters, 175–176

P

Paget's disease, 17, 85, 351

The Paget Foundation, 356

pain

about, 233–234

effect of depression on, 237–240

effect of stress on, 234–235

positive thinking, 240–244

prayer and spirituality and, 244–245

as a symptom of rheumatoid arthritis (RA), 43

Type A personality and, 235–237

pain management

about, 157

acute pain compared with chronic pain, 158–161

arthritis pain, 158

medications for, 168–169

noninvasive therapies, 162–168

organizations for, 360

surgery for, 169

pain relievers, herbs as, 280–282

papaya, 176

passive movement, 166

Patient Assistance Programs (PAPs), 333

The PDR Pocket Guide to Prescription Drugs, 10th Ed., 100

Pediapred (prednisolone sodium phosphate), 134

pellagra, 188

pelvis, lifting, 203

Penicillin, 134

Performance Health, 362

pericarditis, 45

pesudogout, 61–62

Peterson, L.S. (author)

Mayo Clinic Guide to Arthritis: Managing Joint Pain for an Active Life, 363

pharmacies, 335, 336

pharmacist, 161, 339–340

pharmacy discount cards, 333–334

Pharmacy Verified Websites Program, 336

physical exam, 47, 104–106

physical shape, for surgery, 155

physical therapist, 160, 167, 340

physical therapy, 50, 351

pilocarpine (Salagen), for treating Sjögren's syndrome, 83

placebos, 316

Plaquenil (hydroxychloroquine), 135

platelet-rich plasma (PRP), for knee osteoarthritis, 318–319

pleurisy, 45

polarity therapy, 264, 297–298, 351, 360

polyarthritis, rheumatoid factor-negative or -positive, as a symptom of juvenile idiopathic arthritis (JIA), 63

polymyalgia rheumatica (PMR), 17, 84–85, 351

polymyositis, 19, 88–89, 352

positive thinking
  about, 239–240
  biofeedback, 241
  breath control, 242
  cognitive behavioral therapy (CBT), 243
  guided imagery, 242
  hypnosis, 242
  laughing, 243
  meditation, 241–242
  pain and, 240–244
  programmed relaxation, 241–242

postoperative care, 155

posture points, 228

potassium ions, 161

prayer and spirituality, 244–245

prednisone
  for bursitis, 80
  for dermatomyositis, 90
  for polymyalgia rheumatica (PMR), 84
  for polymyositis, 89
  for pseudogout, 61

pregnancy, 251

prescriptions, saving money on, 331–336

pretzel posture, 209

Preventing & Reversing Heart Disease For Dummies (Rippe), 54

primary care physician, 338–339

primary osteoarthritis, 33

primary Raynaud's, 82

primary Sjögren's, 83

processed meat, 182

professional help, 337–343

programmed relaxation, 241–242

prolotherapy, 309

proteoglycans, 30, 33

pseudogout, 15, 352

psoriatic arthritis
  about, 15
  defined, 352
  new drug treatments for, 315–317
  as a symptom of juvenile idiopathic arthritis (JIA), 63
  zinc for, 188–189

psoriatic arthritis (PsA), 66

psychiatrist, 161

psychologist, 161

psychotherapy, 360

R

rash
  as a symptom of dermatomyositis, 89
  as a symptom of discoid lupus erythematosus (DLE), 72
  as a symptom of Lyme disease, 77
  as a symptom of reactive arthritis, 76

Raynaud's phenomenon
  about, 18, 81–82
  defined, 352
  niacin for, 188
  as a symptom of systemic scleroderma, 74

reactive arthritis
  about, 17, 75
  defined, 352
  diagnosing, 76–77
  symptoms of, 75–76
  treating, 76–77

recovery plan, 156

"Red Flags" (Conn), 101–102

reflexology, 264, 298–299, 352, 361

Reflexology Association of America, 299, 361

registered dietitian, 341

Rehabmart.com, 362

reiki, 264, 293–294, 352, 360

Reisdorf, A. (author)
  21-Day Arthritis Diet Plan: Nutrition Guide and Recipes to Fight Osteoarthritis Pain and Inflammation, 363

Relafen (nabumetone), 135

Remember icon, 3

Remicade (infliximab), 52, 135–136

remission, 62

remittive drugs, for rheumatoid arthritis (RA), 51

Renoir, Pierre-Auguste (artist), 27

repetitive motion injury, secondary osteoarthritis and, 34

resources, 355–363

rest, for rheumatoid arthritis (RA), 49–50

rheumatism, 8

rheumatoid arthritis (RA)
  about, 15, 41
  causes of, 45–46
  compared with osteoarthritis (OA), 55–56
  defined, 352
  diagnosing, 47–49
  effects of, 42–43
  janus kinase (JAK) inhibitors for, 313–314
  Mediterranean-style diet and, 176–178
  signs and symptoms of, 43–45
  treating, 49–55
  vagus neurostimulation for, 320–321
  victims of, 46
  vitamin D for, 187
  zinc for, 188–189

rheumatoid factor (RF), 45, 109, 352

rheumatoid factor (RF) test, for rheumatoid arthritis (RA), 47–48

The Rheumatoid Arthritis Healing Plan: A Holistic Guide and Cookbook for Inflammation Relief (Samson), 363

rheumatologist, 99, 338

Rheumatrex (methotrexate), 136

Rinvoq (upadacitinib), 52, 136–137, 314, 317

Rippe, James W. (author)
  Preventing & Reversing Heart Disease For Dummies, 54

risk factors
  for heart disease, 54
  for osteoarthritis (OA), 35–36
Rituxan (rituximab), 52, 137
robotic-assisted surgery, for hip replacements, 321–322
Rolf, Ida P. (biochemist), 295
rolfing, 295
rotating ankles, 206–207
ruta graveolens, 286

S

sabina, 286
saddle joints, 12–13
S-adenosyl-L-methione (SAMe), 189–190, 352
salicylates, 166
sambucus, 286
Samson, C. (author)
  The Rheumatoid Arthritis Healing Plan: A Holistic Guide and Cookbook for Inflammation Relief, 363
sarsaparilla, 279
scans, 106–107
scleritis, 45
scleroderma, 17, 352
Scleroderma Foundation, 357
ScriptSave WellRx, 334
secondary osteoarthritis, 34
secondary Raynaud's, 82
secondary Sjögren's, 83
secukinumab (Cosentyx)
  for ankylosing spondylitis (AS), 68
  for psoriatic arthritis, 66
sedatives, 280
selective co-stimulation modulators, for rheumatoid arthritis (RA), 52
selenium, 185
self-treatment, for treating osteoarthritis, 39
serotonin-norepinephrine reuptake inhibitor (SNRI), for treating osteoarthritis, 37
sex life, 250–251
shortness of breath, as a symptom of systemic scleroderma, 74

shoulders, 201–202, 228
shuffle-off-to-Buffalo, 213
side, stretching, 202–203
Simponi/Simponi Aria (golimumab), 52, 137–138, 315–316
SingleCare, 334
Sjögren's Foundation, 357
Sjögren's syndrome, 18, 43, 83–84, 352
skin problems, as a symptom of systemic scleroderma, 73
sleeping, 231–232, 249–250
slow-acting drugs, for rheumatoid arthritis (RA), 51
snake posture, 207–208
social workers, 161, 341–342, 361
soft tissue rheumatism, 353
SoftFLEX Computer Gloves, 363
spasms, as a symptom of Raynaud's phenomenon, 81
spinach, 176
spinal twist, 210–211
splints, 86, 166–167
Spondylitis Association of America, 357
sports massage, 296
statistics, of arthritis, 16, 21–23
steroids
  about, 24, 118–119
  for bursitis, 80
  defined, 353
  for dermatomyositis, 90
  for discoid lupus erythematosus (DLE), 72
  for polymyalgia rheumatica (PMR), 84
  for polymyositis, 89
  for pseudogout, 61
  for reactive arthritis, 76
  for rheumatoid arthritis (RA), 53
  for tendonitis, 81
  for tenosynovitis, 81
stiffness
  about, 19
  as a symptom of ankylosing spondylitis (AS), 67
  as a symptom of infectious arthritis, 64

as a symptom of osteoarthritis (OA), 32
as a symptom of psoriatic arthritis, 66
stinging nettle, 281
strained muscles, as a cause of pain, 158
strength training, 198–199, 217
strengthening exercises, for treating osteoarthritis, 38
stress
  controlling, as a treatment option, 26
  effect on pain of, 234–235
  preplanning travel to reduce, 325
stressed joints, as a risk factor of osteoarthritis, 35
stretching exercises, 199–200
stride, 229–231
subchondral bone, 35
subchondral cyst, 35
substance P., 161
subtle energetic sensations, 298
Sulfinpyrazone, 138
sun avoidance, for discoid lupus erythematosus (DLE), 72
supplements
  about, 173–174, 183
  aloe vera, 189
  boron, 186
  bromelain, 190
  capsaicin, 190–191
  chondroitin sulfate, 192–193
  flaxseed oil, 191–192
  folic acid, 186–187
  free radicals, 184–186
  ginger, 192
  glucosamine sulfate, 192–193
  grapeseed extract, 191
  hydrolyzed collagen, 187–188
  niacin, 188
  oxidants and, 184–186
  reviewing before travel, 324–325
  S-adenosyl-L-methione (SAMe), 189–190
  tips for taking, 183–184
  as a treatment option, 25

treating *(continued)*

polymyalgia rheumatica (PMR), 84–85

polymyositis, 89

pseudogout, 61–62

psoriatic arthritis, 66

Raynaud's phenomenon, 82

reactive arthritis, 76–77

rheumatoid arthritis (RA), 49–55

Sjögren's syndrome, 83–84

systemic lupus erythematosus, 71

systemic scleroderma, 74–75

tendonitis, 81

tenosynovitis, 81

treatment group, 316

treatment philosophy, 96

treatment team, 160–161

Tremfya (guselkumab), 139, 316

trigger finger, 353

trigger point therapy, 296, 353

Trilisate (choline magnesium trisalicylate), 140

trochanteric bursa, 79

tumor necrosis factor (TNF), 353

tumor necrosis factor (TNF) inhibitors

about, 118, 314

for ankylosing spondylitis (AS), 68

for rheumatoid arthritis (RA), 52

tumor necrosis factor-alpha (TNF-alpha), as a cause of arthritis, 21

Turner, Kathleen (actress), 27

21-Day Arthritis Diet Plan: Nutrition Guide and Recipes to Fight Osteoarthritis Pain and Inflammation (Reisdorf), 363

Tylenol (acetaminophen), 140

Type A personality, pain and, 235–237

U

ultrasounds, 106–107

undifferentiated arthritis, as a symptom of juvenile idiopathic arthritis (JIA), 63

United States Trager Association, 361

urethritis, 76, 353

uric acid, 58–59

uric acid crystals, 353

urine testing, 111

U.S. Pain Foundation, Inc., 360

U.S. Social Security Administration, 333

uveitis, 62

V

vagus neurostimulation, for rheumatoid arthritis (RA), 320–321

valerian, 280

vasculitis, 45

vasodilators, 353

victim talk, 239

vitamin B6, 186–187

vitamin C, 185

vitamin D, 187

vitamin E, 185

Voltaren (diclofenac sodium), 140–141

W

walking, as exercise, 197

warm-up, 217

Warning icon, 3

water

about, 176

cartilage and, 30

exercising in, 197–198

water therapy, 164–165

weight control, for treating osteoarthritis, 39

weight gain, 23

weight loss management, 365–370

whole grains, 176

wild yam, 279

Williams, C. (author)

Meals That Heal: 100+ Everyday Anti-Inflammatory Recipes in 30 Minutes or Less, 363

women

arthritis and, 22–23

rheumatoid arthritis (RA) and, 46

workout programs, designing, 216–219

workplace, managing arthritis in, 256–257

wrist, stretching, 201

X

Xeljanz (tofacitinib), 52, 141, 314, 316

x-rays

about, 106

for diagnosing Paget's disease, 85

for rheumatoid arthritis (RA), 48–49

Y

yoga, 207–211

yourself, taking care of, 248–251

Z

zinc, 188–189

Zyloprim (allopurinol), 141

About the Authors

Barry Fox and Nadine Taylor are a husband-and-wife writing team living in Los Angeles, California.

Barry Fox, PhD, is the author, coauthor, or ghostwriter of numerous books, including the New York Times number one best-seller, *The Arthritis Cure* (St. Martin's, 1997). He also wrote its sequel, *Maximizing The Arthritis Cure* (St. Martin's, 1998), as well as *The Side Effects Bible* (published by Broadway Books in 2005), *What Your Doctor May Not Tell You About Hypertension* (Warner Books, 2003), *What Your Doctor May Not Tell You About Migraines* (Warner Books, 2001), *Syndrome X* (Simon & Schuster, 2000), *The 20/30 Fat and Fiber Diet Plan* (HarperCollins, 1999), and *Cancer Talk* (Broadway Books, 1999). His books and over 160 articles covering various aspects of health, business, biography, law, and other topics have been translated into 20 languages.

Nadine Taylor, MS, RD, is the author of *Natural Menopause Remedies* (Signet, 2004), *25 Natural Ways To Relieve PMS* (Contemporary Books, 2002) and *Green Tea* (Kensington Press, 1998; rev. ed. 2021), as well as co-author of *Runaway Eating* (to be published by Rodale in 2005), *What Your Doctor May Not Tell You About Hypertension* (Warner Books, 2003), and *If You Think You Have An Eating Disorder* (Dell, 1998). After a brief stint as head dietitian at the Eating Disorders Unit at Glendale Adventist Medical Center, Ms. Taylor lectured on women's health issues to groups of health professionals throughout the country. She has also written numerous articles on health and nutrition for the popular press.

Dedication

Dedicated to Nina Ostrom Taylor, world's greatest mom and mom-in-law.

Author's Acknowledgements

Nadine and Barry thank Arnold Fox, MD, for providing us with a great deal of information on arthritis; Jinoos Yazdany, MD, for her invaluable contributions to the previous edition's text; and of course, the editorial staff at Wiley.

Publisher's Acknowledgements

Acquisitions Editor: Tracy Boggier

Development Editor: Daniel Mersey

Managing Editor: Kristie Pyles

Technical Reviewer: Samantha C. Shapiro, MD

Production Editor: Saikarthick Kumarasamy

Cover Image: © spukkato/Getty Images